"Anyone who has ever set foot in a hospital—or might in the future—would do well to read this book. With page-turning prose, Robbins pulls back the curtain on a world rife with joy and challenge. It's brutally honest, emotional, and, most of all, a paean to nurses—the people who help us live, die, and survive every day."—RACHEL SIMMONS, author of *Odd Girl Out*

"Nurses are the unseen warriors of the hospital system, part of a 'secret club' of heroes with its own rules and codes. They're also strong-willed, flawed human beings made of flesh and (unafraid of) blood, rendered here in stunning detail. This fascinating and compulsively readable book even has a few tricks that could save your life. First tip: Don't get sick in July."—MICKEY RAPKIN, author of *Pitch Perfect*

"A funny, intimate, and often jaw-dropping account of life behind the scenes . . ." —*People*

"A detailed, sympathetic, and eye-opening portrait of how nurses work . . ." —*Kirkus Reviews*

"Robbins narrowed her focus to the personal narratives of four nurses. . . . Their stories are compelling in every way."—*BookPage*

"Dishes eye-opening material."—*Publishers Weekly*

"*The Nurses* is exciting and honest . . . shows the inner workings of emergency rooms, offers golden advice, and explains behind-the-scenes events, and why nurses deserve way more kudos than they get."—*New York Daily News*

"A rich, fast-paced book about heroic, neglected professionals . . . editor's recommendation."—Barnes and Noble

"A fascinating and somewhat alarming examination of the contemporary nursing profession. . . . Robbins not only shows, she tells in this revealing exposé of the modern-day state of nursing. It is an eye-opener not to be missed."—*EarlyWord*

"I would recommend *The Nurses* to anyone who wants to understand what nurses really do. If we want American health care to improve, Robbins's advice should become our mantra: Treasure nurses. Hire more."—*Working Nurse*

"5 out of 5 stars—Anyone who is a nurse, who knows a nurse, or who might one day need a nurse, should read this book."—*The Book Nurse*

"A lively, fast-paced story and a riveting work of investigative journalism . . . a captivating book filled with joy and violence, miracles and heartbreak, dark humor and narrow victories, gripping drama, and unsung heroism."—*Bookreporter.com*

"Exciting and honest, from admission to release. *The Nurses* contains good stories, but it's also helpful. In short, it's a reader's McDream."—*New York Daily News*

"A compulsively readable book because of the narrative force of these stories . . . a must-read for anyone interested in nursing as a subculture, a calling, or a vital part of our health-care system."—*Biblionomad*

"Written with heart, detail, and honesty, *The Nurses* is an eye-opening look at the frustrations and joys of this undervalued profession."—*Book'd Out*

"Exceedingly well written."—*Amie's Book Review Blog*

"Robbins does a fantastic job showcasing the profession, giving readers an accurate, honest, and timely glimpse. This book is not only for nurses—it's a good read for everyone and could make the difference between life and death for a patient. The perfect blend of real-world examples, hard data, emotional tension, and clinical accuracy, this book is the real deal."—GAIL INGRAM, NP, *NurseGail.com*

"If any of my children were to express a desire to become a nurse, I would definitely put Robbins's *The Nurses* at the top of their prerequisite reading list."—*Luxury Reading*

"*The Nurses* truly captured my profession. I felt like someone had followed me around for my career and took notes."—*The Nurse Teacher*

"I had a hard time putting it down. . . . *The Nurses* is a brilliantly told narrative providing readers with critical takeaways that could save their lives or ensure better hospital care for themselves and their families. Robbins's skills as both storyteller and reporter are on full display as she gives voice to the millions of nurses who until now have been ignored."—*Agriview.com*

"An honest and heartfelt read, this book is a reminder for us all within the profession to feel honored that we are able to call ourselves 'nurse.'"—ELIZABETH SCALA, author of *Nursing from Within*

"If you're ever looking for poolside nonfiction, she's the one you want. She manages to both inform and entertain."—October book club, Wander & Whine

PRAISE FOR ALEXANDRA ROBBINS'S PREVIOUS BOOKS

"Readers . . . will find themselves guided by an excellent stylist and a first-rate mind."—*Houston Chronicle*

"Alexandra Robbins writes reality TV in book form."—*New Jersey Star-Ledger*

THE
NURSES

THE NURSES

A YEAR OF SECRETS, DRAMA, AND MIRACLES WITH THE HEROES OF THE HOSPITAL

ALEXANDRA ROBBINS

WORKMAN PUBLISHING
NEW YORK

Library of Congress Cataloging-in-Publication Data is available.
ISBN 978-0-7611-7171-3 (HC)
ISBN 978-0-7611-8925-1 (PB)

Design by Becky Terhune

Cover photo by Kurhan/fotolia

Workman books are available at special discounts when purchased in bulk for premiums and sales promotions as well as for fund-raising or educational use. Special editions or book excerpts can also be created to specification. For details, contact the Special Sales Director at the address below, or send an email to specialmarkets@workman.com.

Workman Publishing Co., Inc.
225 Varick Street
New York, NY 10014-4381
workman.com

WORKMAN is a registered trademark of Workman Publishing Co., Inc.

Printed in the United States of America

First paperback printing April 2016

10 9 8 7 6 5 4 3 2

To my family, past and present, with love

CONTENTS

PREFACE

It is astonishing that in the twenty-first century, nurses must continue to battle not only for respect but also for the right to speak.

In a segment about the talent portion of the 2015 Miss America pageant, for example, two cohosts of *The View* mocked Miss Colorado, Kelley Johnson, the pageant's second runner-up. For her talent, Johnson, valedictorian of her nursing school class, appeared in her scrubs and sneakers (common nurse footwear, but you have to admire a pageant contestant who wears sneakers) and delivered a moving monologue about how her work with an Alzheimer's patient reminded her that she is more than "just a nurse."

The next day, Michelle Collins, cohost of *The View*, laughingly insinuated that Johnson wasn't talented, and Joy Behar, watching a clip, asked, "Why does she have a doctor's stethoscope?"

While *The View* segment likely was intended to poke fun at the pageant, the hosts were deeply misguided in their choice of subject to denigrate. It's mind-boggling to suggest that, say, pageant singing or bikini-wearing are more valuable talents than saving lives and giving hope. Here was a contestant who, rather than take the safe route with a traditional talent (she's also a pianist), used her brief moment in the national spotlight to warmly pay tribute to a vital profession.

Nurses quickly went after *The View* with a change.org petition and a #NursesUnite hashtag went viral. Later that week, the cohosts issued a nonapology, claiming their comments were "taken out of context" and suggesting that angry nurses heard them wrong. "Did they hear the conversation?" Raven-Symoné wondered. Whoopi Goldberg cautioned the audience to better "listen" to the show.

Nurses heard them loud and clear over the beeps of the monitors, the demands of their administrations, and the moans of the patients they were tending. It's a nurse's job to listen. That's what they use their stethoscopes for. And by the way, nurses use stethoscopes more often than doctors do.

Whether or not the cohosts' slights were intentional, their comments reflect a general misunderstanding of and disrespect for what exactly nurses do. I wrote this book partly to correct those misperceptions. It's the public who must now "listen" to nurses. Because in many cases what nurses have to say could save our lives.

One of the most important things that nurses have been trying to tell us is that rampant nurse understaffing is causing patients to suffer. California is the only state in the country with hospital-wide safe-staffing nurse-to-patient ratio laws, which means that in any other state and the District of Columbia, hospitals can overload nurses with more patients than the safe maximum. And far too many do. Since the original hardcover publication of this book, nurses continue to report offenses. In a 2015 survey of Massachusetts nurses, 25 percent said that understaffing was directly responsible for patient deaths, 50 percent blamed understaffing for harm or injury to patients, and 85 percent said that patient care is suffering because of the high numbers of patients assigned to each nurse.

Why hasn't there been public uproar over such a glaring cause of preventable deaths and harm? It seems that some hospitals are silencing nurses who try to spread the word. According to the New York State Nurses Association, in 2015 Jack D. Weiler Hospital (of the Albert Einstein College of Medicine) in New York threatened nurses with arrest, and even escorted seven nurses out of the building because, during a breakfast to celebrate National Nurses Week, the nurses discussed staffing shortages. (A spokesman for the hospital disputed this characterization of the events.)

It's not unusual for hospitals to threaten and intimidate nurses who speak up about understaffing, said Deborah Burger, copresident of National Nurses United, the country's largest union of registered nurses. "It happens all the time, and nurses are harassed into taking what they know are not safe assignments. The pressure has gotten even greater to keep your mouth shut. Nurses have gotten blackballed for speaking up. They're considered troublemakers because it's bad for business. It can be cutthroat."

It's appalling that some hospitals are not only refusing to hire enough nurses to treat patients properly but also muffling the nurses who protest.

Nurses are patient advocates. They try to spread awareness of these issues because they want to provide better patient care.

The landscape hasn't always been so alarming. But as the push for hospital profits has increased, important matters such as personnel count, most notably nurses, have suffered. "Every day in every hospital in our state and probably throughout the nation, [hospitals] are deliberately putting patients in danger," said David Schildmeier, a spokesman for the Massachusetts Nurses Association. "Hospitals are ignoring the research and patients are suffering greatly. The biggest change in the last five-to-ten years is the unrelenting emphasis on boosting their profit margins at the expense of patient safety, lives, and the well-being that their mission calls upon them to provide. Absolutely every decision is made on the basis of cost savings."

The research referenced in *The Nurses* clearly shows that increasing nurse staffing leads to better patient outcomes. But experts have said that many hospital administrators assume the studies don't apply to them and fault individuals, not the system, for negative outcomes. "They mistakenly believe their staffing is adequate," said Judy Smetzer, vice president of the Institute for Safe Medication Practices, a consumer group. "It's a vicious cycle. When they're understaffed, nurses are required to cut corners to get the work done the best they can. Then when there's a bad outcome, hospitals fire the nurse for cutting corners."

As this book illustrates, nurses are the key to improving American healthcare. Nurses are unsung, underestimated, underappreciated heroes who are needlessly overstretched, overlooked, and overdue for the kind of recognition befitting champions. Don't silence them. Honor them. Because Johnson is right: No nurse is "just a nurse." We couldn't survive without them. And it takes a heck of a lot more talent to earn the scrubs and stethoscope than it does to mock a hero.

Alexandra Robbins
January 2016

PROLOGUE

Four hospitals stand within a fifty-mile radius of a major American city. On the surface, they are as different from one another as fairy-tale sisters.

Pines Memorial Hospital is a pleasant-looking cream-colored building with a sixteen-story tower and broad, welcoming windows overlooking a quiet tree-lined suburban avenue. After decades of independence, the neighborhood's favorite hospital was bought out by Westnorth, a large healthcare corporation, which is slowly diluting the local flavor. With 190 beds, Pines Memorial serves a highly educated, wealthy population with a large percentage of academics, retirees, and nursing home residents. Because it is close to a major highway, Pines' emergency room, which has approximately 60,000 visits per year, often treats victims of major-impact car accidents. Nurses joke that the hospital should be called Highway Memorial, because the risks of the highway are far more relevant to the medical staff than the quiet red pine forests outside of town.

Several miles away, South General Hospital occupies a mostly gray edifice curved away from the road, as if to shield its inhabitants from the gang violence that occurs frequently nearby. The Level-1 trauma center—designated as such because it has the resources to treat every stage of injury, from prevention through rehabilitation—has 300 beds to serve one of the most indigent areas outside the city. South General's ER sees 95,000 ER patients annually. The reputation of "The South" is like that of the proverbial kid from the wrong side of the tracks, hoping to keep up with her peers, but unable to overcome the disadvantages of living on the poverty-stricken south side of town.

Forty-five minutes west, in a peaceful corner of the city, Academy Hospital, proud and prestigious, inhabits several white-pillared, brick structures that wind around courtyards and patios, reflecting the storied architecture of its surrounding university campus. With approximately 425 beds, Academy treats a ritzy demographic of young and middle-aged residents in the nearby million-dollar homes and the students at the elite university. The Academy ER treats fewer than 45,000 patients per year, partly because it simply does not have the building space to expand its emergency department walls.

And Citycenter Medical, a longtime teaching hospital, is split between two dusty beige high-rises, perhaps representative of its dual personalities: a stalwart institution with top-notch doctors and an ER so poorly managed it is considered dangerous by many of its own staff. A 390-bed Level-1 trauma center, Citycenter has an emergency department that is crumbling beneath the weight of the 85,000 annual patients it does not have enough nursing staff to treat properly. While Pines Memorial treats more blunt force, multisystem traumas because of the car accidents, Citycenter's traumas are typically isolated injuries, such as gunshot wounds. Easily reached by public transportation and in the heart of a densely populated city, Citycenter is a destination of choice for homeless people, drug-seeking addicts, and the uninsured.

In each of these disparate institutions, pale blue curtains shroud pods of frightened people. In each, seasoned healers perform routine procedures and medical feats behind bleached sterile walls. And in each, tracking invisible undercurrents through hallway mazes, nurses connect doctors to patients, carrying out copious orders in synchronized steps, entwining themselves intimately in convalescents' lives.

THE
NURSES

WHAT IT'S REALLY LIKE TO BE A NURSE: The Joy and Heartbreak of the "Secret Club"

"Emergency nurses practice in an environment that has been called permanent whitewater, where constant change, challenge, and crisis are the reality. Amazing stories occur each day and some of these stories may never be acknowledged or written."
   —EMERGENCY NURSES ASSOCIATION, AWARD RECOGNITION PROGRAM

"In the hospital, we're truly a family and we have fun together. ER nurses have the raunchiest jokes, foulest mouths, and grossest stories. Because we're working in such close proximity there are always inappropriate jokes, comments, and teasing. Occasionally it escalates to a one-night stand between a nurse and doc, but mostly that happens off hospital grounds."
   —AN EAST COAST TRAVEL NURSE

"It's like high school, except for the dying people."
   —SAM, A NEW ER NURSE

MOLLY   PINES MEMORIAL, August

Molly raced toward the nurses station, dodging other fast-walking staff, weaving through stretchers lining the corridors. Traffic was stopped ahead; another nurse pushing a patient bed had gotten stuck because the halls were barely wide enough for two stretchers to pass each other. Molly had no time for this. No one did. The Pines Memorial ER was overloaded with patients, many of them moaning in pain or calling for the nurses who scurried through the brightly lit department.

After ten years as a nurse, three of them at Pines, Molly had learned to tune out the voices, and the cacophony of constant monitor chirps, high-pitched call-bell dings, and low-toned beeps of alarms from patients not her own. She didn't even notice the smell anymore, a blend of cleaning spray, urine, and, depending on the number of intoxicated patients, alcohol.

Molly ducked under a stretcher, scooted in front of the traffic jam, and helped the nurse lift the bed slightly to extricate the wheels. When the nurse smiled gratefully, Molly flashed a thumbs-up and hustled to the station.

There, Erica, the senior charge nurse, caught her eye. "I've been trying to call a Code Purple for hours, but Charlene won't budge!" Erica said. Friendly and smart, Erica struck just the right balance for a manager: She was firm but fair, and the nurses respected her. It was unusual for her to be rattled like this. A Code Purple—closing the ER to ambulances and rerouting patients to other hospitals—meant less profit for Pines Memorial, which would explain the administration's resistance. But the ER desperately needed relief.

Charlene, the nursing supervisor, stomped into the nurses station. Erica urgently called out to her. "Charlene! We need to call a Code Purple."

"No way," Charlene said, shaking her long blonde hair.

"Every room is full. Everyone has more than the usual number of patients. Even the hallway is full. We don't have beds to move these people to," Erica insisted. "Where are we going to put any other ambo patients who come in?"

"I'll get back to you." Charlene left the room.

Erica shot a worried look at Molly.

The medic phone rang. Medic phones, which kept Emergency Medical Services in touch with hospitals, resembled walkie-talkies attached to police scanners. As Molly pressed the radio button, the other nurses nearby groaned. "What's this one going to be?" one nurse sighed.

Molly answered the call. "Pines. Go ahead."

A medic's voice crackled over the speaker. "We're bringing in a seventy-two-year-old male. Working code. Five-minute ETA."

"Crap," Molly muttered after she released the button. No time to waste. A working code meant that CPR was in progress.

"We have to make room for a code, y'all," Molly said, in her unmistakably Southern drawl. Erica didn't have time to reply before the phone rang again.

Molly reached over and hit the button. "Pines."

"Medic forty-two en route to your location with a fifty-eight-year-old female in respiratory distress. We have her on BiPAP." Bilevel positive airway pressure was a method of assisted breathing. The patient probably would have to be intubated.

"What's your ETA?" Molly asked.

"Ten minutes."

Erica summoned Charlene again. "Charlene! We're getting *two* working codes."

As the nursing supervisor during a shift when higher level administrators were not in the building, Charlene had the authority to reroute ambulances. But today, she appeared to be more interested in impressing the higher-ups with an enormous patient load than in making sure the patients were safe and the nurses were able to do their jobs.

Charlene gave Erica a long look. "Okay, you can go on purple."

"Can you fill out the justification form? I have to prep for the codes," Erica said, already moving toward the supply closet. To call a Code Purple, the ER had to list the number of patients in the ER and waiting room, the longest wait time for patients, and the number of beds available. Charlene would have to explain the financial loss to hospital administrators.

Charlene backed away, palms up. "Oh no, *you're* the one who has to justify this closure." She turned on her heel and strode off.

Erica looked at Molly in disbelief. Molly fumed. *This place is exploding,* she thought. *We're expected to work at max capacity with no breaks and no acknowledgment or assistance from administration.*

At least it was a weekday. One of the more ludicrous hospital policies dictated that on nights or weekends, the nursing supervisor had to page the administrator on call to get permission for a Code Purple. That administrator could be anyone on senior management, including IT or finance personnel. A major medical decision could be made by someone with no medical training whatsoever. At Molly's previous hospital, the finance director was on call on a day when the ER was flooded with new arrivals. Focused on billing as many patients as possible, he had refused to call a Code Purple even when the physicians insisted that the number of patients was unsafe. A patient easily could have suffered or died because the staff was so busy checking on others. Eventually, an irate ER doctor yelled at the administrator until he agreed to divert the ambulances.

As Erica texted "Code Purple" to the staff and notified EMS and hospitals countywide, Molly and three other nurses scrambled to make room for the incoming patients. They lifted people off hallway stretchers and into standard chairs dragged in from the waiting room. They moved patients from rooms into beds in the hallway. The patients hated being in the hallway because it was a fish tank: Everyone could see you, hear you, rush by you, and knock into your bed. But the nurses had no other choice.

The first code, the 72-year-old man, would be Molly's. She wheeled a crash cart into a newly vacated room and paged the respiratory therapist on call: "We have a Code Blue coming in. ETA three minutes. And another patient coming in on BiPAP."

Molly opened an intubation bag to check that it contained all of the necessary supplies. She went to the medication room to retrieve the drugs needed to paralyze and sedate a patient before intubation, in case they would be needed. She set up the cardiac, blood pressure, and oxygen monitor, then visited each of her four patients to ensure they had easy access to a call light. "I'm about to be tied up for a long time with a critical patient," she told them.

The double doors at the ambulance entrance opened. Two medics raced down the hall, pushing a gurney on which another medic kneeled, rhythmically pressing all of his weight onto the patient as he performed CPR.

The recorder nurse, who documented the proceedings and kept track of time, guided them into Room 5, which nurses had cleaned only seconds before. Molly was glad to see Clark Preston follow them. Handsome and flirtatious, brash and irreverent, Dr. Preston was loved by some nurses and hated by others. Molly thought he was funny—and decisive, which was important in a code.

When the medics entered, the group quickly arranged themselves on either side of the gurney, hoisted the patient onto the ER stretcher, and whisked the gurney out of the way. As Molly hooked up the patient to the monitor, a technician started an IV.

One of the medics addressed the room: "Seventy-two-year-old male. Witnessed cardiac arrest while eating dinner at a restaurant. En route he was given three epi, two atropine. We bagged him because we were unable to intubate." Bagging referred to a plastic mask attached to an oxygen source. Squeezing the ambu bag caused the mask, which covered a patient's nose and mouth, to force air into the lungs.

The respiratory therapist had the intubation supplies ready. "Give me a 7.0 tube," the doctor said. He intubated the patient, and said, "Molly, listen."

Molly ducked under the medic, who was still performing CPR, now standing on a foot-high step stool. She reached under the medic's arms with her stethoscope. She squeezed her head beneath the medic, and listened to the patient's torso for air movement; air in the stomach meant the intubation tube was in the wrong spot. Then she listened to the lungs.

"Equal bilateral breath sounds," Molly said.

The respiratory therapist attached a CO_2 detector, bagged the patient, and watched. "Positive color change on CO_2 detector."

The clatter of the gurney carrying the second critically ill patient echoed from the hallway.

"Secure the tube," Dr. Preston said. "Let's run an ISTAT." The tech quickly drew blood to test whether the patient had a chemical imbalance that could be corrected.

"When was the last epi?" the doctor asked.

"Four minutes ago," said a medic.

"Give another round of epi. Let's give two amps of bicarb and an amp of calcium," Dr. Preston said. "Hold CPR."

The medic stepped down from the stool, trading positions with a new tech. Because CPR was physically strenuous, CPR providers switched off with every pulse check, two to three minutes apart.

Molly quickly felt the patient's femoral artery at the groin. "I don't feel a pulse," she said.

"Continue CPR," Dr. Preston replied. The tech resumed compressions. "Bring me the ultrasound machine."

Dr. Preston swiped gel on the patient's chest. "Hold CPR," he said. He passed the ultrasound wand over the patient's heart.

"I do not see any cardiac activity. What is the total downtime on this patient?" he asked.

"We worked him for forty minutes prior to arrival," said one of the medics.

The recorder nurse reviewed her clipboard. "We've worked him for twelve minutes."

Dr. Preston looked around the room, making eye contact with each of the four staff members. Not all physicians did this. The staff appreciated that Dr. Preston treated them like part of a team. "Total downtime: almost an hour. There's no cardiac activity. Does anyone have any other ideas?" The group agreed that they had tried everything.

Dr. Preston removed his gloves. "Time of death: 18:04."

Erica stepped into the room. "Clark, the next one's ready." The doctor, nurses, techs, and medics dispersed.

Molly was left alone with the deceased. When she turned off the monitors, the room went startlingly silent. Dealing with patient deaths like this usually didn't bother Molly; she didn't even know this gentleman's name. She imagined the deaths were much more difficult for floor nurses, who took care of patients for days, weeks, or months.

This was not to say that each death on a nurse's watch didn't mean something to her. Births and deaths, miraculous saves and sudden tragedies—all were expected outcomes in the microcosm of hospital life, and their frequency both intensified the experiences and desensitized the staff. But deaths were still sacred to the nurses, who were committed to respecting and preserving the dignity in dying.

Molly unhooked the patient from the monitor. He was still warm. She tidied the room in preparation for the family, trashing the plastic wrap from the intubation supplies and the empty glass medication vials. The room looked much more chaotic than the procedure had been. ERs had specific protocols, and everyone on staff worked from the same playbook; if the heart has this rhythm, give this medication; if the heart has that rhythm, shock the patient. Although they had not been successful this time, the staff had worked smoothly together.

Molly thought about how strange it was that she knew this man was dead, but his family did not. She tuned out Dr. Preston's instructions in the next room, where he had plenty of assistance. She could have followed the action, but just because this man had died didn't mean he wasn't her patient anymore. There were still things she could do to help him. Molly wiped the man's face and closed his eyes to make him presentable for his family. Families usually wanted to see the deceased one last time. Molly liked to make the patient and the room look serene.

Moments later, the registration clerk came to tell Molly that the man's family was waiting in the private family room. When Dr. Preston was finished with the other patient, he came to get Molly, wearing his white lab coat. He usually shunned medical coats, but Molly had told him once about a report that people believed doctors wearing white coats were more trustworthy and professional. He had donned the coat for family notification ever since. The moment he left the family room, though, that coat came right off.

When Molly and the doctor opened the door, the family members were seated and crying. "Did he make it?" one of them asked. This was almost always the first thing a family member said. Molly had difficulty avoiding eye contact with the family; she couldn't let them read her sympathy. She kept her eyes trained on Dr. Preston.

As usual, Dr. Preston started at the beginning. "When EMS picked up your father, he wasn't breathing and his heart wasn't beating," he said matter-of-factly, his bright blue eyes sincere. "So they started CPR and transported him to us. When he got here, he still wasn't breathing and his heart wasn't beating. We put in a breathing tube, continued with CPR, and gave him medications to try to restart his heart. I'm sorry to tell you that we weren't able to do that. Your father has died."

Dr. Preston offered his condolences. After a few beats of silence—rarely did a family say something right away—it was Molly's turn. "Do you have any other questions for the doctor? I'm going to stay with you and let you know what happens next." The man's widow and her daughter shook their heads. Dr. Preston left the room.

Doctors and nurses told the family together so that after the doctor left, the nurse could deal with the emotional breakdowns and walk the family through the next steps. Many doctors first explained how they tried to save the life, before revealing that they were not able to, because, Molly said later, "It's easier for them to have that gradual letdown. Once you say, 'He's dead,' they're not going to hear anything else. We want them to know how hard we tried." Doctors specifically used the words "dead" or "died" so that loved ones couldn't misinterpret the message.

Molly's nursing school had offered no instructions on how to talk to the family; her psychology rotation covered only mental illnesses. The one official rule Molly had learned was that staff first had to notify the next of kin before letting nonrelatives know. When a patient collapsed in the workplace, coworkers often sat in the lobby for hours without knowing the patient was dead, because the ER staff couldn't tell them before locating the family.

By watching physicians like Dr. Preston, who presented the news well—and, equally as helpful, those who did not—Molly had learned what the bereaved needed to hear at this crossroad. Many nurses hated this task. Molly didn't mind it, particularly when she was paired with a doctor who was not good at it. She considered it her responsibility to soothe and assist the families, much as she had done with the patient.

Molly sat down next to the widow, who sobbed on her shoulder. Families usually wanted some physical contact with the nurse. Molly typically put her hand on a shoulder and let the person guide her from there. If the family member needed more comforting, she would lean into Molly's shoulder or reach for a side hug. Molly remained quiet during these interactions. At this point, people didn't want to hear, "It's going to be okay."

When the woman's cries subsided, Molly spoke gently. "Next, you'll need to contact a funeral home and let the hospital know which home you'll be using. Your husband will be in our mortuary until you make that decision. Take all the time you need. Whenever you make that decision, Registration will make the arrangements to have him transferred over there."

The widow looked up at Molly, still stunned. "Next week he was going to help drive his granddaughter to her first day of college," she said.

Almost every family told Molly something specific about the deceased, as if subconsciously trying to prolong his life for just a moment longer. Molly always tried to come up with something positive and personal to say, so that the family would know that the hospital staff saw the deceased as a human being rather than a patient. "He must have been so proud that his granddaughter is going to college," she said.

The widow and the daughter both nodded, smiling through their tears.

As soon as a nurse on the 7:00 a.m. to 7:00 p.m. shift got off work, she was supposed to "give report," a recitation of her patients' status for the incoming nurse. Molly already had been working for more than twelve hours without a break. She hadn't even eaten. Nurses at Pines almost never got time off for lunch. There was rarely a chance to go to the cafeteria, break room, or simply outside for thirty minutes. Only once in the past two years had Molly been able to leave the department for a break. The usual scenario involved eating while working at the nurses station, which was an Occupational Safety and Health Administration (OSHA) violation.

Hospitals were required to give nurses breaks, yet the constantly short-staffed Pines nurses never had time for them. Technically, nurses were prohibited from bringing food or beverages to the nurses station to prevent them from contaminating patient labs and vice versa. Priscilla, the nursing director in charge of supervising every nurse in the ER, let the OSHA rule slide because the odds of getting caught were low. When The Joint Commission—the governing body and accreditation group for hospitals—sent inspectors, they had to check in at the front desk. Immediately, a hospital-wide page would announce, "Pines Memorial would like to welcome the TJC inspectors." Molly said the announcement meant "Hide your food!" She explained, "After the announcement, we have about ten minutes before the inspectors get to us. It's so obvious, like, 'Warning! Mayday! All the stuff that shouldn't be out—hide it!'"

Priscilla let many rules slide, actually. She seemed to try to look out for the nurses as best she could, which couldn't have been easy because she also had to enforce the new policies thrust upon them by the Westnorth Corporation, the giant healthcare system that had taken over the hospital six months earlier.

At 7:20 p.m., the charge nurse assigned Molly to put a Foley catheter in an obese paralyzed patient, a somewhat time-consuming procedure that required assistance. Molly walked to the nurses station, where five nurses were giving report to the oncoming shift. "Y'all, can I get a little help in Room 3 with the Foley?" she asked. The nurses ignored her. They didn't even make eye contact with her.

These weren't generally uncivil nurses; they were just busy. The outgoing nurses were determined to give report and go home, and the incoming nurses didn't want to be bothered with someone who was not their patient. The nurse Molly would give report to was already working on a trauma patient. Molly knew that if her friend Juliette had been on duty, she would have been at Molly's side in a heartbeat.

Molly looked over each of the nurses with her piercing green eyes. A tall, striking brunette, she was hard to miss. Five people were ignoring her—and she was not a quiet person. She had hoped that one of them would sense her frustration and offer to assist. But she would not badger them into helping her out.

Typically, many of the nurses at Pines worked well together, giving aid when needed, knowing they were in it together. Erica, for example, was constantly assisting her coworkers at bedside on top of her supervisory duties, as she was today. Ever since the buyout, however, the atmosphere had changed. The morale was as low as Molly had ever seen it. People were just too tired and angry to help each other out. The staff knew why Pines had allowed the buyout: Independent hospitals across the country were having trouble turning a profit because new insurance guidelines made getting reimbursement for medical care more difficult. Westnorth had instituted several changes that angered the nurses, including cutting their weekend overtime pay and slicing vacation accrual in half.

One of the worst new policies forced nurses to pay for parking at the hospital while techs and physicians could still park for free. The nurses who didn't want to pay for the covered garage would have to park at a satellite garage that was a shuttle bus ride away from the hospital. To catch the bus, nurses would have to get to work thirty minutes before their shift began and wouldn't get back to their cars until at least thirty minutes after their shift ended, effectively adding an unpaid hour to their workday. *What kind of company wants to make money off its employees like that?!* Molly had wondered, dismayed.

The hospital takeover had directly and indirectly affected patient care, too, which was evident when Molly ended up struggling to insert the Foley alone. The procedure took longer than it would have if another nurse had helped to lift the obese patient. ER staffing was supposed to be determined by the number of patients who came in. The number had increased drastically enough to justify an additional staff nurse for every shift, but Westnorth had refused to hire anyone. Consequently, waiting time to get into the short-staffed ER had increased from an average of thirty minutes to three hours.

That night, on the drive home, Molly cried with frustration. She was known as being thick-skinned rather than a crier. She was so tough that once while playing pickup basketball, she tripped and broke her arm, but waited hours before going to the hospital because she was having too much fun to stop playing. Now she cried because the once tight-knit hospital no longer seemed to care about the welfare of its nurses, and her usually co-operative coworkers were so worn down that they "acted like I was invisible."

As Pines Memorial's treatment of nurses deteriorated under Westnorth, Molly had toyed with the idea of leaving the hospital. Earlier in her career, she'd worked as a nurse for an agency that assigned her shifts at different hospitals. As an agency nurse, she could choose which days she worked, and the pay was slightly higher. To return to the agency, where she was a nurse in good standing, all she had to do was fill out paperwork and send in her latest certifications.

Molly had stayed at Pines because she enjoyed learning from her experienced colleagues. But lately, there had been too many days like today. That night, she called Priscilla and left a voice message about the day's events. "I have gone home angry and in tears more in the last two months than I have in my whole career. If I leave work angry again, I will not come back." It may not have been the best way to let her boss know that she was close to quitting, but she was too frustrated to care.

The next morning, Molly, the designated trauma nurse, was able to focus exclusively on her patients without having to deal with politics, or so she thought. A middle-aged woman had multiple injuries from a car accident, and the operating team would have to repair her ruptured spleen. Molly's job was to keep her stable in the trauma room until the OR was ready. As Molly connected the patient to a monitor, a nurse sitting at a computer called out from the nurses station.

"You're going to love this one, Molly," she said. "Now we're going to have to pay for fancy uniforms!"

Molly froze. "What?" She breathed deeply. She had a patient to take care of. "Just a minute. Let me finish what I'm doing and I'll come over."

While Molly continued to work on the patient, the other nurse read aloud the policy, which administrators had posted on the employee website without notifying the ER nurses. All staff would now be required to wear a standard uniform. But only the nurses would have to pay for the uniforms out of pocket.

"What about the doctors and the techs?" Molly asked.

"Nope," the nurse replied. "They're covered."

That was the last straw. It wasn't the uniform, specifically. It was what the uniform expense represented: Pines didn't appreciate its nurses. Furthermore, management gave employees little motivation to work hard. Hospital employees weren't held accountable for their actions, and the supervisors were either too wimpy to enforce important hospital rules (Priscilla) or played favorites (Charlene). Too frequently, certain nurses and techs called in sick, then posted vacation pictures on Facebook. Or they were unprofessional: Lucy, the laziest tech in the unit, had refused to do lab work on patients she deemed too "gross" to touch. As Molly said, "There are no consequences for poor work ethic and no rewards for good work ethic."

Later that morning, Priscilla gathered the ER nurses to tell them about the new uniform policy. While the group splintered into side conversations, Priscilla brushed her dark bangs off her face and put a hand on Molly's arm. "I got your message," she said.

"This place is coming apart at the seams," Molly told her.

"I know."

"I'm holding to my word on my message yesterday."

Priscilla nodded, placating.

"I'm not changing my mind," Molly said. "I'm giving you one month's notice. The uniform is just the last straw." She could call the agency tonight, start the re-registering process, and begin orientation within weeks. She was giving Pines Memorial ample notice because she didn't want to leave her coworkers even more shorthanded.

Throughout the rest of the day, nurses complained about the policy. "They're kicking us when we're down," they said. "The changes are making things worse." They looked at Molly because she was one of the most outspoken nurses.

"Doesn't matter to me," she said. "I just quit." Her coworkers laughed dismissively. "No, I actually did, y'all. I gave notice."

Generally, Pines Memorial's schedules were flexible and fair, and Molly had come to value the nurses' intelligence and ability to stay cool under pressure. But, she thought, *I can't be angry at work every single day.*

Molly had originally decided to make the career switch from occupational therapy to nursing after her mother had passed away. While in mourning, Molly received several letters from her mothers' coworkers. The letters "talked about her being the best nurse they had ever known, how much fun she made work, and how much the patients and her coworkers respected her," Molly remembered. Inspired, Molly became a nurse, too, at the age of 27—ten years ago. "I'm not that touchy-feely, but I truly love nursing. It's a meaningful career, I'm good at it, and it's flexible," she said. "You can find work any time of day, any day of the year, which makes it mom-friendly."

Molly had wanted to be a mom for as long as she could remember. After three years of trying to conceive with her police officer husband, Trey, she had finally scheduled an appointment at a fertility clinic. As an agency nurse, she would be able to arrange her schedule around her clinic appointments.

More experienced colleagues kept telling Molly that once she worked at several other hospitals, she would realize that Pines wasn't that bad. "Will I find out from working at other places that that was really as good as it gets?" she wondered. Experiencing hospital life at various institutions was the best way Molly could discover whether anybody was treating both nurses and patients right.

She gave herself a year to find out.

LARA   SOUTH GENERAL HOSPITAL, August

On her way to the staff locker room, Lara stopped in her tracks. The half-used vial of Dilaudid, a narcotic five to ten times more powerful than morphine, lay on a counter. It seemed to shimmer with energy and promise. *You deserve it*, coaxed a voice she remembered well. *You've been working fourteen-hour days. Your mom just died. She died in your arms. It will make you feel better. It's sitting right there. No one will know. You want it. Take it.*

Lara had been a drug addict. It had started so innocently. Nine years ago, as a single 26-year-old nurse, Lara was chatting with the other nurses on the night shift about paying off school loans, when one of them said, "Did you know you can get four thousand dollars per egg if you donate them? We should all go together."

"That's kind of cool," Lara had said. "I'm young, I'm healthy, and it's easy money."

The next morning, the four nurses went to a clinic for the screening process. Lara, with her blonde ringlets and fair skin, was the only donor selected. After the multi-week process of egg retrieval, the doctor handed her a check and a prescription for Percocet.

The pill was the first narcotic she had ever taken. Within minutes, she was simultaneously giddy and calm, suffused with warm happiness, the world's best buzz. She couldn't stop giggling. Nothing bugged her. Her insecurities—about her dating life and her skinny boy's body, which was never fit enough for her standards—dissolved. The next day, she took another pill. She didn't think twice about it. It was her prescription, it energized her, and there were no side effects.

At work she was chattier and also more mellow than usual, and she managed to stay cheerful even while dealing with ungrateful patients and tedious charting. She skipped lunch breaks. When she finished the pills, a girlfriend who didn't need her prescription anymore offered the pills to Lara. *Why not?* Lara thought. That week, she took three pills at a time.

A few days after the bottle emptied, Lara started to feel sick. That afternoon at work, she remembered that she had morphine in her pocket, 1 milligram left over from a patient. Back then, hospitals weren't as vigilant about counting the "waste"—the surplus drugs left over from patients' prescribed doses. Nurses went home, shrugged off their scrubs, and dumped their pocket contents into the trash.

She fingered the vial, running her thumb along the smooth, cool glass. *If the Percocet made me feel that good, maybe morphine will, too,* she thought. She returned it to her pocket to use at home. There was no inner voice asking her what she was doing, no angel on her shoulder imploring for restraint. It was just a little shot in the arm to take the edge off the day. She would never actually take narcotics at work, she told herself.

For the next several months, Lara conveniently "forgot to waste" left-over narcotics. Instead, she brought them home and stashed the Percocet, morphine, or Dilaudid in her underwear drawer. In the beginning, the drugs popped into her mind only occasionally, an elated realization like finding a twenty-dollar bill at the bottom of a purse: *Oh! I have extra narcs in my pocket!* She brought home vials about twice a week. It was too easy. Even once her hospital began requiring nurses to dispose of the excess in front of a colleague, the drugs were there for the taking. "Hey, I'm wasting this milligram of Dilaudid," Lara would say, and the nearest nurse would hardly look up as she scribbled a signature. No one bothered to watch whether Lara actually threw out the vial, a procedure intended to prevent exactly what Lara was doing.

Not only was she able to do her job while taking the drugs, but she also had more energy than she knew what to do with. She worked additional hours for overtime pay. She justified the drug use by telling herself that her increased energy made her a more productive nurse. "You've heard about soccer moms being able to do everything on Ritalin? That was me. I could work! I could do ten thousand things and no one suspected why."

Within months, Lara's tolerance increased and her main concern at the hospital became collecting more drugs to bring home. One milligram wasn't enough to spark a buzz, and she felt fatigued if she tried to go more than a day without taking something. So she signed up to work every day—zero days off—to get access to the meds because she didn't want to feel tired. She was often sick to her stomach, but didn't make the connection between her stomachaches and the drugs.

If you had asked Lara before she donated eggs what she thought about people who took narcotics, she would have responded, "Why on earth would someone do that?" Now it did not occur to her that she had become one of those people. It didn't even occur to her that she was doing drugs (as opposed to taking medicine), let alone stealing them.

Lara was a superstar nurse, energetic without being perky, unfailingly positive, and constantly volunteering to help other nurses. Nobody questioned her, nobody told her it wasn't healthy to work seven days a week. There was always a need for more hands. She would call the nurse manager and ask nonchalantly, "Hey, can I come in for four hours this afternoon?" Nobody ever said no.

About a year after she took her first Percocet, the workday started to seem longer. Lara was eager to get home so that she could inject herself. The first time she shot up in a staff bathroom, a voice broke through her thoughts: "It's getting bad if you can't even wait to get home." *I have a hard job and it's a long day*, she told herself. *If other people saw what I see at work, they'd need something to take the edge off, too.* "You've crossed the line you drew for yourself." *I can stop at any time.*

Lara took sixteen-hour shifts, sailing through them with midday bathroom breaks to insert an IV, eventually injecting up to 8 milligrams of Dilaudid at a time, an enormous dose, but, for Lara, just enough to keep her alert. Once, she put a heparin lock in her foot to give her quicker access to a vein. She wore it the entire workday, attending meetings and caring for patients. She told coworkers she was limping because she had dropped a weight on her toes.

Because the medications helped her to excel at her job and to work extended hours, Lara didn't admit to herself that what she was doing was dangerous.

One afternoon, she realized that she hadn't wasted a single narcotic in five consecutive workdays. Somehow, over the past several months, her maneuvers had shifted from secretive to sloppy. Surely, she worried, someone would catch on to her. She took a swig of Pepto-Bismol to calm her stomach, which was shaky as usual. She blamed her nerves, because she was applying for a position as a flight nurse on a medical trauma helicopter, her ultimate career goal since nursing school. *Ugh, if I could just get another vial, then I won't feel sick.* Then it hit her. *Oh my God, it's not because I'm nervous.* It had taken her that long to see, or accept, the link between her stomachaches and her addiction.

Many addicts say that there is often no single defining event that leads them to want to stop using. For some, there simply comes a point when they are ready to admit to themselves that they have a problem and they don't want to have that problem anymore. That's how it was for Lara. That day was no different from the day before, except that a layer of her denial suddenly lifted. Later, she would be amazed that she had ignored the signs of addiction for so long.

Once it clicked, she was petrified. She was ashamed of herself and afraid of what people would think; she didn't know which was worse. She vowed to do everything she could to quit her addiction. Lara tried calling in sick to force herself into withdrawal. *Okay, I kicked this. It's cool,* she would say to herself after a few days. But then she would return to the hospital to find that her desire for the drug was stronger than she was. After hours of trying to tough it out, she would grab a vial and a needle, so easy, so irresistible, and run to the bathroom.

She attempted to discourage herself by calling her brother, whom she didn't want to disappoint. She wrote herself letters: "This isn't how you want to live your life." She tried stipulating that she could shoot up only at night to help her sleep, or she could use only morphine so she wouldn't get as sick. She told her roommate, Angie, a fellow ER nurse she loved, so that someone else could hold her accountable. Lara and Angie had been

ER nurses together for six years. Angie was the type of strong nurse that other nurses wanted in the room with them. When they started out as new nurses together, they had leaned on each other to endure the ER sink-or-swim craziness the way many nurses did if they were lucky enough to find a competent, likeable partner. Lara and Angie had combined their strengths and pulled each other through stints at two hospitals.

Angie could not believe it. She was sympathetic but appalled. She wouldn't turn Lara in, yet couldn't persuade her to stop using for long. Each time Lara tried to stop, within twenty-four hours she slid from being able to glide through her shift and an invigorating workout at the gym to feeling too sick and depressed to function. She felt like she had the worst flu possible, a debilitating illness that could vanish in moments after an injection. So she kept injecting. She didn't know that there were narcotics addiction treatment programs specifically for medical professionals. She didn't know what else to do. *I need to stop feeling so sick*, she told herself. *I'll take something today and then I'll stop tomorrow.* She said this for four more months.

Eighteen months after her first Percocet, Lara was offered the dream job that she had applied for: a flight nurse for a hospital system. Flight nurse opportunities, prestigious within the field, were rare. When Lara saw the helicopter she would be working on, she couldn't contain her exhilaration. She ran her hand along the airframe, climbed inside, and sat in the nurse's seat, incredulous that she was exactly where she wanted to be.

The next day was a Thursday. Determined to get clean, Lara checked into the drug treatment program at her hospital. She thought she simply needed to get over a few days of drug withdrawal. She'd let the profession-als get her clean over the weekend, and she'd leave on Monday, the drugs gone from her system, her body free from their grasp. Lara assumed her hospital was so large that no one would see her. She didn't turn herself in to her ER bosses because she figured she would quickly get this sorted out. Still in some measure of denial, Lara thought that she could conquer any treatment plan they gave her. After all, she was strong. She was deter-mined. She still didn't realize she was that sick.

That weekend, when Lara was feverish from narcotics withdrawal, Angie called from the ER. The director told Angie that the department had been aware of Lara's problem for months. "The ER knows what's going on," Angie said. "They know you're stealing drugs and I think you should turn yourself in."

I'm an idiot, Lara thought. *Who goes in for drug treatment at the same hospital where they work?* She raced to turn herself in, hoping the consequences would be lighter if she admitted she had a problem and was desperate for help. She dashed out of the building and down the sidewalk in the sweatpants she'd worn for two days straight and a long-sleeved shirt covering the marks on her arms that she didn't want anyone to see. She sprinted the block between the treatment center and the ER and barreled into the director's office.

Before the ER director had a chance to speak, Lara unloaded. "I have a problem and I can't stop and I'm trying to get help and I'm in treatment now," she blurted through tears. "I don't want to live like this anymore."

The director had been one of Lara's favorite people to work with. A former nurse, she came into the unit and helped when the staff was overburdened. Unlike Lara's previous administrators, who would either sit comfortably in their back offices while their nurses drowned in work or stand imperiously on the floor telling staff what not to do, this director rolled up her sleeves, pushed stretchers, and ordered food for her employees.

The director reluctantly pushed a large stack of papers across her desk. The file documented instances when Lara had taken narcotics under a patient's name. Lara had never taken medications *from* a patient, but she had taken larger vials than patients needed in order to increase the leftovers. The administration had tracked her for approximately eight months.

"You're under investigation," the director told her sadly. "We're going to have to fire you. For a long time, I didn't do anything because I just couldn't believe it."

Lara was scared. She didn't know what would happen next. Would she go to jail? At the same time, she felt a tremendous sense of relief. *This is over now and I can move on*, she thought. *Whatever happens is going to be better than where I've been. Now that it's in the open, I don't have to fight this battle by myself anymore.*

Lara never found out why administrators didn't report her to law enforcement. Perhaps it was because she had voluntarily turned herself in and had entered a drug treatment program. Or perhaps they didn't want to derail the career of an exceptional nurse. Lara reported herself to state nursing board officials, who said that to keep her license, she would have to enroll in the Medical Drug Intervention program.

MDI (a pseudonym—most states have their own program) was an intense multiyear program designed to help nurses and other health professionals. Even after the initial thirty-day rehabilitation, patients were not allowed to work in any medical field, so they could focus exclusively on getting clean. MDI administrators decided when to allow a nurse to take a job. Lara met nurses who had been kept out of work for a year.

The thirty-day rehab program was a beast. Lara was the sickest she'd ever been. She had flu symptoms, sweats, chills, extreme fatigue, aches, and unimaginable joint pain. She couldn't brush her teeth because it hurt too much to close her fist around her toothbrush. For weeks, the agony was unrelenting, but Lara was determined to take no medications to ease her through it. She attended her assigned meetings and classes, where program leaders introduced her to Narcotics Anonymous and forced her to examine her demons.

Lara didn't need a therapist to explain to her why the drugs were so tempting. Her divorced parents had been physically and mentally abusive. She remembered vividly the days she arrived at school bruised from beatings, and the times her parents called her fat, ugly, and stupid or told her she would "never be smart enough to be a nurse." Her mother was a mean drunk by night and a sweet woman by day, with no memory of her behavior the night before.

The program also taught Lara that she had been turning to narcotics to escape something else. Lara had believed she was strong enough to ably manage the horrors she saw in the ER—the dying babies, the grisly traumas. Her hospital allowed no time for debriefing; following a tragedy, nurses were expected to get right back to work. Lara had been repressing these images and experiences for years. She hadn't realized they were eating away at her still.

Three months after Lara completed rehab, MDI placed her in a medical advice job. She had gone from working as a Level-1 trauma center nurse to answering an advice hotline. Mortified, she cried during her drive to work for the first two weeks. Every morning before 8 a.m., seven days a week, Lara had to call a 1-800 number to check whether she would be randomly tested. On testing days, within two hours of the call, she had to give a urine sample at a lab (and pay $55 for the test). If she missed the test, she would be kicked out of the program and lose her license permanently, no excuses.

Lara had slogged through the misery of withdrawal. She regularly called her case manager to complain. "I hate you guys!" she'd say. "I'm not doing this. You can take my license." Ten minutes later, she would call back, contrite. "No, never mind! I didn't mean it!"

The program was so strict that Lara met many fantastic nurses who gave up their licenses rather than stick with it. But she was determined to tough it out. "MDI will back you up when you reapply for your license. They want to know how serious you are," she explained. "Now that I can look back, they did know what was best for me when I didn't. I wanted to go back to the ER. But they had to approve the job."

After two years, MDI allowed Lara to resume patient interaction by working at a doctor's office for eighteen months. Finally, MDI let her interview for an ER job at a different hospital. Her résumé was still impressive. She breezed through the interview until the end, when she was required to mention the program. Every month, her employer would have to fill out forms asserting that Lara was not impaired at work.

Another nurse in the program had given Lara advice: "Just look them straight in the face and say, 'I'm doing the right thing now, and have been for a long time.' Don't apologize. You made a mistake. You're moving on." So she did, unflinchingly looking the interviewer in the eye.

"I'm impressed that you're so honest with me," the interviewer said. She told Lara later that she gave her the job because she was so forthright.

Lara had done so well with her recovery that her mother asked her to take her to an AA meeting. Her mother never drank again. Soon, her brother made the same request. Before long, Lara's family was sober. But Lara's battle wasn't over; it probably would never truly end.

After twelve months in the ER position, Lara was considered an official graduate of the program. She would not have to disclose her drug issue or treatment again.

Years later, when she applied for the job at South General Hospital, she didn't mention the addiction. She considered herself fortunate for many reasons, one of them being that the coworkers and friends she did tell about her addiction didn't judge her. She felt secure knowing that her friends, including Angie from one ER and Molly and Juliette from another, were supportive.

One of the great aspects of nursing was that it could forge lasting bonds. Working so closely with coworkers on matters intimate and important created the kinds of forever friendships that could buoy a nurse through long hospital days. Molly, a straight shooter, and Juliette, a loyal pal, fell into that category. "When nurses get to know each other, we have each other's back. We really will do anything for each other," said Lara, who worked every Christmas holiday shift for thirteen years straight before she had kids so that other nurses could celebrate with their children.

Despite the facts that nine years had passed since her first Percocet and Lara was married now with two beautiful children, at South General narcotics tempted her every day. There were even more drugs available here than at her first ER. Nurses constantly left half-full vials on the counters and the protocol for disposing of them was often ignored. *Oh, look at that, there are some narcotics sitting right there*, a little voice would nudge Lara.

She knew that the relapse rate for narcotics addiction was extremely high. To keep herself in check, she attended three Narcotics Anonymous meetings a week. She could count on dozens of friends she had made through NA who would help in an emergency. "In a way the addiction is a huge blessing because I have real strong people in my life now and they help me," Lara explained. "I would have never thought that such a horrible situation would turn so positive."

Lara had been doing pretty well resisting temptation, all things considered. Until six days ago, when her mom, long suffering from emphysema, died in her arms. She was 65. Lara was devastated. She didn't know how to cope with the loss of a parent.

Now, on her first day back at work since the funeral, Lara stared at the vial in front of her. The narcotic promised her security, comfort, confidence, and a happy buzz that would dull the pain of her mother's death.

She wanted it so badly she could barely breathe. *It will make you feel better. No one will know. You want it. You deserve it. Take it.*

The Secret Club

Nursing is among the most important professions in the world.

In no other profession do people float ably among specialties, helping to ease babies into being, escorting men and women gently into death, and heroically resurrecting patients in between. There are few other careers in which people are so devoted to a noble purpose that they work twelve, fourteen, sixteen straight hours without eating, sleeping, or taking breaks and often without commensurate pay simply because they believe in the importance of their job. They are frequently the first responders on the front lines of malady and contagion, risking their own health to improve someone else's. Nursing is more than a career; it is a calling. Nurses are remarkable. Yet contemporary literature largely neglects them.

At 3.5 million strong in the United States and more than 20 million worldwide, nurses are the largest group of healthcare providers. The women who comprise 90 percent of the workforce are a unique sisterhood whose bonds are forged through the most dramatic miracles and traumas as well as the tedious, routine tasks necessary to keep human bodies functioning. Nursing, for brave men and women, is "like a secret club that holds immense emotional joy and fulfillment in spite of shared tragedies," a Michigan nurse practitioner told me. Nurses call the profession a secret club because their experiences are so novel, their jobs so intimate and occasionally horrifying, their combination of compassion and desensitization so peculiar, that they imagine nobody else could understand what it is like to work in their once-white shoes.

Pop culture would have us believe that nurses play a small, trivial role in healthcare; medical television programs tend to show doctors lingering at patients' bedsides while nurses flit and intone "Yes, Doctor" in the background. But this is not the case. As a Minnesota agency nurse said, "We are not just bed-making, drink-serving, poop-wiping, medication-passing assistants. We are much more."

They are, for example, reporters. They discuss and document patient status, serving as the main point of contact for doctors, surgeons, therapists, social workers, and other specialists. They are watchmen, keeping vigil, meticulously monitoring vital signs, deciphering patients' individual trends and patterns, painstakingly double-checking dosages and medications. They are detectives, investigating deviations, asking questions, listening carefully, searching for clues. They are warriors, called to serve at the first sign of outbreak, fighting infection, containing disease. They are gatekeepers, turning staff members away when patients need a break from procedures, a nap, or a moment to digest their circumstances. They are scientists, constantly learning, tackling sociology, psychology, physiology, anatomy, pharmacology, chemistry, microbiology. They are advocates, lobbying physicians for or against procedures, for pain assistance, for a few more minutes of time. They are teachers, educating people about their condition, demonstrating home healthcare to patients and parents: how to suction a tracheostomy, change an airway, inject a medication, breastfeed a newborn. They are the muscle, holding patients down to insert or remove tubes or needles, pushing people to get out of bed following surgery, breaking a sweat when performing CPR, lifting, moving, pushing, forcing, turning. They are confidantes, protectors, communicators, comforters, nurturers; easing fears, offering solace, cradling babies whose parents can't be there, consoling loved ones who feel that all hope is gone. They are multitaskers: supporting, coordinating, and inhabiting all of these roles at once. And they are lionhearted diplomats, helping a patient die with dignity in one room, facilitating a recovery in the next, keeping their composure even when they are shaken to the core.

• • •

To examine what it is like to be a member of this secret club, I interviewed hundreds of nurses in the United States and several other countries. Essays based on their perspectives of the behind-the-scenes realities of nursing support stories that follow a year in the life of four ER nurses in an unnamed region of this country. Most of the people and hospitals in this book have pseudonyms and/or identifying details changed or omitted to protect their privacy. Some chronologies have been shifted.

The nurses I chose as main characters illustrate a variety of triumphs and struggles common in the profession. Confident, funny, and charmingly bossy, Molly is well loved by both patients and staff. When Pines Memorial's anti-nurse policy changes lead her to quit her job, she signs with an agency instead. Molly has given herself one year to find a hospital that treats nurses and patients well enough that she would want to join its staff. At the same time, she begins fertility treatments that place her on the other side of the curtain.

Lara, an able, trustworthy, committed ER nurse at South General, continues to battle the temptations of prescription drugs that are preposterously easy to steal, and doesn't know that the coming year will bring major events that could trigger her downfall. Juliette, an ER nurse at Pines, is a hard worker who doesn't hesitate to advocate loudly for her patients even when it is not in her own best interest to do so. Her blunt outspokenness does not endear her to many of her colleagues. Subsequently, she feels unwelcome in a workplace where patients' lives depend on collegiality and communication among staff. And at Citycenter Hospital, Sam is a new nurse, young and awkward, whose introversion can come across as unprofessional. Sam is discouraged by her doctors' and administrators' overall lack of respect for nurses, but she has to overcome other hurdles, including rumors about her promiscuity.

These four women and the other nurses I interviewed voice a rallying cry for their colleagues. Through their stories and others', this book presents an extensively researched snapshot of a subculture as well as an investigation of the medical industry's treatment of the nursing profession. Physicians grapple with some of the same problems as nurses, and countless skilled and compassionate doctors treat patients, solve medical mysteries, and save lives. Physicians' voices are already heeded, however. This is not their story. As such, some doctors may be depicted negatively in the stories to follow, but this book does not intend to denigrate doctors, techs, or, for that matter, patients. It is meant to represent nurses' perspectives and to celebrate them.

In doing so, this book does not romanticize the career. Nurses want the public to know the truth about nursing. It can be a difficult, exhausting, exasperating, and dangerous job in which they are often overworked and understaffed. But it is also joyous, rewarding, challenging, fascinating, exciting, and meaningful. Nurses want current and future patients and their families to know the healthcare secrets that can save their lives. And they want potential future nurses to know how deeply and passionately they love what they do. "Nursing is not a job. It is a life," a Kansas nurse manager said. "It is who you are."

The nurses who shared their thoughts and stories for this book invite you to peer behind the Staff Only door at the controlled chaos beyond: the jubilance and heartbreak; the temptations, drugs, lies, and violence; the miracles and wonders; the dark humor and innuendo; and most of all, the people who care for us when we are at our most vulnerable and bolster us on what could be the worst or best or last days of our lives.

"Doctors breeze in and out. They do not share the most intimate moments with the patients, but they are the 'important' ones who get the media accolades," a New Jersey nurse practitioner said. "It is the nurse who holds the hand of a patient without a family, who talks to them while they take their last breaths, who aches for them while they die alone. It is the nurse who cleans the patient's body, wipes away the blood and fluids, and closes his eyes. It is the nurse who says good-bye to the patient for the last time," she said. "Our story needs to be told. We want to be heard."

They will be. And you will never view healthcare the same way again.

JULIETTE   PINES MEMORIAL, August

When she left the patient's room, Juliette retrieved an alcohol swab from her pocket and began to wipe down the pen the man had used to sign his discharge papers. Then she thought better of it. The patient was crazy and probably didn't bathe often. She threw out the pen, stripped off her gloves, and trashed them, too. Back at the nurses station, she scrubbed her arms, hands, and neck with hand sanitizer, even though she had been wearing a yellow contact isolation gown.

Juliette's husband made fun of her for being a germaphobe nurse, but she didn't care. She sanitized her hands so often they were red and chapped. All day long she saw sick patients who didn't wash their hands, who touched their faces (or worse), and then touched everything in the room. She reminded patients to cover their mouths when they coughed or sneezed, and still, they sprayed the triage booth unapologetically. The first couple of years she had worked as an ER nurse, she was constantly sick with respiratory or GI illnesses. Now she rarely got sick, but she was determined to protect her family from those germs. Even at home, Juliette made her daughter, Michelle, wash her hands constantly. Molly—the opposite of a germaphobe—teased Juliette that she bathed her child in Purell.

The ER felt different without Molly. In the three weeks since Molly had left, the unit had been noticeably quiet and boring. Without Molly's witty sarcasm and infectious laugh, it was harder to deal with Charlene, the insufferable nursing supervisor. Without Molly, Juliette was lonely at work.

Socially, Pines Memorial hadn't panned out as Juliette had hoped. At Avenue, the hospital where Juliette, Molly, and Lara had worked together before, the nurses had formed a lasting bond. They were together constantly, at and outside of work. When the Avenue nurse manager, whom Juliette had adored, left, and a disorganized, inexperienced manager took over, the nurses scattered to various hospitals across the region. But they had grown so close that three years after leaving Avenue Hospital, they still gathered a few times a year for parties and called each other for advice or comfort. Juliette and Molly were particularly tight. Neither woman was afraid to speak her mind.

When they left Avenue, Juliette and Molly had worked briefly for an agency that had sent them to Pines, where they eventually signed on to work full-time. At Pines, they had joined an ER that was dominated by a clique of beautiful nurses. Pines was known for its attractive nurses and dreamy doctors, but the ER nursing clique outshone the rest. They were a group of nine women who lived in the same town and scheduled frequent social events, including playdates for their children. They invited Molly, who did not have children. They did not invite Juliette, who did. For years, Juliette had tried to gain entry. She often complimented various members of the clique and she frequently mentioned her 7-year-old daughter.

It didn't work. They chatted about their get-togethers at the nurses station, right in front of Juliette. They posted on Facebook, arranging outings and rehashing them afterward, even though Juliette could see every exchange, every ebulliently posed photo. They were pleasant enough in the ER, but they never made her feel included. They acted, and looked, like a sorority.

The clique loved Molly—everyone did—but she didn't hang out with them. Instead, she was a loyal friend to Juliette. Juliette was 42 years old, and it still hurt to be left out. She wondered if they rejected her because she was six feet two inches tall and overweight. Between her size and her bright auburn bob, she couldn't have looked more different from the clique. Juliette wasn't looking for best friends. She just wanted to feel like part of a team. And the fact that Priscilla, the nursing director, was part of the clique made Juliette feel even more excluded.

Didn't they already have something in common, something that could supersede the bonds of colleagues in other professions? They were healers, all of them, whose job was to reach people, to connect with them, to make them whole. Why couldn't they be as compassionate to each other as they were to their patients?

"You don't need them. You have me!" Molly would say.

But not anymore. Molly's resignation was a blow to Juliette and to the ER in general. Dr. Preston, himself a large personality, had told Juliette that Molly's leaving was a major loss to the department. Clark, who had light blue eyes and curly white-blond hair, was loud and hilarious, livening up the ER. He was one of the few doctors to insist that nurses call him by his first name, which seemed to soften the medical hierarchy. He could often be found joking around with the nurses, particularly the cute ones. Although he was a risk-taker with his patients, he was also straightforward, which patients and nurses appreciated.

Once, a successful high school sprinter had come to the ER with a badly fractured ankle. "He can't race tomorrow," Dr. Preston told the boy's parents, who were obviously overbearing and competitive.

"What will happen if he races?" the boy's father asked, prioritizing the sport over his son's health.

Dr. Preston smiled. "He'll lose."

Right now there wasn't time to dwell. In addition to four other patients, Juliette had two rapid heart rate patients who needed constant monitoring. She was also precepting—training—a new nurse, which meant having someone at her heels and explaining everything she did throughout her shift. Juliette enjoyed precepting because she liked teaching and working closely with another nurse, but it did add to the busyness of the day.

Juliette and her precept, a freckled girl named Noelle, had just transported a complicated stroke patient to the Intensive Care Unit, when Charlene assigned them another extremely critical patient, a 60-year-old man who had fallen in the shower and hit his head. As Juliette and Noelle worked him up, Charlene told her, "We have another LOC [loss of consciousness]. Room 18. Brain injury."

Hurrying down the hall, Juliette saw that Room 8, which was directly in front of the nurses station, was empty. Andrea, the nurse assigned to that zone, was idly surfing the Web. *Why is Charlene giving me so many critical patients when Andrea has none?* she thought. Suddenly, the monitors started beeping from Room 18. The new patient was crashing, unable to maintain his vitals.

When Juliette entered the room, she saw a neurological physician's assistant frantically attempting to insert an IV into the brain injury patient. "I can't get IV access," the PA said. She had to prepare the patient for a central line, an IV line going into the major vein near the groin. Sometimes central lines could be difficult to place.

Charlene had overloaded Juliette with critically ill patients as if the preceptee were an assistant, rather than extra work for Juliette. Trainees were supposed to be learning directly from a preceptor, not thrown into the deep end as full-fledged nurses. Quickly but gently, Juliette instructed Noelle how to help. "Go check on the patient with the cardiac drip. Ask him if he's having any further chest pains, and then check to see if the cardiac drip needs to be titrated based on his chest pain. Check on Room 16's level of abdominal pain. Then come back here to see what else we can do for this brain injury patient before we assess him again."

The PA tried again to insert the IV, but couldn't. The pressure was getting to her. "Get me an ICU nurse! We need more people in here," she hollered.

Juliette rushed to the hall to ask Charlene to check on Noelle and Juliette's other critical patients. Charlene was nowhere to be found.

Scatterbrained and prone to favoritism, Charlene spent much of her day gossiping in her office, rather than making sure that patients received proper attention. She was hard on Juliette for coming into work five or ten minutes late when traffic was particularly bad, but said nothing to clique nurses who arrived half an hour late without explanation. She was overly focused on getting patients out the door as quickly as possible, so she could bring in more patients and increase hospital profits. And she certainly didn't prioritize the overall safety of the ER. Recently, when a loud bang sounding like a gunshot occurred near the nurses station, Charlene shoved another nurse out of the way and bolted out the front door. For weeks, the nurses made fun of her for abandoning staff and patients to save herself, especially because the noise turned out to be a harmless equipment malfunction.

Charlene thought she was part of the clique. The nine nurses kissed up to her so that she would give them the plum assignments, and the ploy worked: Charlene blatantly favored Andrea and the other dominant clique members when it came to scheduling. But Juliette had heard them laugh about Charlene behind her back. The childishness of this behavior exhausted Juliette, who did not want juvenile social maneuverings taking up brain space that she hoped to devote to patient care.

Juliette's patient was now completely unresponsive. His Glasgow Coma Scale, a range from 3 to 15 used to measure consciousness, was a 3: He was not opening his eyes to painful stimuli, talking, or moving any extremities. Without the central line dispensing medication, he couldn't be intubated.

Finally, the tech got the line in. Juliette immediately started the medications to prepare the patient for intubation.

When the respiratory tech arrived to take over, Juliette and Noelle made sure their other patients were stabilized. Then Juliette stripped off her gloves, sanitized her hands, and found Charlene at the nurses station, where Andrea was still shopping online. "I'm done. I'm going to minor care for the rest of the day," Juliette said. "I'll meet you there," she told Noelle.

"Okay," Charlene said. "But you have to give report to ICU."

"Andrea can do that," Juliette said, frustrated. Charlene should never have assigned her three ICU-bound patients simultaneously when each of them required a nurse's undivided attention.

Andrea scowled at Juliette.

"Never mind. I'll do it," Juliette said. She wiped down the phone with an alcohol swab before picking it up.

Later, Juliette found Charlene in the break room. "Why didn't you give that patient to Andrea?" she asked.

"Because it was fine for you and your preceptee to take him. You guys could handle it together," Charlene said. "And it was wrong of you to tell Andrea to call report."

Juliette looked Charlene in the eye. "Sometimes I feel like Andrea does a lot more talking than working, and I took it out on her."

"I understand," Charlene said, matter-of-factly. "I do that in my work assignments sometimes."

"Sounds like you're admitting to favoritism," Juliette said.

Charlene rolled her eyes.

The next day, Charlene assigned Juliette four seriously ill Cardiac Care Unit–bound patients, while other ER nurses had only the relatively low-maintenance run-of-the-mill ER cases, none of whom would be admitted to the CCU.

Juliette was a first-rate nurse, and could handle difficult patient loads. But every ICU and CCU patient needed a nurse who could spend time with them one-on-one. On a personal level, Juliette could ignore that Charlene and some other coworkers didn't like her. She knew that stressful working conditions affected how she spoke to people. However, she worried about how tensions and exclusions, power trips, and freezing out among the nurses could impinge on patient care. Perhaps that was why the clique's snubs bothered her so much. They weren't folding sweaters here. Juliette took great pride in being a hardworking nurse who cared intensely for her patients.

Oh, who was she kidding? Of course she took the rejections personally. Between her weight and family issues, she had been socially insecure her entire life. Maybe what bothered her most was that people could lower her self-esteem in an arena in which she felt confident that she was good at what she did.

SAM   CITYCENTER HOSPITAL, August

Just don't kill anyone, Sam thought, taking deep breaths as the charge nurse distributed assignments. *You'll be okay. Just don't kill anyone.*

She could see herself in a mirror across the hall, her arms self-consciously wrapped around her ample chest. Petite and slender with long, dark hair usually tied back in a ponytail, Sam had large gray eyes framed by delicate wire-rimmed glasses. She was sure her normally olive skin had a green tint this morning.

Since she had awakened at 4:30 a.m., 24-year-old Sam had been fighting the nausea that accompanied her nerves on her first official day as a nurse. It wasn't that she was inexperienced. She had interned here at Citycenter Hospital for three months after graduating from nursing school. Before nursing school, she was an ER technician at Pines Memorial. But this was different. Now she would be held personally responsible for potentially fragile lives.

Sam sighed with relief when the charge nurse assigned her to Zone 3. The Citycenter ER was divided into a minor care area for stitches and breaks, and three treatment zones: Zone 1 for the sickest patients, Zone 3 for the least sick. She would be less likely to accidentally kill a patient who wasn't too critical to begin with. As the charge nurse wrapped up the meeting, Sam mentally ran through the phone numbers she had memorized. New nurses were given cards with phone numbers for the charge nurse, lab, radiology, computer help desk, and tube station, a pneumatic labyrinth of tubes that sent specimens and paperwork through the walls to various departments of the hospital. Sam had learned as an intern that if the staff believed a nurse didn't know what she was doing, they gave her a hard time. She had worked her tail off to get here. She wasn't about to lose any respect on her first day because she had to look up a phone number.

Sam went to the nurses station to check the computer for the outgoing nurse's report. Because the night shift nurse's patients all were discharged, triage had assigned a new slate of patients. "Room 12: Lac of unknown area." A laceration sounded easy enough. Sam walked into the patient's room. He—or she, it was difficult to tell—started talking before Sam had a chance to ask questions.

"I didn't tell them at Registration, but I was really tired of this whole situation, so I decided to take matters into my own hands," said Lou, whose chart identified her as female, pointing downward. "I went online and read about this banding procedure. I got hair ties, tied the hair ties around it, took some sterilized scissors, and I untied it, and I cut it off. But there was a lot of blood, so I tied the hair ties back around it."

Sam didn't know what the patient was talking about. "Oh, okay," she replied. "Well, let's just see what we're working with here." She lifted the gown. Her mind went blank except to register, *Uh, there should be balls there.* She cleared her throat. "Are you in pain?" she asked.

Lou's voice was shaky. "Yes."

"Okay, well I'll definitely get you some pain medication, probably some antibiotics. I'll go see what the plan is," she said. She speed-walked to the nurses station, her thoughts reeling. Self-inflicted ball-removal had definitely not come up during nurse training.

She quickly checked the computerized board, which listed the patients, their chief complaints, their room, their nurse, and the residents or attending (the doctor in charge), as well as a small section for comments. Kathleen, a new physician's assistant, was assigned to this patient. Sam found her in the hallway.

"Uhhh, Room 12?" Sam asked.

"I *know*. Urology's coming," Kathleen snapped, without making eye contact. "Someone else will deal with that."

Sam had heard other nurses say that Kathleen was uncomfortable treating patients with more than minor injuries. She must have picked up Room 12 because triage had listed the chief complaint as "lac." Some laceration. Evidently, the patient had told triage "I cut myself" without explaining the important details.

Lou wasn't going to bleed to death, but her condition was serious nonetheless. Sam wasn't about to let her wait in pain while Kathleen passed the buck. She found the attending ER physician outside another patient room. Bernadette Geiger was an African American woman with a high, childlike voice and a reputation for being extraordinarily compassionate. Sam knew she wasn't supposed to approach an attending directly, but she didn't know who or where the resident was and she worried the patient would suffer in Kathleen's care.

"Um, could I please get pre-op labs, antibiotics, and pain meds for the patient in twelve?" Sam asked, her heart pounding.

"Sure." The doctor smiled and wrote the orders.

Sam retrieved the medications quickly, then gave them to the patient intravenously. She tried to make conversation. If she kept Lou talking, she could distract her from the pain until the morphine kicked in. Keeping her calm and in the present moment would also help prevent her from going into shock. "We need to fix you up here, friend," she said.

"You know, it's still bathing suit season and I can't wear cute little bikinis when I have stuff down there," Lou said.

Sam tried to be understanding. "Oh yeah, I know. Bathing suit season sucks. I'm a big fan of board shorts because they offer more coverage."

"I hadn't thought about board shorts," Lou said. "They're probably not my style."

Sam kept the patient stable until she wheeled her to the OR, about an hour later. Sam was pleased that she had kept her cool during a relatively shocking case for a new nurse on her first day when the PA had been no help at all.

Sam had started volunteering as an EMT when she was 16. Every Friday night during her junior and senior years of high school, she slept at the firehouse, on call for the overnight shift. She always did more than was expected of her, always stayed later than her shift. The girls at her private Catholic school didn't know what to do with her; she wasn't "popular," but neither was she an "I'm-going-to-eat-my-hair-in-a-corner person." After college, Sam volunteered at a local rescue squad while she considered her career options. One night during a stop at Pines, she asked an ER nurse with whom she'd become friendly, "What am I going to do with my life?"

"This is what you're going to do," the nurse told her. "You're going to get your second degree in nursing and some experience under your belt. Then you're going to get your NP and be able to call your own shots. That's what I'm doing." Sam liked the idea of becoming a nurse practitioner, which required a master's degree. So she followed her friend's advice. She went right into nursing school, graduated, and interned. She hoped to apply to master's programs after working in the field for a couple of years.

As a nursing intern at Citycenter, Sam had learned that being an introvert would not help her quest. Sam wasn't much of a talker. She preferred to observe her surroundings quietly so that she could soak up as much information as possible. Her goal in most situations was to learn; there was always a way to improve her knowledge base. When she did speak, she was blunt, with a dry wit, and she spoke succinctly, which could unintentionally come across as curt or stiff. To her continued puzzlement, men had somehow interpreted this mannerism as mysteriousness, as if she were being coy. But Sam saw herself as just plain awkward.

During the first month of her internship, she had a patient who couldn't stop vomiting. Sam needed an order for antinausea medication, but was intimidated by Dr. Spiros, the 35-year-old senior resident on duty. He was a tall, exceedingly good-looking man with tousled hair as dark as Sam's ponytail. Sam had heard him speaking with other nurses in the halls about his interest in teaching medicine to doctors in developing countries. The other nurses swooned over Dr. Spiros, who was smart, sexy, and obviously smooth. Sam was not a swooner, but she could be painfully shy around suave men.

Instead, Sam approached Renée, the charge nurse: "My patient's puking his brains out. Can I give him Zofran?"

"Go ask Dr. Spiros," Renée said.

Sam pursed her lips and approached Dr. Spiros, who was looking over the board. She nudged her glasses up the bridge of her nose. "Um, can I get some Zofran for Mr. Nathan?"

"I don't even know who that patient is," he grumbled. "Ask someone else."

Geez, it's only Zofran, Sam thought, her face growing hot. It had a tendency to do that at inopportune moments. She returned to Renée, a Citycenter veteran. "That pompous guy wouldn't give me Zofran!" Sam said.

Renée looked incredulous. "What are you talking about? Dimitri's so nice!"

"That's what you think," Sam said.

Renée approached Dr. Spiros. "Hey, Dimitri, I need Zofran for Mr. Nathan."

Dr. Spiros smiled at her. "Sure, anything you want," he purred. "How's it going?"

Sam's gray eyes widened. *Jerk*, she thought. *It's a shame that such an attractive guy has to be such a douchebag.* She managed to avoid Dr. Spiros for the rest of her internship and hoped she wouldn't run into him again.

There were other annoying carryovers from her internship whom she now wouldn't be able to avoid. On the interns' first day, someone had asked if there were any questions. An intern named CeeCee asked, "You guys! Where do we get highlights done in this town?" Of all the questions. If Sam had been outgoing enough to ask a question, she would have chosen, "Where's the bathroom?"

CeeCee was an overly peppy 22-year-old with meticulously crimped hair. She was a former cheerleader prone to doing celebratory high kicks. Her relentless chatter had a passive-aggressive edge. She and two of her sexy nurse friends made backhanded remarks with toothy smiles.

During the internship, Sam happened to mutter to a tech that CeeCee drove her crazy. She didn't usually talk about people behind their backs, but CeeCee's insincere perkiness, fringed with entitlement, was grating. Within days, CeeCee texted Sam. "Someone told me you talked trash about me and said I'm dumb."

Ugh, drama. Sam tried to avoid drama. She didn't have the time or the personality to deal with it. She hadn't told anyone other than the tech that CeeCee drove her crazy, and she hadn't said anything more. Sam had never insulted CeeCee's intelligence, nursing skills, or work ethic. "Those matter more to me than whether I like someone or they like me," Sam explained. "And, if I put myself in her shoes, I'd say there's no connection between whether you like me and whether I'm a good nurse. Either she somehow equates 'she drives me crazy' with being dumb, or someone exaggerated what I said."

Sam replied with as upbeat a message as she could muster: "I'm sorry anyone said that because it's just not true! I think you're smarter than some of the more experienced nurses here!"

Not everyone at Citycenter was annoying. Sam's preceptor as an intern was gorgeous—a chiseled, 30-year-old African American man with kind, hazel eyes. Intelligent and calm, William was just her type. But she had made the mistake of dating someone at her last hospital, and that had not ended well. In any case, William had a long-distance girlfriend, a nurse many Citycenter nurses had met and spoke of with admiration.

William was one of only two full-time murses (nurse-speak for male nurses) in the ER. He often went out of his way to help his coworkers. Sam knew she could go to William with questions and he'd answer without making her feel uncomfortable or naïve for asking. That was, if she could get to him. He always seemed busy at the nurses station with any number of nurses, engrossed in private conversations that Sam was hesitant to interrupt even with valid medical questions. Women flocked to him for advice, safe flirtation, and to squeeze his impressively sculpted biceps.

By the end of her internship, Sam was comfortable enough with William to barge in on his nurse station conversations. He listened to Sam, as if the few times she spoke up meant that she was saying something particularly important. He was too friendly to intimidate her, and remained unflappable no matter how dire the situation. "Plenty of people in medicine get worked up and freak out over things, so it's nice when someone is reliably even-tempered," Sam said. But just as she got comfortable with her favorite coworker, she was assigned the day shift, while he worked only nights.

The rest of the patients on Sam's first day as a nurse weren't nearly as complicated as the guy who cut off his own balls, but Kathleen made them seem just as bad. She refused to communicate in person, instead writing bitchy comments on the board. Sam wouldn't hear from Kathleen for hours, and the PA would walk silently by her in the halls, but then Sam would go to the computer and see Kathleen's latest comments, directed at her. "Labs drawn????" Kathleen wrote next to one patient's name, though she hadn't told Sam which labs she wanted. In Zone 3, the PA was supposed to act like a physician, but the physicians Sam had known, even the unfriendly ones, would at least tell the nurses what was needed. Kathleen was making Sam feel incompetent.

By 3:00 p.m., Sam, usually cool under pressure, was uncharacteristically shaken because she didn't know the plans for her patients. Kathleen wasn't telling her which patients were being discharged and which were being admitted. Disgruntled patients had been waiting for procedures, test results, or discharge papers, and they were taking out their frustrations on Sam, who couldn't answer their questions.

Embarrassed, Sam talked them down. "We're still waiting for the test results," she bluffed. Or, "The CT scan isn't ready yet."

Sam was too daunted to confront Kathleen directly. She just wanted to get through her first day. Then a patient yelled, "I've been here for *six hours*! I don't know what's going on! You don't know what's going on, no one knows what's going on, and I'm going to leave!"

Nobody wanted that to happen. "I'll-I'll go find out," Sam said, feeling smaller than her five-foot-one-inch frame. "We're still waiting for your test results."

Sam couldn't find Kathleen anywhere. In the hall, she saw Dr. Spiros heading toward the break room. Naturally he was working today, of all days. She was expected to go up the chain of command and he was the next person in line. He was also the only familiar face she saw.

"Umm, I'm having a bit of a problem," she said. Remembering her previous encounter with Dr. Spiros made Sam even more flustered.

"What's wrong?" Dr. Spiros asked, gazing into her eyes.

Sam was surprised that he seemed sincerely concerned. She spoke quickly, ignoring the deepening flush of her cheeks. "I don't know what's going on with my patients. Kathleen's not talking to me, everyone's getting mad, and I don't know what else to do."

Dr. Spiros patted her on the back. "It's okay." He walked her to Dr. Shannon, another senior resident, whom Sam hadn't noticed. *Dr. Spiros's shift was over*, Sam thought, wanting to disappear. "Brad, this is Sam. She needs some help." He patted Sam again and left for the night.

"The foot lady wants more Dilaudid, the guy in six needs his discharge—he's been ready for an hour—the guy in sixteen is still puking and he's already had two rounds of Zofran, and I have no idea what's going on with the fourth patient," Sam said, her voice rising.

Dr. Shannon's voice was soothing, as if he had plenty of time to help her. It was no secret that Kathleen was a difficult PA to work with. "Okay, I can tell you what's going on with that first patient. I will find out about the second and third patients. And discharge papers are being written up for the fourth patient."

As she followed him down the hall, Sam wondered whether she had made a mistake: Maybe nursing was not the right career for an introvert. She decided to try the night shift instead.

MOLLY   September

SOUTH GENERAL HOSPITAL

After quitting her staff job at Pines, Molly immediately signed with a nursing agency. The scheduler, whom she would interact with only over the phone, assigned her to rotate among three different hospitals. Molly chose to work twelve-hour shifts, three to four days per week.

Academy Hospital was a brand-name hospital with first-class doctors and pretentious medical students. Most of the nurses, young and cliquish, were just out of school; Molly dubbed them "baby nurses." Citycenter Hospital was a teaching hospital with a poorly run ER. And South General was a Level-1 trauma center in an impoverished neighborhood. Molly had to leave her house at 4:30 a.m. to get to South General in time for her 6:00 a.m. shift. South General was in such need of experienced nurses like Molly that administrators put her to work after only an hour of orientation, rather than the usual four to twenty-four hours.

During her first week at South General, Molly ran into Dr. Lee, a wonderful trauma doctor who also worked at Pines. Dr. Lee was prone to self-deprecating humor, which was relatively rare among surgeons and a good way for physicians to get nurses to appreciate them. "Molly! Welcome to The South," he said. "I heard you left Pines because of the uniform."

Molly laughed. "You've got to be kidding me. Do you think I'm that big of an idiot?"

Dr. Lee nodded. "I thought that was a little weird. So you left because I'm based at Pines, then?" he joked.

"Ha. The uniform policy was just the last thing I was willing to tolerate," Molly said. "I wanted something different."

"Well, this is different!" he replied cheerfully, and left to check on a patient.

Over the next few weeks, as the agency circulated Molly among hospitals, she came to understand what he meant. South General nurses had nerves of steel. In this particularly disadvantaged part of the state, they saw extreme cases of medical and psychological distress. By contrast, on Molly's first day at Academy, a college-aged patient had a psychotic break. She sat on her bed laughing and talking to an emesis basin that she held to her ear like a telephone. Molly could hear the "baby nurses" whispering, "Can you believe how crazy she is?" "They thought she was the most psychotic person they'd ever seen," Molly said. "My thought was 'That's a big deal to y'all? *That's* crazy?'"

At South General, medics once brought in a homeless guy high on PCP. When they tried to move him from the gurney to a stretcher, he jumped up, ripped off his clothes, ran naked into the full waiting room, and "helicoptered," gyrating so that his noticeably long penis spun like a propeller. "To impress a chick, HELICOPTER DICK!" he shouted. While one nurse called security and gathered staff—it usually took several people to hold down patients on PCP because they had herculean strength—other nurses calmly ushered people to the other side of the large lobby, far from the now naked man.

"The South General nurses were like, 'Hmm, naked man helicoptering in the lobby. Security was called, no big deal.' That's why I like South General," Molly explained. "When he started screaming—'Waaaa!'—and dove out the plate glass window, *then* he became a trauma."

CITYCENTER MEDICAL

On Molly's first day at Citycenter, she felt sick to her stomach. She was not the nervous type, and certainly had never been anxious about a job before, even as a new grad. But she could see that Citycenter's ER was extremely unsafe. First, the entire department was filthy: Blood spattered the walls, full urinals sat on counters in rooms that were supposedly ready for a new patient, and dried urine covered a utility room counter. Second, patient wait times were inordinately high. And because there was no dedicated trauma nurse, a nurse in Zone 1 was expected to drop all of her patients—the sickest bunch in the ER—when a trauma patient came in. Trauma patients could require one-to-one care for several hours, leaving the sickest patients neglected and in danger.

Molly's anxiety was justified. That morning, she was assigned at least seven patients at a time, sometimes nine, which was more than she'd ever had at Pines, and too many for her to care for adequately. "How do you handle this kind of patient load?" she asked the other nurse in her zone.

"We can't," the nurse replied. "People are quitting left and right, which means an even bigger workload for the rest of us."

One of Molly's patients was a 400-pound drug addict who had been running around the city without pants. It had taken nine police officers to bring the man in. The ER staff had shackled him in four-point leather restraints and left him alone in an empty room. When Molly saw the patient, her jaw dropped. As Molly understood it, The Joint Commission instructed that patients in four-point restraints should have a one-to-one staffer who was supposed to document the patient's behavior, note medical interventions, and offer nourishment and toileting every fifteen minutes. If the patient became cooperative, the staff was supposed to release him from the restraints. The patient's chart said that since he had been in the ER, he had been quiet and cooperative, but tied down for hours.

Molly found Sarah, the charge nurse. "Where's his sitter?" she asked.

"There isn't one," Sarah said.

"But TJC recommends a sitter for patients in four-point restraints," Molly pointed out.

Sarah shrugged. "We tie people down here all the time. With the patients we get, we prefer it that way."

The staff was generally competent and dedicated but spread so thin that they couldn't consistently provide quality healthcare. Citycenter, where Molly was scheduled for several upcoming shifts, was in even worse shape than she had expected.

THE FERTILITY CLINIC

The next day, Molly was off from work so that she could attend her first appointment at the fertility clinic. The nurse at the desk showed her the list of tests the clinic wanted for the initial blood draw. Molly scanned it, concerned. Her husband's health insurance covered only up to $10,000 of certain fertility treatments and didn't cover in vitro fertilization. As a nurse, Molly typically made about $60,000 a year before taxes. Trey's police officer salary brought in $77,000 before taxes. They were trying to save for a down payment on a house, but too many out-of-pocket fertility treatment costs would wipe out their savings.

Molly crossed the varicella, rubella, HIV, and hepatitis C tests off the list. She had been tested for all of them within the last two years.

"Why are these crossed out?" the nurse asked.

"I had those tests performed less than two years ago and I only get a certain amount of insurance funds, so I'd like to save money on tests that have been performed recently," Molly said. The nurse shook her head and led Molly to the back room to draw blood.

The nurse frowned as she poked Molly. "You're as tight with your blood as you are with your money," she carped.

Molly ignored the dig. "I didn't know what two of the tests on that list were. Could you tell me?"

The woman didn't answer. After the draw, Molly watched the nurse label the tubes. She pointed. "These two here—what are those?"

"I can't tell you," the nurse said. She didn't even look at Molly.

"Because you don't know or because you aren't allowed?" Molly asked, confused.

"Our policy is to not tell people."

"That doesn't make sense," Molly said. "I'm paying for these. These are elective tests."

"You're a nurse. You understand," the nurse said.

"No, I don't understand. When my patients ask what a test is for, I tell them," Molly said. The woman glowered at her and left the room.

Safe in the elevator hallway, Molly composed herself. Struggling with infertility was difficult enough; why did the clinic have to make the process so unpleasant? Typically, she chose her doctors based on their bedside manner, but she had selected her fertility clinic because of its success rates. Patients here dealt mostly with the nurses until the actual procedures. Still, she couldn't help yearning for "someone to make eye contact, to have some inflection in their voice that shows they care about me, not just keeping their profits up," as she phrased it. "At a fertility clinic, a little warm fuzzy would go a long way."

That experience, and subsequent visits to the clinic, left Molly feeling like a number. On no occasion did clinic doctors or nurses introduce themselves before performing a procedure. As a result, Molly vowed to introduce herself clearly to each of her patients, to show them her badge, and to explain her role. "People aren't taking the three seconds to say, 'Hi, I'm Sandy and I'll be doing a transvaginal ultrasound on you today,'" Molly said. "As a healthcare worker, I'm generally less sensitive to that type of stuff, but the fertility experience is making me feel horrible. My patients see me during an emergency. They're probably more scared than someone going in for routine fertility testing. I will do a better job of putting ER patients at ease."

CHAPTER 2

CROSSING DOCTOR-NURSE LINES:
How the Sexy-Nurse Stereotype Affects Relationships with Doctors and Patients

"I will not be ashamed to say 'I know not,' nor will I fail to call in my colleagues when the skills of another are needed for a patient's recovery."
　—PHYSICIANS' HIPPOCRATIC OATH

"The intimate nature of nursing care, the involvement of nurses in important and sometimes highly stressful life events, and the mutual dependence of colleagues working in close concert all present the potential for blurring of limits to professional relationships."
　—CODE OF ETHICS FOR NURSES, PROVISION 2.4

"Lots of hot residents and nurses rush off to have quickie sex in utility closets during night shifts."
　—A NURSE PRACTITIONER IN VIRGINIA

MOLLY   September

ACADEMY HOSPITAL

During Molly's third week at Academy, a patient arrived at the ER already dead. Molly asked the charge nurse what kind of paperwork she needed to fill out.

The nurse, who was about 22, looked perplexed. "Honestly, I've never had a dead patient so I don't know. Can you ask someone else? I'm not getting patients out of here quickly enough. It's just too overwhelming."

Molly tried not to show her surprise. *How are you in charge without ever having seen a dead body?* she wondered. *Twenty-two-year-olds have no business being in charge of an ER.*

The patient load would have been considered a breeze at Pines; Molly had already come to think of Academy as easy money. Nurses here typically had no more than four patients, few of the patients were critically ill, and patients spent no more than thirty minutes in the waiting room.

Molly wondered whether a recent shift in nurse training contributed to the girl's inexperience. Traditionally, new nurses first had to work on the medical surgery floor to gain experience before moving to the ER and other critical care areas. The nationwide nursing shortage (or in some cases, short staffing) instead punted grads into more difficult areas of the hospital. Nurses were starting their career in the ER, OR, or ICU. "At Academy, some of the baby nurses don't know what they don't know," Molly said. "And there are med students and new doctors who are also on the learning curve. At Pines, there were plenty of times that a doctor put in a wrong medication order, and an experienced nurse was there to say, 'Hmm, that doesn't seem right.' But not at Academy. There's potential for big mistakes with this young staff."

Many of the doctors at Academy were egotistical, but Dr. Cynthia Baron took the cake. Dr. Bitch, as Molly referred to her privately, was a resident who resembled Malibu Barbie, swishing her impeccably blown-out hair as she sauntered down the halls. She rarely deigned to talk to nurses unless she was angry with them or needed something, in which case she treated them like preschoolers: "Hi, pumpkin, can you do me a teensy favor? Thaaanks."

One day, a well-dressed 88-year-old woman came into the ER. Molly was prepping her assigned room when two nurses practically carried the wheelchair in, rickshaw-style, one tipping the chair back and the other holding the woman's kicking feet to the leg rests to prevent the woman from pitching forward. Molly was horrified. *Do you really need to do that to this poor little old lady?* she thought.

"I just want to go home!" the patient cried, thrashing about as the nurses set the wheelchair next to the bed. "I don't want your help!" She tried to walk out of the room, but she was unsteady, and the nurses, assuming the woman was suffering from dementia, returned her to the chair.

Molly, the patient's primary nurse, quietly observed her. Dr. Baron poked her head into the room, saw the commotion, immediately ordered antipsychotic drugs for the patient, and left. Hospitals could hold a patient for seventy-two hours following an assessment, but Dr. Baron hadn't evaluated the patient at all; she based the order on the patient's initial behavior alone.

Finally, Molly spoke to the woman, who was again trying to escape her chair. She gently put her hand on the woman's arm. "May I please speak to you for a couple of minutes?" she asked. "Everyone else, can y'all please leave the room so I can talk to my patient?"

The nurses shrugged and left Molly alone with the woman. Molly's green eyes softened. Occasions like these were important, to nurses and to patients—the moments of exchange with another person on a human-to-human level.

Just because a patient wanted to leave didn't mean the hospital could allow her to go. Where would she go? Who would make sure she got home safely? Molly wanted to learn the woman's story to give her a chance to explain why she was in the ER and whether she would be safe if she were discharged. "So what's going on?" Molly asked. "Why are you so angry?"

The woman sat down and calmly told Molly that her neighbor had taken her to her doctor's office. The doctor told her she was in heart failure, needed new medications, and should probably move into a nursing home. When she rejected the plan, the neighbor drove her to the ER and left. "I've lived a full life," the woman said. "I've outlived my husband and most of my friends. My doctor said I'd die if I didn't take his advice. I'm fine with that. I've lived in my home for forty years. I don't want to leave it. I have help. I don't need doctors telling me what to do. I'm ready to go."

Molly nodded. "That makes complete sense to me."

Molly found Dr. Baron in the hallway and relayed the discussion. The doctor barely looked at her. "She's not competent," she said.

"We just had a very lucid conversation. She wants to go home and let nature take its course," Molly replied.

"She can't make her own decisions," the doctor insisted.

"Come back to the room with me," Molly said.

Dr. Baron followed her and addressed the patient. "What is today's date?" she asked. To determine whether a patient was clearheaded, it was standard practice to ask the patient's name, the date, and the name of the current president of the United States.

The patient was frustrated. "I don't know or care what the date is."

She knew her name and the president's, but Dr. Baron said, in front of the patient, "She is not competent."

"You're so pretty," the patient suddenly told the doctor.

Molly laughed. "Well, I guess you're right," she said to the doctor. Dr. Baron turned on her high heels and went straight to the nurses station to order a psychiatric consultation and a variety of lab tests. Luckily, Dr. Baron's shift ended soon afterward. When the next physician, Dr. Ward, arrived, Molly explained the situation. She liked Dr. Ward. He took the time to listen to the nurses. Molly had seen the doctor respect even a new nurse's input when she knew that a rhythm change on a heart monitor signified that something was wrong, though she couldn't pinpoint exactly what was amiss.

Dr. Ward sat down with the patient to hear the same story she had told Molly. The doctor called the patient's son, who confirmed that the woman was entirely competent and able to make her own decisions. He let Molly put the woman in a cab twenty minutes later.

"If I hadn't advocated for her, she could have ended up being committed to the psych unit for observation while they prolonged this woman's life against her will," Molly realized. "I think a lot of ER docs forget that not everyone wants to—or needs to—be saved."

A few days later, a patient came in with a bad bone infection in his foot. While at home, he had broken his foot by merely putting weight on it, and the already infected area began to bleed. Paramedics bandaged his foot and brought him to the ER. By the time he arrived, the bleeding was controlled but his blood pressure was low.

Molly started an IV and hung fluids to try to increase his blood pressure. Before long, the man looked better, was talking normally, and reported feeling fine. Molly ran a few blood tests to make sure.

When Dr. Baron came into the room, she declared, rapid-fire, "He's hypotensive because of blood loss. We need to transfuse immediately."

Molly shook her head. "I don't think he could have possibly lost enough blood out of a foot wound to be hypotensive. I think he's septic," she said.

"I'm ordering blood," the doctor insisted.

"I just ran an I-STAT and his H/H [a lab that shows blood volume] are normal."

Dr. Baron raised her voice. "Since he started bleeding so recently, his H/H might not reflect the blood loss yet."

"*Or* he's septic," Molly said. "His lactate is elevated."

Dr. Baron couldn't possibly let a nurse upstage her. She called the blood bank and ordered the transfusion, STAT.

Molly reluctantly transfused the blood, per the doctor's orders. The ICU doctor who came downstairs to examine the patient before transferring him looked confused. "Why are you giving blood for septic shock?" he asked Molly.

"You'll have to discuss that with Dr. Baron," Molly said. "I asked the same question."

When Molly complained to the charge nurse, the nurse answered, "We get a lot of complaints about how she treats nurses. She's been reported to the director of the medical staff several times. It's frustrating that no one does anything about it." Most hospitals Molly had worked at had individual doctors here and there who mistreated nurses, but at teaching hospitals like Academy, the overall egotism led to particularly horrendous communication.

One autumn afternoon, Molly was waiting for a call from gastroenterology to find out whether doctors were going to take an ER patient bleeding from the stomach to the OR or to the endoscopy suite, or if he was going to be admitted to a floor. She was at the nurses station talking to the charge nurse about the case when she saw the attending GI doctor, whom she had not worked with before, and a resident pushing a stretcher carrying her patient down the hall.

"Hey, that's my patient!" Molly said.

She hustled down the crowded corridor after the doctors. "Excuse me! Where are you taking this patient?" she asked.

"I'm the *attending*," the doctor announced.

"I understand that," Molly responded, "but I need to know if the patient will be coming back to the ER or if he has been admitted. If so, he can't leave until he has orders. I need to know who is writing the orders."

Molly wasn't trying to engage in a battle of egos; she had to look out for her patient. A patient leaving the ER for another floor needed to have an admitting doctor accept him so that someone was officially taking responsibility and writing orders. Because the patient had not yet been assigned an admitting doctor, once the GI doctor took him to another floor, the patient could potentially fall through the cracks of the hospital system. The charge nurse needed to know whether the patient would be coming back to the ER to be discharged after surgery or whether he would need a room elsewhere in the hospital. Otherwise, after surgery he could be left in the PACU (Post-Anesthesia Care Unit) with nobody managing his care.

The surgeon looked at Molly as if "I had a penis growing out of my forehead," in Molly's words. "How could I possibly question what he was doing?"

He scolded, "All *you* need to know is I'm taking the patient," and continued down the hall.

The nurses and ER doctors within earshot were so accustomed to this behavior that they didn't say a word.

Various doctors displayed this kind of egotism again and again. During another shift, police brought in a 27-year-old who was arrested for drunk and disorderly conduct. The officers had wrestled him to the ground to take him into custody, and he had cut his chin badly in the scuffle. Molly assessed the patient, who was covered in blood. She documented that the patient was calm, cooperative, and responding appropriately.

"I don't have insurance and I don't want a lot of stuff done," he said. "Can we hurry this up so I can get out of here?"

"You obviously need stitches, so let's get you triaged," Molly replied.

In the patient's room, the physician's assistant created a chart for the patient; like Molly, she documented that the patient was calm and cooperative. Then the patient made the mistake of talking back to the doctor, who had a low tolerance for drunk patients. "Doc, I want to get the fuck out of here!" he shouted. "Leave me the fuck alone."

Molly liked this doctor, but he had a habit of giving a psychiatric diagnosis to intoxicated patients who disagreed with him. "This man is a harm to himself and needs chemical restraints," he declared to the PA. "Give him twenty milligrams of Geodon," an antipsychotic that put people to sleep. The PA refused.

"What, are you too lazy to put it in?" the doctor said.

"I don't think it's the right thing to do," she said, uncomfortable. "He's not psychotic. He just disagrees with you."

The doctor was unruffled. "I thought we had a better working relationship than that," he said. Not only did he put the order in, but, worse, he deleted the PA's chart and started his own, in which he stated that the patient was combative and a harm to himself. It was the sort of behavior for which a doctor could lose his license. But even if Molly were to complain to administrators, which she did not, she expected the hospital would ignore her. It was as if the nurses' voices didn't matter.

Doctor Versus Nurse

Molly's experiences with egotistical doctors are not atypical. In fact, they barely scratch the surface of an even more disturbing trend, a doctor-bully epidemic that one doctor described as lurking in the "shadowy, dark corners of our profession."

In news reports and hospital break rooms, stories abound of doctors berating nurses, hurling profanities, or even physically threatening them: shoving matches in the operating room; a surgeon pushing a nurse so hard mid-operation that he left a bloody handprint on her scrubs; physicians throwing stethoscopes, scissors, pens, or surgical instruments. Physical abuse by physicians is on the rise. In Maryland, a surgeon yelled at a male nurse, "Are you stupid or something?" and threw a bloody surgical sponge at him from across the room. A Texas doctor heaved a metal clipboard at an advanced-practice nurse and told her he was going to strangle her. A surgeon threw a scalpel at a Virginia nurse, who said, "He was angry because I didn't have a rare piece of equipment he needed, so he endangered me and several others by throwing a tantrum." North Carolina nurses referred to one doctor as "He-Who-Must-Not-Be-Named," because he got into a fistfight with another doctor and physically assaulted a nurse.

Most nurses have been victims of or have witnessed doctor bullying. The Institute for Safe Medication Practices (ISMP), a nationally respected nonprofit watchdog organization, has reported rampant bullying in healthcare, including verbal abuse, threatening body language, condescension, and, though less common, physical abuse. A 2013 ISMP survey on workplace intimidation found that in the preceding year, 87 percent of nurses encountered physicians/prescribers who had a "reluctance or refusal to answer your questions, or return calls," 74 percent experienced physicians' "condescending or demeaning comments or insults," and one in four nurses had objects thrown at them by doctors. Physicians shamed, humiliated, or spread malicious rumors about 42 percent of the surveyed nurses. As a New York critical care nurse said, "Every single nurse I know has been verbally berated by a doctor. Every single one."

This is a global problem. Significant numbers of nurses in Australia, South Africa, Hong Kong, Canada, and many more countries are bullied by doctors, according to surveys. In 2010, a nurse in India committed suicide reportedly because administrators would not address her complaints about a doctor who was sexually harassing her. A nurse's association president said, "This case has not been taken seriously because the victim is a nurse." In South Korea, a 2013 survey found that more than half of nurses were sexually harassed; the majority of the assailants were doctors.

Doctor bullying has many serious ramifications. A 2013 study found that the more that nurses experience it, the more likely they are to report poor working environments and to quit their workplace and/or the nursing profession. This is not the first study to find a link between doctors' intimidation and poor nurse satisfaction, yet researchers repeatedly have found that most nurses don't speak out against the behavior.

Why is hospital bullying veiled in organizational silence? Nurses are afraid to report doctors because they believe administrators will prioritize and refuse to penalize physicians who generate revenue or garner media accolades. They worry they might lose their own jobs in retaliation, and they fear the stigma of being perceived by colleagues as a whistle-blower.

If precedence is indicative, these fears are justified. A slew of double standards protect doctors' jobs but hang nurses out to dry. Many hospitals have fired nurses for reporting doctors' inappropriate or incorrect treatment of patients, while allowing the doctors in question to continue to practice.

In Florida, travel nurse C. T. Tomlinson saw Lawnwood Regional Medical Center cardiologist Abdul Shadani preparing to insert a stent in a heart patient although the patient's scans revealed no arterial blockages. (A travel nurse is an agency nurse whose jobs are temporary assignments in various locales.) "Sir, what are we going to fix?" the nurse asked, according to a *New York Times* investigative report. Shadani said the patient had a 90 percent blockage and inserted the stent; Tomlinson told the *Times* that other staff in the room did not object. Soon after Tomlinson reported Shadani to HCA, Lawnwood's parent company and the largest for-profit hospital chain in the United States, Lawnwood did not renew the nurse's contract. An internal, confidential memo reviewed by the *Times* admitted the nurse's contract was not renewed because of retaliation. HCA did, however, initiate an investigation that found issues with Shadani's treatment of thirteen out of seventeen patients, including several other unnecessary procedures. Tomlinson was reportedly correct—and an ideal patient advocate, hoping to protect patient safety—but the hospital let him go. Meanwhile, at the time of this writing, Shadani still works at Lawnwood.

In 2009, two Texas nurses filed an anonymous ethics complaint with the Texas Medical Board against Dr. Rolando Arafiles Jr. for conducting dangerous practices that risked patient health, taking hospital supplies to perform at-home procedures, and pushing patients to purchase herbal supplements that he conveniently sold on the side. When the board informed

Arafiles about the nurses' complaint, Arafiles enlisted the help of the county sheriff, a friend and former patient who participated in his supplement business. At Winkler County Memorial Hospital, Arafiles tracked down personal information for the patients listed in the complaint and gave it to the sheriff, who contacted them to determine the nurses' identities. The sheriff obtained a search warrant to seize the nurses' computers, where he found the letter.

A hospital administrator fired both nurses, who had worked at the hospital for decades, and who had not signed their letter because they feared exactly this type of retaliation. They had resorted to filing the complaint after months of unsuccessful attempts to persuade hospital administrators to investigate the doctor. Worse, Arafiles and the sheriff convinced the county prosecutor to take the nurses to trial in criminal court, charging them with "misuse of official information," a felony with a maximum penalty of ten years in prison and a $10,000 fine. Charges against one of the nurses were dropped and the other nurse was acquitted.

In turn, the nurses filed a federal lawsuit against the county, the hospital, the sheriff, and other officials, charging that their First Amendment rights were violated and that their firing and criminal charges had been retaliatory. The women won a $750,000 settlement. State prosecutors then went after the sheriff, who lost his license, was convicted of retaliation, and sentenced to 100 days in jail; and the county attorney, who was sentenced to ten years' probation. Arafiles pleaded guilty to retaliation and misuse of official information and received a sentence of two months in jail and five years' probation. As part of his plea agreement, he surrendered his medical license.

It is confounding that initially, the nurses were fired but the doctor was not. The medical board charged Arafiles with violations including sewing a rubber scissor tip to a patient's thumb, using an unapproved olive oil solution on a patient with a bacterial infection, failing to diagnose a case of appendicitis, and performing a skin graft without surgical privileges. But not until Arafiles was charged with a felony did he lose his license. The Texas Medical Board allowed Arafiles to continue to practice as long as he took additional classes, paid a $5,000 fine, and agreed to be monitored by another doctor.

As a result of this case, the Texas Legislature passed a bill increasing fines against doctors who retaliate against nurses reporting unsafe care, and protecting those nurses from criminal liability. The Winkler nurses' story doesn't culminate in a tidy, happy ending, however. Because of the case, the Legislature passed another law prohibiting the Texas Medical Board from considering anonymous complaints against doctors. Meanwhile, the Texas nursing board still permits people to complain anonymously about nurses. In fact, an examination of policies and calls to nursing boards in every state revealed that doctors in forty-one states can report nurses to state nursing boards without having to identify themselves.

So not only did the two nurses who advocated for their patients by reporting unsafe healthcare get fired, arrested, and criminally indicted (their necessary and heroic actions damaging their careers and their incomes until they won their suit), but future nurses were dissuaded from reporting dangerous practices at all. "It is shameful that nurses don't get the same level of protection as physicians. If nurses face the possibility of being outed and then prosecuted, they will think twice before turning in a dangerous physician," said Alex Winslow, executive director of Texas Watch, a nonpartisan Texas citizen advocacy organization. "The lack of protection for nurses puts patients at risk."

This unequal treatment is ridiculously unfair and glaringly unsafe. Nurses are caught in a terrible conundrum: When they report dangerous doctors, they can be fired. But when they don't speak up, people can die.

The biggest problem with doctor bullying is that hospitals are not a run-of-the-mill workplace, where bullying might simply cause individuals' feelings to get hurt or departmental tensions to rise, which are not trivial matters but are at least self-contained. In hospitals, what The Joint Commission calls "intimidating and disruptive behaviors" can lead to medical errors, increase healthcare costs, and harm patients. These consequences are possible because certain doctors refuse to listen to nurses or because nurses are too intimidated to ask questions promptly, if at all. Nurses have reported that they have caught themselves making mistakes, such as mislabeling specimens, because they were so upset, stressed, or distracted by a confrontation with a physician.

Approximately half of surveyed respondents told the Institute for Safe Medication Practices that doctor bullying had caused them to change the way they react when they believe a doctor has made a medication error. These nurses tend to succumb to pressure to administer the medication anyway or to suggest the doctor give the medication himself. As a result, many respondents admitted that they "had been involved in a medication error during the past year in which intimidation clearly played a role."

A national study of 6,500 nurses and nurse managers conducted by the American Association of Critical Care Nurses reported that many nurses are too intimidated to voice their concerns when doctors make mistakes during surgery. Despite mandatory safety protocols like checklists, more than 80 percent of nurses are still worried about "dangerous shortcuts, incompetence, and disrespect" at their hospitals. Of the nurses who admitted that patient harm or "near misses" occurred because of a doctor's safety violation, 83 percent did not report the violation.

While any staff member might badger another, researchers say that doctors bullying nurses are most likely to jeopardize patient safety. Botched communications appear to be the leading cause of avoidable surgical errors. More than two-thirds of medical professionals say that disruptive behaviors have caused medical errors or patient deaths. Separately, The Joint Commission has found that in healthcare organizations nationwide, 63 percent of cases resulting in patients' unanticipated death or permanent disability can be traced back to a communications failure.

How long will these preventable tragedies continue? Researchers have proven these links as far back as the 1980s, when a study of Intensive Care Units revealed that "the most significant factor associated with excessive mortality was the degree of nurse-physician communication." When nurse-doctor relations are poor, patients die unnecessarily. More recently, the Workplace Bullying Institute reported that the mother of a toddler hospitalized for burns thought her daughter was thirsty because she was frantically sucking on wet washcloths. The mother called nurses into the room twice during the night, but the nurses only repeated the doctor's insistence that the girl was fine. The toddler died of dehydration, according to the institute, because the nurses were too intimidated by the doctor to question him.

The story is shocking, but it's only one of countless examples of patients suffering because of healthcare providers' failure to communicate effectively. Consider this anecdote, which nurses reported in a 2010 survey jointly conducted by the Association of periOperative Registered Nurses and the American Association of Critical Care Nurses. During the surgical safety checklist, nurses saw that a surgery was erroneously scheduled for one side of the patient while the patient-verified permit listed the other side. When the nurses tried to stop the plastic surgeon, he told them the permit was wrong. "The patient was already asleep and he proceeded to do the wrong side against what the patient had verified, which had matched the permit. We could not get any support from the supervisor or anesthesiologist. The surgeon completed the case. Nothing was ever done. We felt awful because there was no support from management to stop this doctor. . . . We felt absolutely powerless to being an advocate for the patient." (No further information was provided.)

Alan Rosenstein, the medical director of a nonprofit hospital alliance, is one of the leading researchers of physician bullying. He has surveyed thousands of medical professionals, many of whom reported outcomes such as the following, which he disclosed in a *Journal of the American College of Surgeons* article:

- "Failure of MD to listen to RN regarding patient's condition. Patient had postoperative pulmonary embolism."
- "Cardiologist upset by phone calls and refused to come in. RN told it was not her job to think, just to follow orders. Rx delayed. MI [heart attack] extended."
- "Communication between OB and delivery RN was hampered because of MD behavior. Resulted in poor outcome in newborn."

In a presentation at an annual meeting of the Pacific Coast Obstetrical and Gynecological Society, researchers described similar issues among labor and delivery staff:

- "When a nurse reported to the physician that her patient was highly anxious and had shortness of breath, the physician told the nurse to give the patient some Ativan and take some herself. Later that evening the patient was admitted to the ICU with congestive heart failure."

- "A nurse reported that the final sponge count was incorrect after a difficult tubal ligation. The physician was sarcastic and said that an expensive X-ray would be ordered because the nurse obviously suffered from obsessive-compulsive disorder. A sponge was found in the patient."

- "Doctor's behavior has been hostile, aggressive, threatening, and escalating in the past months . . . including raging at charge nurses and unit director. . . . [L&D] nurses are working in a hostile environment and fear for their safety and well-being."

It is important to note that these types of behavior are exhibited by some doctors, not all, and that incidents should be viewed in proper context. Tensions run high in life-or-death situations, and doctors may not have time to temper their tone or monitor their language when their priority is saving a life. The doctors considered the worst offenders are the specialists whose work is consistently urgent and carries the highest stakes. Doctors and nurses have reported that the most frequent bullies are general surgeons, cardiovascular surgeons, cardiologists, orthopedic surgeons, neurosurgeons, and neurologists. The hospital departments most likely to host doctor bullying are ORs, medical surgery units, ICUs, and ERs. In the OR, attending surgeons are more than twice as likely as anesthesiologists and nurses to exhibit this kind of behavior.

An American College of Physician Executives survey found that three-quarters of doctors are concerned about "disruptive physician behavior"; virtually all of the respondents said that it affects patient care. Yet "despite the best efforts of many, our profession is still plagued by doctors acting in a way that is disrespectful, unprofessional, and toxic to the workplace," ACPE CEO Barry Silbaugh observed.

Ultimately, these issues can be attributed to a fundamental lack of respect between doctors and nurses, who should be considered separate but equal, yet too often are treated as master and handmaiden. To wit: When an attractive, young female East Coast ER doctor didn't even try to save a man who coded in the ambulance on the way to the hospital, the nurses in the room complained to the hospital's medical director. The director dismissed the nurses' complaints patronizingly: "You're just saying that because she's young and pretty."

In Arkansas, an anesthesiologist told a Certified Registered Nurse Anesthetist, "I could teach a monkey to do your job." CRNAs are advanced-practice nurses with master's degrees who provide anesthesia either autonomously or under a physician's supervision. They are "the sole anesthesia providers in nearly all rural hospitals, and the main provider of anesthesia to the men and women serving in the U.S. Armed Forces," according to the American Association of Nurse Anesthetists. CRNAs told me they are stuck between doctors and nurses. "The medical profession perceives you as a glorified nurse and the nursing profession perceives you as a nurse trying to be a doctor," said the Arkansas CRNA. "The general public is not aware of what a nurse anesthetist is or that we provide seventy to eighty percent of all anesthesia in the United States."

The doctor–nurse hierarchy is rooted in the past, in traditionally ingrained remembrances of outdated roles. Up until the mid-twentieth century, nurses were expected to stand when a doctor entered the room, offer him their chair, and open the door so that he could walk through first, in chivalric reverse. Nurses were expected to await instructions passively without questioning the physician. By the 1960s, nursing schools were still teaching that, as one nurse described it, "He's God almighty and your job is to wait on him."

In 1967, psychiatrist Leonard Stein described the nurse's role in an essay entitled "The Doctor–Nurse Game." The object of the game, he said, was for a nurse to "make her recommendations appear to be initiated by the physician. . . . The nurse who does see herself as a consultant but refuses to follow the rules of the game in making her recommendations, has hell to pay. The outspoken nurse is labeled a 'bitch' by the surgeon. The psychiatrist describes her as unconsciously suffering from penis envy."

Since then, "Nurses have spent the last half century fighting to overcome the stereotype that they are defanged doctors. It's a division rooted in education, income, and gender. Doctors—men, affluent, with a professional education—reigned supreme in the hospital," pediatrician Rahul

Parikh wrote in a *Salon* article: "Do doctors and nurses hate each other?" In present-day North Carolina, a physician still expected the medical/surgical nurses to rise from their seats when he entered the unit. "A couple of the nurses staged a sit-in," a nurse from that unit told me. "He eventually got the point."

The current doctor–nurse divide cannot be strongly attributed to gender, however, because some female physicians, like Dr. Baron, can be just as disrespectful as the men. "Female doctors are working in a predominantly male-centered world," said a Washington State ER nurse. "They want to be respected and heard, but aggressiveness can be confused with assertiveness. They seem to not like to be questioned. A married doctor couple in town is known by the nurses as 'Bitch and Bitchier.'"

Nurses have continued to battle the stereotypes even as their profession has evolved. They developed specialties and expanded their scope to include more medical tasks. Nursing schools shifted from hospitals, where doctors oversaw the students, to universities, where the instructors are nurses. "Nursing school was now independent of doctors," *New York Times* nurse columnist and author Theresa Brown told Parikh in a dialogue for his *Salon* article. "Yes, we are taught to be patient advocates, but we are also taught to be a check on the doctor. The problem with that is we're only taught to see docs as adversaries." Nurses "never get a good understanding of the stresses and strains of what it's like to be a physician." If nursing schools don't share doctors' perspectives and medical schools don't teach nurses' perspectives, then "how do doctors and nurses learn to behave and negotiate with each other?" she asked.

Many physicians trace doctor bullying to behavior they learned in medical school. Kevin Pho, the physician who runs the popular medical blog KevinMD.com, has argued, "Blame should be directed toward the physician education system, rather than doctors themselves. The hierarchical culture that perpetuates bullying goes back as far as medical school, when as students, future doctors are trained in a pecking order not unlike the military. It's no wonder that some carry that attitude into the workplace."

In a 2011 survey, doctor bullies blamed a heavy workload and behavior they had learned in medical school and residency. Indeed, Rosenstein has written, "Surgeons have learned that disruptive behavior can intimidate others into doing what they want, and surgical residents seem to learn this behavior by observation."

If medical school helps to ignite what the ISMP calls a "culture of disrespect among healthcare providers," then some hospitals and health officials help to perpetuate that hierarchy. In October 2014, when Texas Health Presbyterian Hospital nurse Nina Pham contracted Ebola from a patient, Dr. Thomas Frieden, the head of the Centers for Disease Control and Prevention, seemed quick to appear to blame the victim. "Clearly there was a breach in protocol," Frieden told *Face the Nation*. "Infections only occur when there's a breach in protocol."

But Pham's colleagues said that was not the case. National Nurses United, the country's largest nurses' union, spoke to the nurses and issued a statement asserting that the hospital neither trained the nurses nor established protocols to begin with. Supervisors told nurses that certain protective masks were unnecessary, hospital authorities resisted a nurse supervisor who demanded that the patient be moved from a non-quarantined zone to an isolation unit, and the nurses' protective gear left their necks exposed, according to the NNU.

While, amid an uproar from nursing communities, Frieden later said his remarks were misconstrued. "There's a lot of outrage about Frieden's comments," American Academy of Nursing president Diana Mason told NPR. "It's blame the nurses again."

Some health organizations place nurses on the front lines, and then fail to protect them, let alone treat them like the heroes they truly are. On a lesser scale, many hospitals develop policies that blatantly set nurses apart from other staff members. WSMV-TV Nashville reported that at Vanderbilt Medical Center in 2013, administrators cut costs and risked cross-contamination by forcing nurses to perform housekeeping duties, including emptying garbage cans, changing linens, sweeping, and mopping patient rooms and bathrooms. At other hospitals, nurses were the only employees who were charged for parking. A lighter but still legitimately irritating example occurred at a northern California hospital, where administrators announced that they would no longer provide half-and-half for nurses and other staff, but would continue to have it available for doctors and administrators. The staff responded by planting a "Will

Work for Half-and-Half" jar in a break room, in which coworkers deposited donations of half-and-half containers.

These administrators' message is clear: They value doctors more than they value nurses and treat them accordingly. They might also prioritize some doctors over others. In one study, nearly 40 percent of doctors said that administrators are more lenient with the physicians who generate large amounts of money for their organization. Hierarchies like these do not promote patient care; rather, they enmesh doctors and nurses in territorial fights that can make them lose sight of what matters.

The controversy over the doctorate of nursing practice degree (DNP) is emblematic of the professions' crossed signals. As of 2015, nurses wishing to become nurse practitioners—who are able to diagnose and treat patients in ways similar to a general practitioner—must go beyond master's level training to earn a doctorate, and can therefore add "doctor" to their title. Nurse leaders say the additional education is important to expand nurses' expertise, enhance their qualifications for hospital administrative jobs, and gain more respect in the medical field.

But physicians have turned the debate into a turf battle over the "doctor" title that some NPs, as they are known, would use, claiming that the degree threatens the medical doctors' position as healthcare leaders. They argued that nurses calling themselves "doctor" will confuse patients and is an attempt to equate their status with physicians, who have thousands more hours of medical training. The American Medical Association loudly protested the Doctor of Nursing Practice designation, calling it "title encroachment," and proposed a resolution to restrict the "doctor" title in medical settings to physicians, dentists, and podiatrists. Eventually, the AMA instead adopted a resolution to "advocate that professionals in a clinical healthcare setting clearly and accurately identify to patients their qualifications and degrees attain(ed)" and to "support state legislation that would make it a felony to misrepresent one's self as a physician."

Nurse practitioners say they are looking to develop their knowledge, not to take over the field. In general, they have more time than physicians to spend with patients and charge less for their services. A major study found that nurse practitioners' patients have "essentially the same" health as physicians' patients. At the time of this writing, nineteen states and the District of Columbia allow nurse practitioners to practice independently. Nurse-owned practices are a growing component of healthcare; in 2011 (the most recent year for which data is available), 100,585 advanced practice registered nurses billed $2.4 billion in services to 10.4 million Medicare patients—32 percent of the Medicare fee-for-service population. Those numbers are expected to grow. With a looming physician shortage in the United States by 2020, nurses with advanced degrees offer an additional option to patients, particularly in rural areas where access to doctors is scarce.

Effective 2009, The Joint Commission required hospitals to have a "code of conduct that defines acceptable and disruptive and inappropriate behaviors" and a process for managing those behaviors. Since then, studies have shown "moderate improvement" in doctor bullying and nurse reporting of this behavior. In 2005, only about 10 percent of critical care and OR nurses spoke up if they were bullied by a doctor or if they felt patient care was compromised; by 2010, this number had increased to about one-quarter of these nurses. TJC continues to receive reports of intimidation, and medical researchers say "there are still large, disconcerting gaps between what we have been able to achieve and where we need to go."

Some healthcare providers have devised helpful strategies to handle intimidation. In one surgical department, when any staff member in the room feels that tensions are rising, he or she can call out, "Tempo!" as a reminder for everyone to calm down. (That safe-word strategy would not work in all hospitals.) A Southern hospital keeps red phones at each nurses station; if a physician is berating a nurse, she picks up the phone and an administrator quickly arrives to assist her. Similarly, nurses in a New Brunswick, Canada, hospital began a practice known as "Code Pink" when they got fed up with a particular doctor bully. When the doctor lambasts a nurse, other nurses spread the "Code Pink" alarm and stand beside her in support. The practice has expanded; at another hospital, a mistreated nurse can page a "Code White" to the same effect.

Still, these codes go more toward treating a symptom rather than preventing problems in the first place—perhaps fitting in an American healthcare model. Rather than collaborating with each other, too many groups of healthcare providers view their roles as practically adversarial. Some doctors equate "nurse-friendly" hospitals with "doctor-*un*friendly," as if what's good for the nurse can't possibly also be good for the doctor.

Nurses have earned their place at the table. Is it possible to have a chain of command without implied levels of superiority? To view the various scopes of practice as complementary rather than hierarchical? One strategy is to rework administrators' perspectives and doctor–nurse relationships so that all staff members view each other as part of a team. Obviously, this won't work for every pairing. As one ER pediatrician told me, "If I have a shitty nurse, it affects my entire day." But it is imperative that the professions acknowledge that every member of the team deserves a voice.

In his 2011 commencement address at Harvard Medical School, surgeon Atul Gawande said, "We train, hire, and pay doctors to be cowboys. But it's pit crews people need." He explained to the graduates that the hospitals that achieve the best medical performance results are not the most expensive, but rather, the places where "diverse people actually work together to direct their specialized capabilities toward common goals for patients. They are coordinated by design. They are pit crews."

To get there, healthcare organizations are going to have to force stakeholders to agree on the most effective role for a twenty-first-century nurse. As a Canadian ER nurse posted on KevinMD.com, "The issue boils down to whether the healthcare industry can tolerate highly educated, vocal, critically thinking, engaged nurse-collaborators who, in the interest of their patients, will constructively work with—and challenge, if necessary— physicians and established treatment plans. Or does the industry just want robots with limited analytical skills, who blindly and unthinkingly collect vital signs and carry out physician orders? More importantly, which model presents the best opportunity for excellent patient care?"

SAM   CITYCENTER HOSPITAL, September

Before Sam's first night shift, she guzzled a grande nonfat mocha from the hospital's twenty-four-hour coffee shop. As a morning person, she wasn't sure how to handle her sleep logistics to remain alert for a 7:00 p.m.

to 7:00 a.m. shift. She had awakened at ten that morning, unable to sleep later. She was scheduled to work three night shifts in a row.

Sam arrived early, wiped down her glasses, tied her long hair back in its usual ponytail, then went to the outgoing day-shift nurse for report. She had heard that the beginning of night shifts were the craziest part of the twelve-hour period. She expected to have several patients initially, and then taper down to two or three. She didn't expect the outgoing nurse to list six patients immediately, more than a full load. Sam rushed around the department, taking each patient's vitals. Her ER cell phone buzzed. "Your drip is here," the secretary said.

"What drip?" Sam asked.

When she got to the nurses station, she looked at the patient's name on the bag of Cardizem, a heart and blood pressure medication that the pharmacy had premixed. It was unfamiliar. She looked at the computer, and there he was, a seventh patient—and the sickest one—whom the other nurse had forgotten to mention. Sam rushed to the room. The patient, who had come into the ER with an irregular heart rhythm, was in danger of a blood clot traveling to his lungs or brain. Sam hung the drip and prepared the patient for the Cardiac Care Unit, where he would be monitored closely.

By 2:00 a.m., the ER was quieter, but Sam felt like she was going to keel over. She was distracted from her vaguely unsettled stomach only by the piercing headache behind her gray eyes. All she wanted to do was lie down on a stretcher to nap. As she slugged down the hallway, her eyelids drooping, the charge nurse called out to her. "You just gotta keep moving, sweetheart, you just gotta keep moving." Sam revisited the coffee shop and drank another mocha.

Still, she did not regret her decision to work nights. During the following weeks, she learned that the night staff was more laid back, less harried. By day, the ER was loud; it was hard for Sam to hear herself think. At night, under the fluorescent glow of emptier hallways, it was more peaceful. Only the people who truly needed to be at the hospital were present at night. If a chief resident came down to the ER during the day, he would be accompanied by a fellow and four medical students. At night, the resident visited the patients alone. The ER felt like more of a team that had to pull together to get things done. The night shift was better for introverts, too. In this smaller community, it was easier for Sam to get what she needed for her patients. Gradually she began to learn how and when she needed to be assertive to get something done.

The only drawback to night shifts was that they wreaked havoc on Sam's social life. As a new nurse, she was given the least desirable schedules, which rendered her entire week useless for nonwork matters because she slept until 5:00 p.m. She wasn't a party girl to begin with; she spent much of her free time babysitting her brother's young daughters. But when she did date, she found that people outside the field of medicine usually didn't understand her. She would tell a guy about seeing a rare disorder or amputation, and his response would be, "That's nice, but did you see the basketball game?"

A week after a date that seemed to go well, Sam hadn't heard from the guy and was debating whether to text him. Working a slow night, Sam ran into William, her attractive former preceptor. "Hey, how's it going?" he asked.

Sam unleashed on him. "Guys suck!" she growled. "I had a date last week. I had a good time and he didn't seem like he was having a terrible time, either. But I haven't heard a word. If you say you're going to call, call. If you don't want to call, tell me."

William smiled, his kind eyes crinkling. "Yeah, I've never understood that. That's not my M.O.," he said. "But most girls aren't like you, so guys might not be used to someone with no pretense. You're not one of those girls who acts dumb or creates drama. You're quiet, but if someone says something stupid, you let them know."

"I just wish guys would be straightforward."

"Some guys are nervous, I guess," William said, shrugging his broad shoulders. "They don't want to hurt your feelings. But, Sam, you're a great girl. You're like the opposite of a damsel in distress."

Another nurse came over to talk to William and Sam scurried away. She realized that William was usually surrounded by nurses because he was a good listener who made people feel better about themselves. He seemed to know everything that was going on in the department but he didn't spill secrets.

Sam was just getting settled into the hospital when a new ER director came on board. The staff despised Victoria almost immediately. She would sit in her office or go out for meals when her nurses were struggling with excessive patient numbers. She sent annoying mass emails announcing the ways nurses and other staffers were "*really* supposed to" do their tasks or they would be written up, but she wasn't willing to expend the resources needed to execute those policies. When a trauma came in, for example, nurses were "*really* supposed to" don plastic gowns to protect from blood spatter, which sounded fine on paper, but usually there was no time to waste, there weren't any gowns in the ER, or there were only size XLs, too large for most of the nurses to use safely.

On multiple occasions, nurses went into Victoria's office to ask a question or to voice a concern, and exited the office either fuming or sobbing. One nurse quit within minutes of leaving Victoria's office. She had gone in to tell the director that the nurses were short-staffed and needed help, and Victoria had answered, "Pull yourself together, put your big-girl panties on, and do your fucking job." Within four weeks of Victoria's arrival, twenty of the fifty-eight full-time nurses at Citycenter had reportedly quit because of her. The ER was nearly always extremely short-staffed now, which meant higher patient-nurse ratios and longer wait times.

With fewer nurses, it became impossible to dodge CeeCee. She was everywhere, chatting, flirting, bubbling, high-kicking. CeeCee seemed to take a particular liking to William. Any chance she got, she sat next to him, at meetings, at the nurses station: "Oh, William! I need your help." "Oh, William! Listen to this." She would sashay to the busy nurses station and toss passive-aggressive barbs at Sam, like, "Oh my God, I have so much work to do. Sam, you're sitting down; what have *you* been doing?" as if Sam were relaxing. Sam bit her tongue.

One night, a young woman came in with severe pain from endometriosis and repeatedly falling blood pressure. She was potentially septic from pelvic inflammatory disease, which meant she was in danger of a systemic infection. Sam monitored her, noting that her blood pressure would drop significantly over a couple of hours, then rise slightly in response to the saline that the resident kept ordering to replace the volume in the blood vessels. In fuller veins, the blood pressure was supposed to go up. In sepsis, however, other factors could cause the blood vessels to dilate; flooding the patient with saline would not fix the problem.

After a few hours, per the resident's orders, Sam had given four liters of fluid (the body has room for approximately four to five liters), but the pressure was still low.

Sam sought out the resident, a first-year. "Um, something is obviously going on here. Her B.P. is low and I've just given her four liters of saline," she told him. "I think we need to do something about this blood pressure instead of overloading her with fluid."

"Let's get a CT scan and see what's going on," he said.

The results revealed that the woman had fluid in her lungs. *That's probably from the fluid that I already gave her*, Sam thought. But the attending physician insisted that because the blood pressure was still low, Sam had to administer two more liters.

Sam was getting frustrated. The woman's heart rate was still elevated, indicating that she was either in pain or experiencing another type of physiological distress. Meanwhile, the attending physician was relaxing at his desk, surfing the Web. He had not spent five minutes with the patient.

Sam found William at the nurses station and relayed the scenario. "The attending said the patient probably lives low [normally has low blood pressure]. So we're not giving her any pressors." Pressors would constrict the woman's blood flow, thereby raising the pressure. "But I'm not comfortable with these orders."

"Your thought process is right," he said. "Document everything."

When Sam talked to the resident about the attending's orders, he also seemed uneasy. But he was new, and seemed to trust that the attending knew what he was doing.

At dawn, the woman spoke. "I feel puffy," she said. Her eyes were extremely swollen, and she was pale and lethargic. The fluid bags had emptied. Sam took her blood pressure. 85/50. That was low.

Sam approached the resident again. "At what point do we want to start getting concerned about this?"

The resident paused for several moments. "Eighty systolic." (Systolic refers to the top number of a blood pressure reading.)

Twenty minutes later, the woman's blood pressure had dropped further. "She's at eighty over forty," Sam told the resident.

"Okay, I'm worried now." He went to talk to the attending.

When the resident returned, he pulled Sam into the hallway and told her that the attending didn't want to do anything about the blood pressure and had given no explanation why. The doctor had ordered them to give the woman another liter of fluid, for a total of seven, and then hopefully a bed would open up in the ICU.

"Are you kidding me? We have to do something!" Sam said, gesturing to the patient.

"He's my boss; I can't do anything about it," the first-year said. Sam would eventually come to know the attending as a doctor who didn't excel in situations in which a patient had no clear diagnosis. But for now, the resident was too green to question a superior, and Sam was too new to tell an attending that she thought he was doing something wrong. Sam updated the notes in the patient's chart, making sure to add, "No new orders per MD." After leaving for the change of shift, she never found out what happened to the patient.

That was typical for ER nurses: Each patient's story continued, at home or on another hospital floor, but the nurses were left with only a caption of the patient rather than the whole of the person, a full narrative life shrunken down to a room or a diagnosis: "Remember that patient in Twelve?"

Medicine asked something extraordinary of nurses: to forge intimate connections with another person for hours, weeks, or months, to care thoroughly and holistically—and then to let that individual suddenly go, often never to be heard from again.

That was just life in the hospital.

LARA · SOUTH GENERAL HOSPITAL, September

Lara sprinted on a treadmill at the gym, sweat dripping off of her chiseled abs. *I want my mom*, Lara thought, pushing herself to run faster. *I do not want the drugs.*

Since the day at South General when she'd nearly taken the vial of Dilaudid, Lara had attended more than her usual thrice-weekly NA meetings to bolster her support. She had increased her interactions with her sponsor and sponsees, all of whom were looking out for her. And she went to the gym as often as she could. She knew full well that she had replaced her painkiller addiction with an exercise addiction. She went to the gym every day for boot camp and spin classes. At home, she religiously exercised to Beachbody Insanity DVDs, a hard-core cardio workout.

She rationalized that exercise was an acceptable outlet which, unlike the drugs, wouldn't kill her. Besides, it helped. "I think too much about the bad stuff I see: children who have died, a teenager who died in a motorcycle accident. I can't help thinking about their parents' faces," Lara said. Exercising "helps me release some of that negative energy. It allows me to think about it without breaking down and becoming incapacitated. Before, I wasn't facing things going on. Drugs helped me to stuff it down more. Exercise helps me process it."

She had been able to put down the Dilaudid in August because she reminded herself how painful withdrawal had been. She had suffered through weeks of sleeplessness, night sweats, diarrhea, vomiting, and terrible nausea. "The withdrawal from narcotics is a living hell. I felt like my skin was crawling. All you want to do is sleep and you can't. That's why you hear about heroin addicts who can't get clean. It's because they're like, 'I know what will make this go away for just a little bit,'" Lara said. "I do not ever want to go through that again. Could you imagine feeling like that and having to take care of your kids?"

When she got to work after the gym, a loud drunk woman came into the ER shouting vulgarities. "That motherfucker!" she screamed. "My brother's going to cut his dick off and shove it up his ass!" She was so out of control that the nurses couldn't calm her down.

Lara took report from the medics. The woman claimed that someone followed her home from a party and raped and sodomized her. Unfortunately, she had showered afterward, which likely washed away much of the evidence for her case. While she waited for South General's designated sexual assault nurse to arrive, Lara had nowhere to put the woman but the lobby.

Patients in the waiting room were loudly gossiping about the woman, whom they assumed was a typical ER drunk. "What's her problem?" they complained. "Just let her go home," a security guard muttered. Gradually, patients yelled back at her directly: "Shut the fuck up!"

Lara couldn't tell them not to judge. And she didn't want the woman to go home; she wanted her to get the help she needed. She brought the woman back to triage with her, depositing her in a room where nurses did blood work and EKGs. The waiting patients were angry at Lara for not sending the still-ranting woman home and the woman was angry because she said it hurt too much to sit down. Lara tried to ignore the glares coming at her from all directions, reminding herself repeatedly, *This is not about me.* She didn't know why, but she believed the woman.

At first, Lara had been slightly nervous to work at South General, where violence, including murder and rape, touched many patients' lives. Now, South General was her favorite hospital. While some patients had been initially leery of the curly-haired blonde nurse assigned to them, they soon changed their minds. "Once they lose their attitude against me, they see I'm there to help them and we build a rapport," Lara said. "I respect them, I'm taking care of them, I'm not judging them. I can give them a pillow or blanket or five minutes of my time to really listen, and they're grateful. Sometimes I'll even get a hug from a patient after they're discharged." That didn't happen elsewhere.

Lara also liked working with her colleagues, despite racial tensions that separated the black nurses from the few white nurses. She was the only white nurse whom many of the black nurses treated the same way they treated each other. A veteran ER nurse named Rose, in particular, had gone out of her way to welcome Lara since she had first arrived at South General. Rose was a sweet woman with no edges. If any nurse needed help of any kind, Rose was there for her without hesitation. She kept an eye on her coworkers so that if one of them was struggling with her patient load, Rose would step in, offering to take a patient for a CT scan or an admitted patient upstairs. She was a true team player.

When the sexual assault nurse finally arrived to evaluate the still-ranting patient, she spent more than an hour examining the woman.

Afterward, she told Lara she was right to keep her in the ER. The woman's injuries corroborated her story.

Lara was a self-assured nurse, skilled and experienced. She'd been confident ever since she had made the correct call on her own child. When Lindsey was four months old, Lara happened to be taking a pediatric advanced life-support class. She was reviewing her textbook in bed and decided to quiz her husband. "Hey, John, what would you do if one of our kids was choking and I wasn't home?" she asked.

He answered correctly. "And where would you take a pulse on a baby?" John didn't know that one.

Lara went to Lindsey in her crib and pressed her fingers on her upper arm. She counted. "Sixty?" she said. "That can't be right." She did it again. "Oh my God, her heart rate is sixty and it should be one-forty!" She ran to the book to show John the page. "It shouldn't be sixty! Something's wrong!"

"You're overreacting. Lindsey's fine," her husband said.

The next day, she took her daughter to the pediatrician, who said that Lindsey's heart rate was normal. "Umm, maybe she has a cold," the doctor said.

"What does having a cold have to do with her heart?" Lara asked. There was no reply.

Unsatisfied, Lara made an appointment with a cardiologist. The morning of the appointment, Lara weighed whether to cancel it. "I feel like the freaky know-it-all mom. I don't want to go there and have them look at me like I'm crazy," she told her husband.

"You might as well keep the appointment since you made it."

At the cardiologist's office, even before Lindsey's EKG results had finished printing, the doctor told Lara, "Your daughter is in heart block and needs a pacemaker this week." Heart block referred to a dangerously slow heart rate because the electrical signals that caused the heart to contract were partially or totally blocked. Lindsey had a pacemaker inserted during open heart surgery. Two months later, she went into complete heart block, saved only by the pacemaker. The cardiologist told Lara that if she hadn't detected the problem, Lindsey "would have been one of those babies who was put to bed one night and didn't wake up."

Lindsey, who still had the pacemaker, was now a healthy 5-year-old. The experience bolstered Lara's faith that she was "supposed" to be a nurse. Between the pacemaker and Lara's addiction recovery, "Weird things have happened to me. I look at them as ways to grow," Lara explained. "I am a stronger, more confident woman now. I tell my patients all the time to listen to their gut. I tell parents who seem self-conscious or unsure, 'You know your kid better than we do.'"

She wished she were as confident in her marriage, but John was making that difficult. His own addictive personality led him to relate to and help her with hers, but dealing with his gambling and cheating—he said he had a sex addiction—added to her stress. He loved her, she knew, but he said he couldn't curb his behavior. She stayed with him because Lindsey and her 6-year-old brother, Sebastian, were young. Lara and John made a good living together; at least, they had, until he got laid off from the heating and air conditioning company. They led separate lives anyway, with their own interests and friends. "I have a beautiful home, beautiful babies, and a good life, just a ridiculous husband," she said. "When my mom got sick, I didn't have time to focus on his stupidity."

She remembered during her mother's illness, she was working full-time, taking care of her children, and shuttling back and forth to her mother's home twice a day. The week she put her mother in hospice care, her husband was cheating on her in Vegas. When Angie, Lara's former coworker and roommate, asked Lara why she put up with it, Lara had replied, "I don't have time to focus on John right now. My mom is dying and she is my focus."

Lara still wasn't ready to address her marriage. For now, she had plenty of other distractions. She was taking college classes toward her bachelor's degree, and she was hoping to volunteer once a week as an elementary school nurse to spend more time around her children and their friends. Volunteering was also an outlet to express her gratitude. She said, "I've messed up so much in my life, and this is a way to give back. I made a lot of mistakes and God kind of let me off."

JULIETTE PINES MEMORIAL, September

While Priscilla, Charlene, and Erica managed the ER nursing staff, in that order, rarely did all three work the same shift. The day's supervisor directly affected Juliette's workload: Priscilla and Erica were fair, Charlene was not. Juliette wished her work life weren't so tied up in her feelings about her coworkers, but nursing was a deeply interpersonal profession in which people had to depend on others—doctors, techs, fellow nurses—to do their job well.

Erica made Juliette want to be a better nurse. As senior charge nurse, she advocated for fellow nurses: If a doctor talked down to a nurse, Erica would march up to him or her and announce, "You can't talk to my nurse that way." She was a good charge nurse, a good manager, and a good teacher; she had taught Juliette how to be a good charge nurse, too.

Juliette was eager to please her supervisors because positive reinforcement inspired her to work harder, perform better, learn more. At Avenue Hospital, the ER director had made clear that she appreciated Juliette. Every few months, she emailed Juliette a positive message: "The charge nurse told me what a great job you did last night" or "We're so happy you're part of our staff."

At Pines, Juliette had been dismayed to learn that Priscilla, the nursing director, was a member of the exclusive nurse clique (and that Charlene thought she was part of it, too). Juliette cared so much what her manager thought of her that she shared personal secrets with Priscilla, wanting her to understand everything she could possibly need to know about her. That way, like the Avenue director, Priscilla could encourage her to be the best nurse she could be. Priscilla appeared supportive of Juliette and had a good rapport with several of the nurses. Juliette had made an extra effort to show Priscilla that she was a hard worker, hoping to get the same positive reinforcement that she had received at Avenue. She was still waiting for it.

On a warm September morning, Juliette walked into the building thinking, as usual, *Please don't be Charlene, please don't be Charlene.*

It was Erica. "Yay! Erica, I'm so glad to see you!" Juliette exclaimed.

"I'm glad you're here, too!" Erica said. "We're staffed well today. Where do you want to be, with Mimi?"

Erica assigned her to a zone with Juliette's favorite tech, Mimi. A good tech could make an enormous difference to nurses; procedures went smoothly and nurses could use their time more efficiently. Mimi, a Filipina woman in her forties, was a conscientious tech who had been at Pines for twenty years. Mimi would do whatever a nurse needed without hesitation. It wasn't uncommon for techs to stand around reading magazines when new patients were wheeled in, despite knowing that when a patient with chest pain arrived, for example, he needed an IV, EKG, and a monitor. Nurses had to ask most of Pines' techs to do each task. They didn't have to ask Mimi for anything.

When a patient arrived in the ER with mild chest pain, Mimi ran an EKG. The patient had been waiting awhile. He was 55, the pain was on his left side, and he was sweating. Juliette made an executive decision to test his troponin levels, which could indicate damage to the heart muscle. At Pines, nurses were allowed to run advanced treatment protocols like this without waiting for doctor's orders, if the doctor hadn't yet seen the patient.

When Dr. Preston came in, he reviewed the patient's chart. "I wish you hadn't run troponins on him. His EKG didn't show any changes."

Clark Preston was an efficient doctor. He didn't order more tests than necessary. He decided quickly on a patient's diagnosis, then focused his testing on that diagnosis rather than conducting a broad spectrum of tests to make sure. This was easier on the nurses, who knew that his diagnoses were likely to be correct. But the nurses, who looked out for him because he was fun to work with, still worried that sometimes he was too brazen, too quick to assess. So far, he had not been sued. In this case, he wanted to examine the patient before running cardiac labs. Based on the EKG and the patient description of the pain, the problem could have been GI-related.

Forty-five minutes later, the lab called Juliette. She found Dr. Preston in the doctors' back office. "Troponins came back positive," she told him. The patient likely was having a heart attack and required further cardiac evaluation.

Dr. Preston leaned back in his chair, palms up, content to give Juliette credit. "Well," he said with a disarming grin, "I'd rather be proven wrong than have to explain a dead guy."

Juliette laughed, and went to administer the patient's cardiac medications and reassess his pain and vital signs.

Midshift, Erica switched Juliette to triage to help improve patient flow. Knowledgeable, experienced nurses were more efficient at getting patients the right care. Soon afterward, someone from the Employee Health Department wheeled in a young, red-haired woman who was weeping uncontrollably. Juliette recognized her right away; she was a secretary who worked in the ICU. When they were alone, Juliette asked her name, per protocol.

"Nancy. You know who I am."

Juliette smiled compassionately. "What brings you to the ER today?"

Between sobs, Nancy said, "I'm stressed and I can't work and it's horrible up there and I just can't take it anymore!"

Juliette handed her some tissues. "What's going on?"

"I'm . . . having . . . boy problems," she said through gasping breaths.

Gradually, Juliette coaxed out the story. Nancy's boy problem was that for nearly a year she had been dating Dr. Fontaine, a sexy charmer who worked in the ICU. That morning, Nancy had learned that Dr. Fontaine was also dating three nurses at Pines, and one of them was pregnant with his child. The pregnant nurse had told Nancy in person. Nancy was heartbroken. She couldn't eat.

As Juliette triaged her, diagnosing anxiety and a panic attack, she offered what consolation she could. "I am so sorry this happened," Juliette said. "Try to relax and we will take care of you. We'll get you a private room in the back so you don't have to see anybody." Juliette was glad that the ER doctor that day was sympathetic. The doctor gave Nancy antianxiety medication and discharged her.

Juliette would never be able to look at Dr. Fontaine the same way. Nurses liked him because he was friendly and didn't order too many ER tests per patient. The ER nurses' goal for ICU patients was to get them quickly upstairs, where they could be stabilized and receive proper care. Many specialty doctors asked the ER nurses to do the initial tests, or they ordered extra labs and tests for the sake of ordering them. Dr. Fontaine usually said, "We can do everything upstairs." *Oh, that's why he didn't order a lot of tests*, Juliette thought. *He wanted to get back upstairs to get busy with all of his girls.*

The Sexy Nurse: From "Yes, Doctor" to "Ooh Yes, Doctor"

The outdated caricature of the sexy nurse—breasts straining buttons on a form-fitting white minidress, shapely legs slipped into fishnets and white heels—remains pervasive and global. Nurses say it also holds the profession back.

A small (and strange) 2012 study published in the *Journal of Advanced Nursing* found that of the top-ten media-generated nurse videos on YouTube, six presented nurses as either sexpots or stupid. In a similar vein, on a 2010 *Dr. Oz* show, several women wearing sexy nurse costumes and red lingerie danced with Dr. Mehmet Oz. This came a few years after nurses objected to Dr. Phil McGraw's on-air pronouncement that "cute little nurses" are husband hunters. Nurses strongly protested both doctors' portrayals of the profession.

Imagery that sexualizes nurses can depict hardworking women as frivolous playthings or present a difficult job that requires significant expertise as nothing more than a provocative cartoon. At times, this portrayal has slipped into the province of actual medical care. Near a Las Vegas diner, where waitresses dressed as sexy nurses push customers to their cars in wheelchairs, a real medical assistant at an actual medical IV therapy practice wears a sexy nurse costume with white fishnets as she ministers to patients. In England, a bus company advertised its route to a hospital by adorning buses with a giant picture of a sexy nurse in a skimpy, figure-clinging dress, captioned, "Ooooh, matron!" Not only was the ad disparaging, but it also implied that patients need only step on board to be transported to the healthcare provider of their fantasies; the ad seemed to beckon, "This way to hot, nursey sex."

Some hospitals aren't above spinning the stereotype, either. A Swedish hospital recruiting nurses to work during the summer of 2012 posted an

Internet ad that instructed, "You will be motivated, professional, and have a sense of humour. And of course, you will be TV series-hot. . . . Throw in a nurse's education and you are welcome to seek a summer job at Södersjukhuset's emergency department." The hospital, which has the largest Emergency Care Unit in the Nordic region, completely trivialized nurses' qualifications, tossing in a nursing degree as if it were an afterthought.

Nurses laugh at the idea that their job is TV-series sexy. Instead of come-hither white dresses, today's nurses wear scrubs that might be stained with blood, urine, or various other un-arousing substances. A male nurse in Virginia said, "We're sweaty and smelly and covered in germs. Plus, we've all had patients die in horrible ways in pretty much every corner of the building. I would never be able to get it on in a hospital." Similarly, former certified nursing assistant Erin Gloria Ryan, news editor of the popular women's issues blog *Jezebel*, remarked on a nurse-related comment thread, "Nothing sexier than someone who is going to record the frequency and consistency of your bowel movements on a chart."

As a Michigan nurse manager pointed out, "Some nurses do fit the naughty nurse persona." And some nurses are often happy to engage in tongue-in-cheek innuendo (or worse; see Chapter 5). But sometimes the sexy nurse seeps into the public consciousness as more than just a joke. Nurses told me about doctors groping them. An Oregon nurse said, "Some of the docs are lecherous old perverts." Gail Adams, head of one of the United Kingdom's largest unions, has noted, "People are happy to sexualize the image of nursing but are then surprised when nurses are attacked or have lewd or indecent comments made towards them."

In 2010, a Dutch nurse union received complaints that male patients were requesting sex and some nurses were complying. Reuters reported that a 24-year-old nursing student told the union that she had seen a 42-year-old disabled man's home care nurses sexually gratifying him. The man, who had a muscle disorder that let him move only his mouth and eyes, told her that his previous seven nurses had done the same. When the student refused his request, the man tried to fire her, claiming that she was unfit for the job. The incident prompted one newscaster to remark, "I've got to get myself a nurse in Holland."

The union launched a campaign reminding the public that sexual services were not part of a nurse's job description. The campaign, "I Draw the Line Here," featured a young nurse crossing her hands in front of her face. According to the union, in response to the campaign, the managing director of a patient interest group argued, in all seriousness, that patients "are free to ask. You are free to refuse."

For now, let's set aside the idea of happy-ending healthcare and tell it like it is. Like men and women in any other profession, nurses have sex. And yes, many of them boff their colleagues. In an unscientific poll for the purpose of this book, I asked more than 100 nurses whether they or any of the nurses they worked with had engaged in a sexual relationship with a doctor, nurse, or other coworker. Eighty-seven percent of them said yes.

Depending on the hospital and the unit, a nurse's relationship landscape can range from "I feel like I'm actually living *Grey's Anatomy*" (Washington State) to "Hospital life is so damn far from *Grey's Anatomy*, it's not even funny. Our doctors aren't that hot, supply closets almost always have two doors and they never lock from the inside. And no one has time to go make out with a doctor anyway, because we're usually behind in charting, haven't peed in nine hours, and are fighting hypoglycemia on a constant basis because we don't get the time to eat" (Colorado).

Nurses describe affairs with married doctors, trysts with residents, techs, and fellow nurses, and certain units that are more infamous than others. "Some places, everyone is banging each other and it's an incestuous circle," said a Delaware nurse. "ERs are notorious. The nurse is hooking up with the medic, who is also seeing the case manager, who just got the physician pregnant. It happens whenever you put young, money-strapped, stressed-out people together for long hours with few breaks."

It also happens on hospital property. Nurses have gotten intimate in on-call rooms, equipment lockers, storage closets, linen closets, family conference rooms, stairwells, visitor bathrooms, libraries, patient rooms, offices, and parking lots.

Nurses offer several reasons for their coworkers' allure, beyond what a Washington nurse who slept with a cardiology tech called the "heady" feeling of conducting an illicit relationship in a taboo place. In any situation when people constantly spend long hours together, they are more likely to consider each other potential romantic partners. "Sexual exploits are bound to happen," said a Virginia nurse practitioner who dated a med student. "When I worked in the ER, there were always residents who'd try to convince younger nurses to join them in the call room at night."

The medical setting adds an intoxicating variable: Surrounded by reminders of mortality and infused with the adrenaline rush of tackling emergencies, medical professionals can get caught up in the enticement of sex and affairs. A Pennsylvania nurse attributed some of her nursing expertise to a mild flirtation with a resident: "I wanted to be in the same room with him, so I tried to predict what cases he would be attending and ask to be assigned. Those were big cases—partial gastrectomy, abdominal aneurysms, thoracic procedures—and I grew as an OR nurse because of that."

Nurses said they hook up with coworkers for the same reason they are drawn to police officers and firefighters: They "get it." Emergency personnel understand what it's like to save a life, to face a trauma, to try to help, to fail. "It's like any kind of trauma: Those who survive the experience have memories in common. It's harder to go home to a spouse who has no idea what the trenches are like," said an advanced-practice nursing professor in Texas. "When people work under stress, they bond, and sometimes the bonding crosses over to sexual activity."

Hospitals carry a longtime tradition of nurses marrying doctors. Years ago, when most doctors were male, "residency was all-consuming, so the only women they met were at the hospital," said a Michigan women's-health nurse who married a resident. "Every year in June, teaching hospitals distribute pictures of the residents. When I was a young nurse, the pictures would become marked with 'M' or 'S' for married or single, so we would all know who was available. Of course, now that more women are residents, doctors marry other doctors."

If colleagues can remain discreet, as in any workplace, are their relationships such a bad thing? "We've gone to a quiet stairwell, or outside when it was dark, listening for someone coming," said an Indiana psychiatric nurse who has dated a security guard and a cafeteria worker at her hospital. "People are able to keep it a secret unless they work directly with one another and act like awkward idiots."

Or unless they're caught in the act. At one East Coast hospital, a camera captured a nurse giving oral sex to a surgeon in the library. "They were both reprimanded and the entire hospital staff found out about it, which had to be the most embarrassing thing ever," said a travel nurse assigned to the hospital. "CCTV is a bad, bad thing for a secret hospital rendezvous."

As happens anywhere, intimate relationships can strain interactions with coworkers, who may feel they have to take sides, keep secrets, or avoid drama. An Arizona oncology nurse's coworker dated several doctors in the same hospital. "She became a joke among the docs," the nurse said. "Everyone in her department lost respect for her. At multiple social events, she showed up clinging to the arm of a different doctor each time. Bad social move, bad career move."

After a Louisiana oncology nurse accidentally walked in on her preceptor having sex with a doctor, the preceptor criticized the new nurse daily until she drove her out of the job. "Usually, it only causes issues when there's a breakup or jealousy. It makes it hard to work when they are fighting," said an Indiana nurse whose unit included two nurses having affairs with three doctors. "We do have fun, but there have been times when it has gone too far. The younger nurses aren't that discreet and can get distracted by drama. A new nurse had an affair with an older nurse's husband, a respiratory therapist, and flaunted it. Needless to say, the new nurse found it difficult to work here and transferred."

The double standard

It takes two (or, in the case of nurses caught having sex in a Scottish hospital's geriatric ward closet, three), but the nurse commonly suffers more consequences than the doctor. Upon learning that a nurse manager was sleeping with a doctor, Virginia administrators fired the nurse and eventually promoted the doctor, even though the couple got married. When a resident and a nurse were caught having sex in an Eastern Maryland hospital supply closet, the hospital gave the resident a slap on the wrist but fired the nurse.

There is an odd dichotomy by which the public seems to want to sexualize nurses yet keep them from having sex; they can be whorish angels but not angelic whores, nor anything in between. In the U.K., a writer remarked, "As Britons, we are obsessed with the 'naughtiness' of nursing."

When a group of nurses posed in their underwear for a calendar, the U.K.'s Nursing and Midwifery Council (NMC) threatened to remove them from the register (roughly equivalent to rescinding their licenses). An NMC spokesperson said, "Nurses are expected to uphold the good reputation of their profession at all times. This is clearly stated in your Code of Conduct, and failure to comply may bring your fitness to practice into question." First, this happened in the same country in which buses advertised a nurse wearing not much more than the calendar models. And second, to expect a nurse to follow an employer's rules "at all times" is ludicrous. The NMC sounded like college sorority officers, vetting clothing, demanding pages' worth of arbitrary codes of conduct, and attempting to govern members' nonsorority activities. Like any other professionals, nurses have independent lives outside of work. Why should a regulatory organization expect to control nurses' lives when there is no comparable oversight for, say, accountants?

The double standard struck again when radiology staff at another U.K. hospital posed nude for a charity fund-raising calendar: *The Nursing Times* reported that there were no complaints. And a London hospital knowingly rented out a ward to a company that shot a big-budget pornographic film inside.

Britons do seem to obsess over the topic. Lord Benjamin Mancroft, a Tory peer (similar to a senator), delivered a House of Lords speech in which he complained that nurses at the hospital to which he was admitted were "promiscuous." (His evidence was that he overheard his nurses chatting about their social lives.) He made this announcement a couple of months after the Council for Healthcare Regulatory Excellence issued "sexual boundaries" guidelines to health professionals, whose failure to comply could result in loss of license. Among other stipulations, the ruling banned doctors and nurses from dating patients.

Nurse-patient sex

Nurse-patient relationships open a new can of controversies. Minnesota's Mayo Clinic fired a male neurology nurse for "maltreatment of a vulnerable adult" because he had sex with a patient several times in her bathroom. But the Minnesota Health Department subsequently determined that the man had not violated state rules because the relationship was consensual.

One in six U.K. nurses know of a coworker who has had sex with a patient, and one in ten think it is acceptable for nurses to have relationships with patients, according to a *Nursing Times* survey. A British nurse received a one-year suspension for having a three-month affair with a cystic fibrosis patient after he was discharged from her hospital and despite his returning for a heart and lung transplant. Hardly discreet about it, she joked to coworkers that she had to increase his oxygen and give him a nebulizer inhaler before they had sex.

In the United States, between 1999 and 2009, state nursing boards disciplined 636 nurses for sexual misconduct. "The actual prevalence, however, is not known. Indeed, 38 to 52 percent of healthcare professionals report knowing of colleagues who have been sexually involved with patients," the National Council of State Boards of Nursing (NCSBN) reported. The NCSBN defines sexual misconduct as "engaging in conduct with a patient that is sexual or may reasonably be interpreted by the patient as sexual; any verbal behavior that is seductive or sexually demeaning to a patient; or engaging in sexual exploitation of a patient or former patient," according to the council's *Practical Guidelines for Boards of Nursing on Sexual Misconduct Cases*. "Any and all sexual, sexually demeaning, or seductive behaviors, both physical and verbal, between a service provider (i.e., a nurse) and an individual who seeks or receives the service of that provider (i.e., client), is unethical and constitutes sexual misconduct."

It's arguable that healthcare employers can hold tighter reins on staff because their stakes are so high. The Oklahoma Nursing Board barred a hospice nurse from practicing for twenty years because she had a sexual relationship with a married patient who was terminally ill. While the nurse argued the relationship was consensual, the board's lawyer told the judge, "It is the responsibility of the professional to say no to the vulnerable patient." The 43-year-old Lou Gehrig's Disease patient attempted suicide after the nurse broke up with him.

When officials try to micromanage nurses' sex lives, the slope slides rather precipitously. In Australia, a 61-year-old nurse faced disciplinary action because of a sexual relationship with a patient who was an old childhood friend she had not seen in decades and whom she ultimately married after they reunited. The Nurse Board nevertheless argued that the nurse had behaved unprofessionally because: "Consent is not an excuse with issues of professional boundaries. The care of a patient needs to be in a safe and trusting ethical relationship."

Headlines in the U.K. exploded in 2010 when the Nurse and Midwifery Council investigated a British nurse whose hospital fired her because of accusations of "inappropriate relationships" with patients' widowers. The resulting headlines—"Cancer Nurse Bedded Three Victims' Husbands"—implied that the nurse had affairs with the men while caring for their wives. In reality, the divorced mother of two said that she began a ten-year relationship with one widower more than a year after his wife died, and later fell in love with the second widower, with whom she was in a year-long relationship that began months after his wife passed away.

It's hard to see how engaging in a serious relationship with a former patient's widower compromises nursing care of other patients (not to mention the dead one). But some states, including Maine, Arizona, and Washington, officially ban nurses from dating patient family members. When you work near your home, you inevitably will encounter people in different contexts. If nurses who spend most of their days working long hours at the hospital can't have a relationship with coworkers, patients, or patients' relatives, then Lord help the small-town nurse who wants to date.

The NCBSN prohibits nurses from sexual activities with former patients, clients, or "key parties" (defined as immediate family, including the spouse, domestic partner, sibling, parent, child, guardian, and others "who would be reasonably expected to play a significant role in healthcare decisions") for two years after the individual is no longer a patient. After two years, nurses still cannot engage in sexual activities with a former patient or a former patient's "key party" if chances are high that the patient will need future treatment or if there is an "imbalance of power, influence, opportunity, and/or special knowledge of the professional relationship."

If healthcare employers can dictate whom nurses date, can they also control whom they befriend? Three weeks after a psychiatric patient was discharged from a Canadian hospital, she saw her nurse at a greenhouse, where the women chatted and exchanged phone numbers. The women eventually decided to rent a place together. The hospital fired the nurse for becoming platonic friends with a former patient. When the nurse took the case to court, the judge sided with the hospital. According to the *Hamilton Spectator*, the judge argued that the nurse should have known better because of the high "return rate" of psychiatric patients to their hospitals as well as their vulnerability and emotional dependency within the nurse-patient relationship.

Certainly, hospital paramours are duty-bound to uphold their responsibilities and maintain professionalism even after the relationship ends. Healthcare workers cannot afford to have "bad blood" between them. But nurses in particular are stuck; they are glorified as sex objects, then punished when they have sex.

In Ontario, after nurse Lori Dupont tried to end a long, rocky relationship with married anesthesiologist Marc Daniel, the doctor, who had a history of inappropriate and unwanted contact with nurses, harassed her at work, according to the *Windsor Star*. When several nurses complained, their manager reprimanded them. The nurses took it upon themselves to protect Dupont, inserting themselves between Dupont and Daniel when they were in close proximity, or sneaking Dupont out of the room.

Administrators were aware of Daniel's physical, verbal, and sexual harassment of nurses. Internal reports list that Daniel suggested he give a nurse a naked, oiled backrub; kissed a nurse who bent over to speak to him; and broke a nurse's finger when grabbing a pillow from her. On a quiet weekend day, Daniel and Dupont were inexplicably both scheduled in the OR. Daniel stabbed her to death, then killed himself.

While the hospital board chairman called the murder-suicide "an unforeseen event," Dupont's family and coworkers said that Hôtel-Dieu Grace Hospital prioritized Daniel's career over Dupont's safety. "When a nurse behaves badly, I'm before a disciplinary hearing and the hospital reports it to the College of Nurses of Ontario. When a doctor behaves badly, nothing happens," nursing union officer Colin Johnston told the *Star*.

Before their relationship began, when Daniel was pursuing Dupont, a single mother, he would grab her and try to push her into rooms. When a friend told her that she should report the sexual harassment, she replied, "He's a doctor. I'm a nurse. You just can't do that. There'd be all kinds of problems."

CHAPTER 3

WHO PROTECTS THE NURSES?
Taking Care of People Who Punch You in the Face

"The nurse takes appropriate action to safeguard individuals when their care is endangered by a coworker or any other person."
    —The International Council of Nurses' *Code for Nurses*

"Almost every single ER nurse I know has been assaulted by a patient at some point. If someone walked into a bank and told the teller, 'Fuck you, you little bitch, now get me my money,' they'd probably be arrested or, at the very least, kicked out of the bank. I'm expected to take no action and, worse, to continue to treat the patient."
    —an ER nurse in Colorado

"If I had a dollar for every horny old man who's tried to grab my ass or tits, I would be a crazillionaire."
    —a medical/surgical nurse in Illinois

MOLLY   October

THE FERTILITY CLINIC

A few weeks after her initial blood draw at the fertility clinic, Molly was in the patient's seat once again for her first intrauterine insemination (IUI). As she lay on the table in what resembled a standard ob-gyn exam room, she was both excited and, to her surprise, slightly nervous. Thus far in her cycle, she had not been fazed by the medications, the hormonal changes, or the diagnostic procedures. She was optimistic that she and Trey would have a baby.

Trey had been a rock throughout the process. He was what Molly called "a man's man," easygoing and even-tempered. He got along with everyone. As loud and brassy as Molly was, Trey was quiet and stoic. So his reluctance to come to this appointment had been unsettling. "This is going to be really awkward," he said as they waited for the doctor to come in to deposit a vial of Trey's sperm directly into Molly's uterus.

"What? You standing next to me while another man tries to get me pregnant?" Molly cracked.

"You're not helping."

When the doctor and a tech entered the room, they hardly said anything to Molly or Trey. The tech put Molly's feet in stirrups and the doctor got to work.

Molly had heard that IUIs were painless, but the physician had difficulty threading the catheter through her cervix. As much as she had tried to make light of what she called her turkey basting, she reached for Trey's hand in discomfort. His palm was clammy. If Trey was uneasy, then so was she.

Abruptly, the doctor got up and left without a word; no "Have a good day," no "Good luck." A tech placed a kitchen timer next to Molly. "Lie still for the next five minutes," the tech said, and she left, too. Molly remained still for ten minutes, her legs in the air.

Normally, Molly would crack more jokes or make conversation to fill the airspace. Disconcerted by the strangeness of this form of conception and overcome with emotion about the possibility of success, Molly and Trey continued to hold hands in silence.

When Molly and Trey left the clinic, the women at the front desk didn't even look up from their chatter.

Molly had not booked agency shifts in advance for the week of the IUI because the clinic didn't schedule the procedure until a few days before. For Molly, the most stressful part of the fertility process so far was that she had to keep changing her work schedule, and she didn't like to bother her hospital bosses.

CITYCENTER HOSPITAL

When she got home, Molly called Citycenter's scheduler, who had two full days available. "Every time I turn around, someone else is resigning. I don't know what's going on," the scheduler said.

I do! Molly thought. *Your ER sucks!*

Of the three hospitals to which the agency had assigned Molly, Citycenter was her least favorite. Since she had started working there once or twice a week, the hospital's quality had declined even further.

When Molly arrived at Citycenter, the charge nurse assigned her to minor care, the ER zone for nonserious injuries. At other hospitals, this assignment was considered relatively low-key; the minor care nurse would assess each patient and talk to the doctor or PA, who wrote orders or treated the patient. The nurse would see the patients two or three times before discharging them. Usually there were no more than ten nonemergency patients at a time.

At Citycenter, however, Molly saw twenty patients on her board. She raced from chart to chart, checking orders and reading the triage nurse's notes to prioritize her rounds. Citycenter minor care nurses were not supposed to assess patients themselves because the hospital wanted to turn the patients over as quickly as possible: more patients, more profit. The minor care nurse was supposed to trust that the triage nurse had accurately separated the urgent care patients from the minor care cases. Based on that quick analysis, patients waited to see the doctor or PA while the nurse attended to one patient at a time.

Molly took a patient with a broken ankle to get an X-ray, discharged another patient, then returned to the first patient to put on a splint. She retrieved crutches from the supply closet, taught the patient how to walk with them, and pulled pain medications from the Pyxis (an automated medication dispensing machine).

As Molly sped down the hall to get his discharge instructions, she ran into Sam, whom Molly had known when she was a tech at Pines Memorial. Molly liked Sam; she was a hard worker always willing to pitch in, and she had no idea that she was beautiful. Molly remembered when Sam had dated one of the murses at Pines. The murse had dished to several coworkers that while Sam was quiet and reserved in the ER, she was, he insisted, a "freak in the sheets."

"What do you think of this place?" Molly asked her. "The patient ratio is pretty scary."

Sam looked beaten down. "A new grad should not have seven or eight patients on her own."

"I have twenty patients in minor care and I've seen two of them," Molly said.

"That's normal here."

Sam told Molly that Citycenter patients were often mistriaged, which meant that sick patients who needed more serious, urgent treatment sat in the minor care area for hours. If a patient had an emergency such as an allergic reaction, the minor care nurse might not know in time to save him. The nurses had the clear impression that, rather than blame understaffing or hospital policies, administrators would let the nurse take the fall for any errors.

After her shift, Molly met with several nurses in the break room. Some of them were crying in frustration because they couldn't properly care for their many patients. Molly had seen this happen during about half of her Citycenter shifts so far. These nurses were petrified because of the combination of patient volume, concern about losing their licenses because they didn't have enough time to keep patients safe, the unhelpful ER director, and patients who treated them horribly and threatened them physically. When tensions ran high and nurses were spread thin, patients could snap and turn violent in an instant. Victoria, the ER director, remained unsympathetic to nurses, which was particularly distressing because she had been a nurse herself.

"No other hospital in the area operates like Citycenter," Molly told the nurses in the break room. "The nurse-patient ratio is insane, the hallways are full of patients, most patients aren't seen by the attending until they're ready to leave, and the policies are really unsafe."

"That's just how Citycenter does things," a nurse replied, resigned.

"Maintaining eight to nine patients at a time isn't safe," said Renée, a veteran Citycenter charge nurse. Molly and the other ER nurses had a tremendous amount of respect for Renée, who had worked in the department for twenty-five years. She was stern but fair, and willing to teach less experienced nurses whenever they asked for help.

"Yeah, for patients or for our nursing license," another nurse muttered.

"I talked to Victoria about the patient ratio," Renée said. "She told me she didn't understand what all the grumbling is about."

"I don't understand how the hospital can completely ignore repeated safety concerns from staff!" Molly said.

"We've all been submitting complaints to The Joint Commission. You should do one, too," Renée suggested. TJC accreditation was required for hospitals to receive federal funds and Medicare/Medicaid reimbursement. To get the accreditation, hospitals had to recertify every three years. Supposedly, TJC inspectors could show up at any time to investigate whether a hospital maintained TJC standards.

At home, Molly reviewed The Joint Commission website: "Joint Commission standards focus on safety and quality of care." *Everything I complain about involves safety and quality of care!* she thought. She clicked to a page where she could register a complaint. The website made it easy: She had only to select a few categories from drop-down menus and fill out a short comment box. "Citycenter's ER is unsafe based on workload," she wrote. "I'm expected to care for nine patients at a time when the standard is four to five. When my partner goes to lunch, I'm required to take care of double that number, even if it's eighteen patients. And minor care consistently has one nurse to twenty patients." She wondered whether the authorities would step in.

ACADEMY HOSPITAL

Molly was working triage at Academy when a fellow ER nurse, upset and disheveled, came in for treatment. She told Molly she was trying to get a patient settled in bed when the patient jumped up and walked out of the room. The nurse called for security, but the officer only watched. "Wait!" the nurse had shouted as the patient continued toward the elevator. The nurse hurried after her. "If you want to leave, I'll take out your IV and get you ready to go!"

The elevator door opened. "Come back!" the nurse said, leaning in the doorway. The patient lunged, grabbing her neck and scratching her multiple times before the security officer finally stepped in.

"You should file charges," Molly told the nurse.

"It's too much trouble. Administration wouldn't like it."

Molly exhaled loudly. This incident had hit too close to home. "If you worked at Macy's and someone grabbed you by the neck and scratched you up, would you do nothing?"

"It's different in healthcare."

"No!" Molly yelled. "Too many people have that attitude! It is not okay to assault healthcare workers. If a nurse thinks that, how can we possibly get anyone else to change their mind? You need to get mad!"

The previous week, a Citycenter patient had thrown her urine sample into a nurse's face. Management had pleaded with the nurse not to report the incident; when she did, the police said the report probably wouldn't go anywhere because "the patient is mentally ill."

Molly was livid. "I can't believe even the cops gave her a hard time," she told a friend. "There's no other career where you can be hit, scratched, spat on, verbally assaulted, have people threaten your life, and you just go about your business like it never happened."

It had happened to Molly two years before. Daryl was a frequent visitor to the ER. In his forties, he lived in a shelter, and when he wanted free meals and time to himself, he came to Pines, claiming to be suicidal. He would refuse all treatment, medication, and therapy, but the hospital kept him for three to five days. He had done this countless times. One day Molly entered his room in the ER's psychiatric area and prepared to take his blood pressure. Within a matter of seconds, Daryl punched her in the eye, yanked her long hair, and scratched her arms and neck. He grabbed Molly's shirt and began to pull her onto the bed. As Molly struggled with him, Daryl bit her arm, breaking the skin. Molly tore herself away and rushed out of the room. Daryl fell to the floor, unharmed.

While Molly washed the bite with soap and water, the psych tech, who was assigned to observe patients from behind a glass window, told her that security wasn't answering her call. Molly could hear the security department's emergency line still ringing. When an officer finally arrived, he escorted another nurse into Daryl's room to take over his care. Molly found out later that Daryl's first words were "I should have bitten her fucking face off."

Because Molly equated going home with "letting Daryl win," she returned to work after Employee Health had documented her injuries. Back in the ER, a doctor recommended she go to a specialized medical clinic for monitoring: Daryl had hepatitis C. She would have to return to the clinic at 6:30 a.m. weekly, then biweekly for a year for blood draws to make sure she hadn't contracted the disease.

That day, Molly filed charges against Daryl. Priscilla supported her, but the Pines Memorial lawyers and risk management team told Molly that if she wanted to pursue a case against the patient, she was on her own. Fortunately, the state took the case. Police issued a warrant for Daryl's arrest.

More than a month after the incident, Daryl filed a restraining order, claiming that Molly had assaulted and intimidated *him*. An officer came to the ER to give Molly a court summons. Suddenly Pines' risk management department wanted to get involved. Molly would never forget the conversation with the hospital administrator.

"He's making some very serious allegations against you," the risk management director told Molly. "When were you planning on telling us about it?"

"This was given to me this morning. My court date is on Tuesday," Molly said.

"We're getting you an attorney and changing your court date."

"I don't want to change the date. I'm ready."

"It's not about you anymore. You don't have a choice in this," the administrator said.

"It absolutely is about me! It's a case against me!"

"Well, you represent the hospital and we're going to get it changed."

"The hospital had nothing to say about it when I filed my charge, but now risk management wants to get involved? I'm not changing the date." Ultimately, the hospital had no right to reschedule the hearing. But Molly was left feeling devalued because Pines' administrators didn't support her until they believed the hospital's reputation was at risk.

When Molly asked the head of security for a copy of the tape from the video cameras in the psych area, he told her that the cameras didn't actually work.

At court, the judge immediately dismissed the charges against Molly because the statute of limitations for Daryl's claim had passed. Nevertheless, for two more months, the state's judicial website—a collection of public records—listed the restraining order against her.

For the case against Daryl, the judge sided with Molly. He sentenced Daryl to one year in jail, as much time as Molly would have to worry about her health. When Daryl was released, one of his terms of parole would be continued mental health treatment.

Not long after he got out of jail, Daryl was back in the Pines ER, enjoying free meals and refusing treatment once again, without consequences. And by the time Molly quit, Pines Memorial still had not fixed the security cameras in the ward.

The Third Most Dangerous Profession

DeAnne Dansby was a travel ER nurse in Sacramento when she experienced the worst patient assault of her career. Medics brought in a hypothermic, unresponsive homeless man whom Dansby and a student nurse were able to revive. Dansby left the patient with the student for a moment. When she returned, the patient had backed the student into a corner. Dansby rushed to protect the girl, holding out her arm so the student could get behind her. The man ripped out his IV and lunged at

Dansby, tackling her so hard that when they fell through the doorway, her head banged hard onto the floor. Feeling an excruciating snap in her neck, Dansby screamed. The man pulled her scrub pants down, bit her inner thighs, and was about to attempt to rape her before several of Dansby's coworkers were able to wrestle him off her.

Shaken and injured, Dansby, crying, told the ER supervisor that she had to leave. "The ER is full and we have no one to take your place," the supervisor told her. "You have to keep working." Because she was able to stand up, Dansby felt she had no choice but to complete her twelve-hour shift.

When she finally was able to see a doctor, Dansby, a mother of two, learned that the man had fractured her neck, severing nerves that ran to her left deltoid and bicep. More than four years after the attack, Dansby still can't feel her left arm or look straight up. She has pain and difficulty swallowing. The surgery to correct the injury was so extensive that it caused her voice to change irreversibly. She has an eight-inch scar because her doctor had to clean out so many bone fragments. "I see that scar every day," Dansby said. "And I see him every time I close my eyes." As far as Dansby knows, her assailant is still free.

When Dansby told her department manager she wanted to call the police, the manager said, "If you are going to work for this hospital, you are not going to press charges." Afraid of losing her job, Dansby agreed. She knew the hospital wasn't bluffing. Two security officers who had come to Dansby's assistance allegedly had been fired on the spot for putting their hands on a patient. Dansby told only the U.S. Occupational Safety and Health Administration (OSHA) and The Joint Commission about the attack. Two months later, she said, the hospital fired her anyway, claiming she couldn't do her job properly.

Today, Dansby is a nurse case manager for a large insurance company. She can't work in hospitals, her true passion, because she can no longer lift anything heavier than a gallon of milk. Certainly, the hospital had reason to keep the assault quiet. Violence in the ER could attract negative press, deter future patients, and damage the hospital's standing in the community. But, like Molly, Dansby believes that if administrators couldn't protect her from the assault, they should have at least assisted her in the aftermath. "The hospital didn't stand behind their personnel. When I scanned my badge and turned on that computer, I was nothing but a number," Dansby said. "Nurses put their lives in danger every time they walk through that hospital door."

It is horrific enough that sick or desperate patients attack the people who joined this demanding profession specifically to help them. But the ways some hospitals treat nurses who are victims of assault may be more chilling than the attacks themselves.

Violence against nurses, also called "ward rage," is on the rise. Nearly nine out of ten ER nurses say they were assaulted at work during the past three years, according to an Emergency Nurses Association national survey. The same survey found that one-quarter of ER nurses were physically assaulted more than twenty times in that period and one-fifth of nurses each had been verbally abused more than 200 times. Several nurses told me that every nurse they know has been physically assaulted by a patient.

Experts have attributed the rise in violence to several factors that have nothing to do with individual nurses. Patients grow frustrated with short-staffed ERs that can't attend to them instantaneously when wait times are long. Some drug-seeking patients become irate when nurses—merely the messengers—tell them they can't have a prescription. Other patients are drunk or come straight from crime or accident scenes. Caregivers might dump patients with mental health issues into ERs unnecessarily. And hospitals like Pines don't always have adequate security measures to protect their staff.

Patients often punch, kick, bite, shove, hit, scratch, or strangle nurses, but typically only the hospital shootings hit the news. Bureau of Labor Statistics data indicate that nursing is the country's third most dangerous profession behind police officers and correctional officers, and OSHA admits that "the actual number of incidents is probably much higher" than we know. Nurses are approximately sixteen times more likely than employees in other professions to be assaulted at work.

Patients' family members are sometimes the aggressors. In a high-profile case, Douglas Kennedy, son of the late senator Robert F. Kennedy, attempted to take his newborn son out of the hospital for some "fresh air." The hospital had not discharged the infant, however, and concerned

maternity nurses simply saw a man trying to exit the ward without autho-
rization. When two maternity nurses tried to block the doorway, Kennedy
assaulted them, according to charges filed by the nurses. "I wanted to
make sure the baby was safe and secure," one of the nurses told the *Today*
show. "He brought his leg up and kicked me, and I went flying through
the air." Kennedy went downstairs, where he was stopped by security. He
was subsequently charged with harassment and endangering the welfare
of a child.

Many nurses said that, as in Dansby's case, superiors tell them not to
report the violence. Nurses who don't keep silent—by complaining about
the incident, reporting it, or seeking help—might be fired. That's what
happened to Tammy Mathews, an ER nurse in Alabama, after a drunk
patient spit in her face and choked her until she couldn't breathe. Her hospital tried to convince her to drop her assault charges. When she refused,
the hospital fired her.

Little wonder that 65 to 80 percent of assaults on registered nurses go
unreported. Even the Department of Labor has warned that "incidents
of violence are likely to be underreported, perhaps due in part to the per-
sistent perception within the healthcare industry that assaults are part of
the job." This is precisely what a Massachusetts judge told a nurse when
he threw out her case against her attacker: Getting assaulted is part of
the job. This attitude, which I'll call the "shrug-it-off culture," can make
nurses feel that reporting an attack will reflect poorly on the nurse as an
individual, as if the violence is a result of their own negligence or weak-
ness. Partly because assaults are so common, the industry has conveyed
that being attacked is acceptable. Because of this message, the violence
goes unreported and unchecked, and continues to rise.

Meanwhile, multiple studies reveal that hospitals that encourage
nurses to report violence have fewer assaults than other healthcare institutions. Even nursing organizations perhaps unwittingly contribute to
the view that nurses may be partly to blame. In a *Preventing Workplace
Violence* brochure, the American Nurses Association lists under the heading "Characteristics of Victims and Perpetrators" the following statement:
"Victims are often untrained staff nurses or newly hired nurses." Tell that
to Molly, who had been a nurse for several years when she was assaulted.

Or Jeaux Rinehart, former president of the Washington State Emergency Nurses Association. In 2007, a drug-seeking patient bashed Rinehart in the head with a billy club, breaking his cheekbone. Rinehart, 51, had worked in ERs for three decades. Nurse assault is "actually getting worse," he told MSNBC.com.

Not all assailants are patients who are mentally compromised. "I don't have patience for the completely lucid adult patients who abuse us," said a Maryland medical/surgical nurse whom patients have hit, kicked, and pinched so hard she developed bruises. "I've had trays, pills, and cups thrown at me. There was nothing done about any of these things. I told my manager and the general message I received was 'This is the way it is. It's just part of the job.' You can call security and they'll maybe tell the patient to stop, and then they'll go back downstairs. There are so many restrictions that make it hard for nurses to stay safe. You can't restrain a patient who is mentally competent, unless they're hurting themselves. Police won't arrest them because they need treatment in the hospital. If you assaulted a police officer or any other professional on the job, you'd be in big trouble. But nurses are assaulted every day and there is little to no protection or justice."

Never mind that many hospitals aren't providing counseling or other resources to help assaulted nurses cope with the distress that lingers after an attack, including insomnia, flashbacks, anxiety, and other symptoms of post-traumatic stress disorder. In nearly three-quarters of assaults against ER nurses, hospital management never even responds to queries from nurses who are attacked (according to those nurses). "They want the nurses to ignore it, partly because they don't want the liability, but mostly because people outside of nursing just assume since the patient is elderly or mentally ill, they don't know any better. Right. Let me sit here and get my ass kicked because 'she doesn't know what she's doing and doesn't mean it,'" Molly said. In hospitals, the shrug-it-off culture forces nurses to endure treatment that would not be tolerated in any other profession.

More assaults occur at acute-care hospitals than any other workplace, according to the Bureau of Labor Statistics, and the majority of these healthcare assaults target nurses. Yet many hospitals don't train nurses how to manage violent people. As an Emergency Department chairman told me, "My residents get more training than my nurses do," even though nurses are assaulted more frequently than doctors because they are more often at the bedside.

Hospital administrators aren't the only people dismissing the victim. In 2012, Tennessee state senators debated a bill to strengthen penalties for people who assault healthcare workers. Senator Ophelia Ford gave an odd, rambling statement in which she complained about "mean and hateful" nurses during her own medical care and not getting a private room. She concluded, "To come before this committee and ask for this kind of thing is ludicrous." The bill passed the committee anyway with a five-to-four vote, but attacking a nurse is still only a misdemeanor in Tennessee and twenty other states.

When workplaces put measures in place to protect their staff, the results can be impressive. The Veterans Administration Medical Center in Portland, Oregon, installed a computerized database to identify patients with a history of violence, so that staff members would know to take additional safety measures, according to the National Institute for Occupational Safety and Health. The program helped to decrease the number of violent attacks by an astounding 91.6 percent.

The prejudice against nurses is alarming and dangerous. In 2006, Brenda Coney, a patient in Jacksonville, Florida, pulled a knife on another patient. The hospital called the sheriff's office, which filed a police report. Two months later, when Coney slapped a nurse twice in the face, the hospital ignored the incident. Later that same month, Coney returned to the hospital, where she shot and killed a pharmacist.

If nurses are ignored, blamed, or laid off when patients assault them, what happens to other hospital staff members? Consider the case of Paul Matera, who worked in Washington, DC. A trauma patient who had been stabbed punched Matera in the back of the neck, rupturing several discs. Matera, who continued treating the patient almost immediately, needed three surgeries (covered by workers' compensation insurance) to repair his own injuries. He didn't press charges because, he said, "He was a young guy under the influence of alcohol and cocaine and under duress from his own trauma, so I felt he likely did not know what he was doing." But

Matera wasn't a nurse. He was an ER doctor. So his hospital didn't fire him or fault him for the attack. Instead, Dr. Matera received an entirely different sort of response: The American Medical Association gave him the rarely awarded Medal of Valor for "courage under extraordinary circumstances in nonwartime situations."

SAM   CITYCENTER HOSPITAL, October

Now in her third month as a nurse, Sam was certainly more confident than she'd been back in August. She enjoyed the work, even if Citycenter's ER was crazy. The patient load was enormous, but as a result, she had treated so many people that she no longer felt like a brand-new nurse. She relished learning something interesting every shift.

By focusing on the work rather than the environment, Sam could even put up with the spontaneously high-kicking CeeCee, whose personality continued to grate on her. Sam tried giving her the benefit of the doubt, because CeeCee was the type of nurse who jumped in to help without being asked (and even if her help wasn't actually needed). Yet the way CeeCee went about helping made it seem as if she were doing so not to alleviate another nurse's workload or to improve patient care but because she wanted her fellow nurses' gratitude and adoration.

That was okay. Sam could let that go. One thing about being an introvert—because you avoided drama, it was easy to let petty matters go. And the other nurses were mostly gracious and willing to teach her. On rare occasions, Sam was lucky enough to share a shift with Shirley, a well-respected nurse practitioner who cheerfully answered any questions Sam had about being an NP. Shirley told Sam that she could do nearly anything in the hospital that ER residents did.

William, in particular, seemed to get a kick out of Sam. "You're so funny, Sam," he told her once. "You're so quiet and then suddenly you speak up—'Screw this!' It's like, tell me how you really feel." Sam was enjoying getting to know him, too. They had several mutual interests outside of medicine, like biking and swimming, and he was easy to talk to.

But Sam was still disheartened by how difficult it was for nurses to find respect at Citycenter. "Nurses are really looked down on by residents. Some residents are amazing, but others you just want to drop-kick," she said.

Dr. Spiros, who pulled ER night duty about every three weeks, continued to fall into the latter category for her, which was frustrating because everyone else seemed to love him. Sam's style of speaking was casual, but Dr. Spiros's was not. So when Sam asked, for example, her cheeks flushing, "Hey, Dr. Spiros, do you mind if I get some morphine for Mr. Neberz?" he was short with her. Half the time, he didn't even look at her. Granted, she tended to run into him when both of them were stressed or tired. And her attempts at nonchalance probably didn't mask how awkward she felt approaching the busy senior resident.

One night, a nurse mentioned that Dr. Spiros had helped her out of a tight spot with a seriously ill patient.

Sam scoffed. "He wasn't an ass?"

The nurse looked at Sam quizzically. "Oh, no, no, no! He's a nice guy who did right by my patient." The nurse told her that Dr. Spiros had gone through a sad divorce the year before. "When he told me about it, he got all teary-eyed and said he just wanted to find the right person," she said, shaking her head sympathetically.

"Really? I just find him pompous," Sam said.

"Oh, but he's so nice. Seriously, he's Mr. Nice Guy."

Sam doubted that. An hour later, when Sam went to the minor care nurses station to document patient information, Dr. Spiros was telling another nurse about his recent trip to Greece. The other nurse brought Sam into the conversation before she left.

"I'd love to go there someday," Sam said.

Dr. Spiros pointed to the surname on her badge. "Where's that name from?"

"I'm Greek, can't you tell?" Sam answered.

"That can't be right," he said.

"My grandparents lived closer to Italy."

Beneath his tousled hair, Dr. Spiros fixed his deep brown eyes on Sam as if she were the only person in the room. "Oh, really. So you're supposed to be pretty fiery . . . " He grinned at her. "And 'Sam'? Not short for Samantha?"

"Salome."

"Salome! It means 'peace.' Fitting." He raised an eyebrow. "So, Sam. Why are you so quiet?"

Sam adjusted her glasses for a moment to avoid the intense gaze of this hunky doctor. Why was she quiet? There were several reasons. She liked to observe her surroundings, to soak them in, rather than to insert herself clumsily into them. Somehow the words in her head rarely exited her mouth as elegantly as she had hoped. She preferred to "feel things out" rather than charge headlong into a situation. And she didn't believe in jabbering only to fill a silence; silence could be beautiful, and illuminating.

When she looked up, Dr. Spiros was still smiling amiably at her. "If I'm talking then I can't listen, and if I'm not listening, I won't learn," she said, sincere.

"You're like a little mystery," he mused.

For the next ten minutes, Dr. Spiros gradually drew Sam out by asking her about local Greek restaurants. He had unknowingly hit her sweet spot. She found it easy to speak enthusiastically about food.

That night, as Sam did her rounds, she reflected on the conversation. *Okay, maybe he is a nice guy*, she thought. *He must have just been off whenever we've interacted before.*

When Sam woke up the following afternoon, she sent Dr. Spiros a Facebook message to reinforce their positive momentum. "Hey! Thanks for livening up the shift!"

He wrote her back quickly. "Likewise. What was the name of that especially good Greek restaurant again? Perhaps we should go there together."

Well, this was interesting. She had not seen this one coming. Dr. Spiros was more than ten years older than Sam and had a strong reputation at Citycenter. She was hesitant to date someone she worked with again. She had dated a murse for four months when she was a tech at Pines, and had later regretted it; the murse was fun but too immature. After she broke up with him, she knew that he had spread rumors about her, blabbing to the staff that she was a wild woman in bed. Hospitals were small worlds. It was hard to command respect in an environment in which people assumed she was promiscuous.

Dr. Spiros had already made the move, though, which meant that she was destined for awkwardness either way. Sam felt obligated to give him a chance because he had asked her. Maybe it could work out. After all, she had apparently already misjudged him as a pompous ass and he had proved her wrong. And she preferred relationships with medical professionals anyway, because they understood her interests and schedule better than anyone else.

During her next shift, Sam did some subtle investigating. Dr. Spiros was supposedly dating a tech, but after some small talk with another tech, Sam discovered they'd broken up. The following day, he asked when Sam was available for dinner and they worked out the logistics.

That night, Sam sought out William at the nurses station. She told him that Dr. Spiros had asked her out. "Is it crazy for me to do this? If this is a bad idea, I don't want to do it," she said. "I'm not in love with him or anything. I don't need to make life tricky for myself."

William gave her a look that she couldn't interpret. "I guess there's no hope for you and me then," he said. For a moment, Sam gazed into his soulful eyes and wondered briefly if he was flirting or joking.

She quickly dismissed the thought. "Get to the point," she said. "We're not talking about you and me." She wished they were. William was the man of her dreams. Sam could see no reason why he would be interested in her. From what she had heard, his long-distance girlfriend was beautiful, generous, and a heck of a nurse.

He had, however, made a point of teaching Sam some valuable nurse tricks, such as a way to outwit the Pyxis in order to get extra medication for a patient without having to wait for the pharmacy. She appreciated his subtle manner of instructing her. He would say, "You can do this your own way, but I like to do it like this." He was the ideal nursing mentor: caring, approachable, and wise.

William exhaled. "It's fine to see Spiros. Just don't go making out in the on-call room." Sam had heard rumors about the on-call room. On a few occasions, while wheeling patients to the elevators, she had heard unmistakable rumblings from behind that door. Hooking up in the hospital was definitely not Sam's style.

JULIETTE   PINES MEMORIAL, October

Nurses were buzzing about a cookout that Anastasia, the leader of the nurse clique, was hosting for hospital staff. Juliette could see Anastasia inviting several of their coworkers and mutual friends on their individual Facebook walls. She waited for Anastasia to invite her. Anastasia was calling it the Pines Memorial Cookout, for Pete's sake. She had even invited Charlene, and Juliette knew that Anastasia didn't like Charlene.

Juliette had considered unfriending Anastasia so that her Facebook posts wouldn't torture her anymore. But everyone at Pines was Facebook friends with one another, and the nurses were constantly Facebooking at the nurses station. Juliette had joined Facebook when she was hired at Pines specifically because the network was an integral part of those nurses' lives.

Juliette's favorite tech noticed that Juliette's mood had dipped. "What's bothering you, Juliette?" asked Mimi.

"The whole Anastasia thing about the party," Juliette said. "I can't believe she didn't even invite me."

"Oh, I wouldn't worry about that," Mimi said.

"I do worry about that!"

"Anastasia's the kind of person who will walk by me and not even say hello," Mimi said.

"Really?" At least Anastasia was cordial to Juliette in person.

"Absolutely. She's just part of that clique," Mimi said, shrugging as she left to check on a patient.

Juliette wished she could ignore the clique's behavior like Mimi did. Then again, Mimi probably didn't have Juliette's insecurities; she was slender and fit.

Juliette rubbed her temple and smoothed her auburn hair off her forehead. She had a terrible headache. She got migraines regularly, headaches that knocked her flat with pain and nausea. She had told only Priscilla,

Molly, and Lara about them. Her primary care doctor didn't believe in prescribing narcotics, but the medications he did prescribe rarely worked. In desperation, Juliette had asked for a Percocet prescription from a PA who had prescribed her antibiotics in the past. With the hours nurses worked, getting prescriptions at the hospital sure beat waiting for a primary care doctor's appointment.

The Percocet soothed the migraines within forty-five minutes, but the headaches returned at least once a month and Juliette's prescription was running out. Percocet was the most efficient, if not an optimal, solution. She did not have time to deal with headaches at work, and she certainly didn't have time to deal with them at home.

Priscilla, Pines' nursing director, was the only person at Pines who knew about Juliette's home life; this was one of several secrets Juliette had confided to Priscilla. Juliette's husband, a data center manager, was an unrepentant workaholic. Juliette knew this when she married him, but the problem had accelerated over the years. Nearly every night after dinner, Tim went back to the office for hours, endlessly stressed about earning enough money. The rest of the day, Tim was an attentive husband and father, smart, interesting, and helpful; he took Michelle to and from school and got her ready in the morning. But his insistence on working nights had put a strain on their marriage.

In the evenings, Juliette would rush around, trying to manage the household herself. She would go to bed later than she should, hit the snooze button in the morning, and fight traffic on the long commute to the ER. She often arrived at work five to ten minutes late.

That afternoon, after giving a patient a dose of Dilaudid, Juliette palmed the half-full glass cylinder. It was the length of her index finger and about 3 millimeters in diameter. *It would be so easy to take this home,* she thought. Prescription costs added up. *No one will know if I take some. It's not like I'm shooting up at work. It would just be a home injection of a med that we were going to throw out anyway.* Patients often came into the ER seeking narcotics, and got them. Why couldn't a nurse who truly needed the medicine have it, too?

When a new patient arrived, Juliette put the Dilaudid in her pocket. She would think about it later. The patient, a middle-aged woman with orange-tinted hair, was complaining of back and neck pain and trouble with urination. She told Juliette and the ER doctor that she had waited for an hour in the lobby. "This can't take very long, because my dog's in the car," the woman said.

"Why did you bring your dog?" asked Dr. Mark Kazumi, a generally pleasant man. Juliette liked working with Dr. Kazumi. Other nurses teased him because he ordered a lot of labs. But Juliette appreciated that he tried to do right by his patients.

"I didn't think it would take very long," the patient said. Many ER patients assumed that service should be like fast food: Get in, get your orders, get out.

"Well, it's going to take a little bit of time," the doctor said. "I can't make it quick for you. I've ordered a urinalysis and a CT scan."

When Dr. Kazumi and Juliette left the room, he turned to her. "Juliette, I need you to check on the dog."

"Are you serious?" Juliette asked. It was a balmy, breezy October day.

"Yeah. The dog can't be left outside alone. It's against the law," the doctor said. "The dog could suffocate out there; it could be stolen. You need to find the dog, and I'm going to call the police on her if it's not okay."

Juliette sighed. "Don't call the police." She returned to the patient's room.

"Where are you parked?" she asked the woman as she wheeled her to radiology.

"In front of the ER."

That was helpful, Juliette thought. "Can you give me more of a description?"

"No. I'm in front of the ER."

"What kind of car?"

"Accord."

"What color?"

"Silver."

While the woman was in the CT room, Juliette went outside. There was no silver Accord in front of the ER. There were, however, several silver Accords throughout the parking lot. Juliette grumbled to herself. *I have four other patients but I'm out here searching for a Bichon in an Accord.*

After ten minutes and eight empty silver Accords, Juliette called the tech in the CT room. "Can you please ask Mrs. Swirsky where exactly she parked?"

Juliette could hear the patient saying, "The dog is fine. I knitted him a blanket and he's sleeping on it."

The tech came back on the line. "She doesn't remember."

Juliette continued to wander the parking lot, her headache now weightier beneath the disappointments of drudgeries that had little to do with her job.

LARA   SOUTH GENERAL HOSPITAL, October

On a crisp afternoon, Lara's friend Juliette called to say hi. After some small talk, Juliette mentioned her migraines and her struggle with them at work and at home. "It's really inconvenient, because my regular doctor won't prescribe narcotics, so I got Percocet from a PA. It wouldn't be a big deal if I took a wasted vial from the ER now and then, right? They're just going to get thrown out. I still have one in my pocket because I forgot to waste it."

Lara froze. This sounded all too familiar. "That would definitely be a big deal. I'm really worried about you," Lara said. "You're talking intramuscular use."

"Oh, it's just occasional," Juliette said. "I was thinking I could give myself a shot of Dilaudid to get rid of my headaches. But only if they're really bad."

"Yeah, but I'm really worried. Narcotics are a slippery slope."

"There's nothing to worry about! It's just for my headaches. You know how bad my migraines get. The Dilaudid would be only point-five milligrams at a time."

"It's still narcotic use and you're talking about stealing," Lara pressed.

"Only one or two times a month," Juliette said.

"Juliette, listen!" Lara said. "You are using drugs. You're using drugs! You're softening it too much. I'm afraid you're going to end up in a situation like I did where you have to have it or else you're sick. When you use narcotics, you get rebound headaches. They're the worst."

"Oh, it's just intramuscular. It's not in a vein," Juliette said.

"That's bullshit," Lara said. "No normal person brings home narcotics and gives themselves shots." The first few times Lara brought narcotics home from the hospital, she, too, had rationalized it as "just occasional." Then she told herself she did it because "I like the buzz." And then "That guy was a jerk." Eventually, she didn't bother with excuses. Lara decided that Juliette had told her about the Dilaudid because she wanted help.

She took another approach. "From my history and experience, I'm afraid for you to go through the same hell I went through. It's a nightmare. I don't want that to happen to you. Throw it out."

Juliette was silent. "Well, maybe you're right," she said. "I have enough issues with eating, anyway. I don't need to have anything else. And I don't want to get in trouble or disappoint Priscilla."

That's the least of your worries, Lara thought. Lara believed Juliette cared too much about what Priscilla thought of her because the nursing director was Juliette's only confidante at Pines. Sometimes Lara wondered if Juliette was confusing Priscilla's managerial tendency to let employee transgressions slide—in Juliette's case, late arrivals to work—with friendship. Lara wished Juliette had more faith in herself. Juliette was a fantastic, knowledgeable nurse who was an unwavering advocate for her patients. She shouldn't need to seek her supervisor's approval to validate her self-worth.

A few days later, Juliette texted Lara. "I've been thinking about what you said. I threw out the vial and I'll go ahead and look into some other options for my headaches."

Relieved, Lara would pray for Juliette, both because she didn't want anything bad to happen to her friend, and because she was grateful. "Listening to her downplay it reminded me I don't want to be there again," Lara said. "The whole Nurse Jackie thing is so prevalent. Not just nurses, but doctors, PAs. One of the NA meetings I go to is specifically for firefighters, nurses, doctors, and policemen. They don't know who can help them watch their back."

CHAPTER 4

WHEN NURSES BULLY NURSES:
Hierarchies, Hazing, and Why They Eat Their Young

"The nurse treats colleagues, employees, assistants, and students with respect and compassion."
— *Code of Ethics for Nurses*, Provision 1.5

"I knew the minute it came out of my mouth that I had just 'eaten my young.'"
— A PEDIATRIC ONCOLOGY NURSE IN ARIZONA

MOLLY November

RIVERPORT HOSPITAL

One day, for variety, Molly took two shifts at Riverport, a highly regarded local hospital, despite another nurse's warning that "some of the charge nurses try to set up agency nurses to fail." Molly didn't mind; the timing worked with her fertility schedule. Her first IUI had been unsuccessful and she was now preparing for her second.

She didn't let the results get her down. Her fertility treatments affected her work life only in that she cared even less about the drama among coworkers. She had always been a diligent, focused nurse, but now that conceiving a child was at the top of her priority list, she wasn't about to spend time or energy getting emotionally involved with non–work-related nonsense. Her goal was to come in, do her job, and go home. At Academy and South General, she could do this well. At Citycenter, it was more difficult because the conditions were so unsafe.

At Riverport, Molly learned quickly that the warning about other nurses was accurate. The charge nurse assigned Molly four critical Priority 1 patients, each of whom needed one-to-one care. When Molly said the patients needed more attention, the nurse snapped, "I just figured you could handle it. I guess not."

Molly gave report that night to an incoming nurse who happened to be someone she had worked with at Citycenter. Molly told her what had happened.

"Yeah, they are such mean girls here," the nurse said. "No one helps anyone out, and there's definitely a social hierarchy."

Molly noticed the hierarchy during her shift the following day. Seven nurses were apparently the "cool" nurses in the ER. They were 22- and 23-year-olds who, as Molly observed, "do their hair and makeup like they're going clubbing."

The cool nurses hung out together exclusively, which was fine with Molly, but the techs wanted to help only the cool nurses, which was not fine. Molly happened to be charting at the nurses station next to Lena, the clique leader. Whenever another "cool nurse" walked by, Lena stopped her.

"Hey, we're going to happy hour tonight, but don't tell anyone, because I only want the cool people there," Lena would say.

Molly shook her head in disbelief. After six cool nurses—and fifteen apparently uncool nurses—passed by, Lena turned to Molly. "I *guess* you can come, too"—she paused—"if you want."

At first Molly was astonished by the nurse's immaturity. She had to remind herself that these were girls, not women, and that they weren't that many years out of high school. She was constantly amazed by the ways that some of these young nurses could act like teenagers one moment, then flip a switch and impassively handle high-pressure patient situations the next. ERs could hire new grads to work on codes when they were doing keg stands a month ago. Molly decided not to call the nurse out on her behavior because it didn't affect her, unlike the charge nurse's attitude toward agency nurses. "I already have plans," she said. She would not return to Riverport again.

Molly had heard that some staff nurses treated agency nurses poorly, but she was surprised now that it was happening to her. "If the agency nurses weren't there, the staff nurses would have a much higher patient ratio," she explained. "We make their job easier, but they're rude and unfair." Another agency nurse had told Molly that one day she had arrived at an ER that had a total of seven patients. The charge nurse assigned her all seven. When the nurse asked why, the charge nurse said, "You're agency. You're getting paid more than us. You can handle it."

Some hospital administrators were partly to blame for creating an us-versus-them mentality. During October's Emergency Nurses week, one of two nurse appreciation weeks during the year (the other is National Nurses Week in May), hospitals usually gave nurses tokens of appreciation. At an Academy Hospital staff meeting Molly was required to attend, the ER manager had given plush blankets with Academy's logo to every nurse in the room except Molly. "Sorry, these blankets are for staff," she said. *How easy would it have been to give out one extra blanket instead of making me feel like I don't contribute to the department?* Molly thought.

Molly cared less about the gifts than the sentiment. Academy supervisors had repeatedly told her that she was a valuable nurse and had asked her to pick up extra shifts. "I probably would've used it as a dog blanket anyway. But really, right in front of me? 'You're agency, so we can't give you one?'" she groused to a friend. "Why are you going to make people feel excluded when we're there to help you? All of the agency people are experienced nurses. Why are y'all trying to create animosity between the two?"

CITYCENTER MEDICAL

By the time Molly finished an exhausting shift at Citycenter, 110 patients waited in the ER, more than many ERs saw in an entire day. That night, Molly vented to Trey about Citycenter. He listened patiently to her, like he always did.

"So stop working there," he said. As usual, a man of few words.

Molly paused for a moment to reflect. Why wouldn't she simply stop working at Citycenter? Academy was easier (though less interesting). "I don't want this job to beat me," she said. "I don't want anyone to think I can't handle it. I don't think any job is too hard for me, and I don't want to walk away."

"If you're getting burned out, just work a day or two every once in a while," Trey suggested. "Lowering your stress level might make it easier to get pregnant anyway."

"That's true, but I'm not stressed. I'm just angry. And full-time Citycenter nurses are putting themselves through those conditions every single day. If I walk away, I'll feel like they are stronger nurses than me."

"You took the agency jobs to see if there are better hospitals than Pines," Trey said, affectionately squeezing her shoulder. As he left the room, he added, "Maybe there aren't."

The next day, Molly had just given report to a night-shift nurse when an ambulance brought in a little old lady who had fallen. She had been assigned to a room, but the Citycenter nurses were swamped with other patients.

As Molly passed by the woman's bed, she noticed that the woman had urinated on herself. Molly was weary and off the clock, but she knew that if she didn't help the patient, she would be sitting in wet clothes for hours. Molly worked up a sweat as she struggled to change the woman's clothes.

The woman was grateful. She said sweetly, "I think anyone who is an ER nurse must really want to be an ER nurse. It's such a difficult job."

"I think so, too!" Molly said.

On her way home that night, Molly reflected that the woman was correct. "As much as I complain about all the B.S., if I didn't want to do it, there are lots of other options in nursing. But I choose the ER. There's a sense of satisfaction that comes with 'fixing' people," she said. "In so many areas of healthcare, people have long-term treatment for things they may not recover from. In emergency medicine, a person comes in with crushing chest pain, gets diagnosed with a heart attack, gets meds, gets shipped to the cardiac catheterization lab, and gets fixed. A person comes in with abdominal pain, gets diagnosed with appendicitis, goes to the OR, and gets fixed. I need to remember that I chose this specialty. The reality is *healthcare* is broken. I need to figure out how to either let it go or decide how I can contribute to fixing it."

Molly had no desire to be a floor nurse. At every hospital where she had worked, there was a rivalry between the ER and the other nursing departments. "We think they're lazy and they think we're bitches," Molly said. One of the most frequent complaints ER nurses had against floor nurses was that floor nurses tried to avoid getting new patients as shift change approached.

Many floor nurses made excuses to Molly and her colleagues for why they couldn't take a patient at shift change. "The room's not clean" was one of them. More than once, Molly had gone upstairs to the floor, found the room to be clean, and called the nurse's bluff. Another favorite was "There isn't a bed in the room," which meant housekeeping would have to bring up a bed. When one floor nurse used this excuse, Molly discovered that the nurse herself had pulled the bed into the hallway to avoid getting a new patient when she wanted to leave work.

During Molly's next Citycenter shift, she called the medical/surgical floor to give report on a patient. The nurse who answered the phone said that the patient's nurse-to-be was on break.

"Okay, I'll give report to whoever is covering for her," Molly said.

"There isn't anyone covering," the nurse said.

Right, Molly thought. *This hospital is so fucked up.* "So if one of her patients needed something while the nurse was at lunch, who would help them?"

"Me," the nurse answered.

Molly didn't miss a beat. "Okay, then you're going to be getting a forty-four-year-old female admitting for intractable vomiting . . ."

LARA   SOUTH GENERAL HOSPITAL, November

In the middle of the nurses station, two nurses were screaming at each other. Lynn, a young ER nurse, was trying to move a patient to the psychiatric department, but the patient's blood sugar was high, at 200 mg/dL, when normal levels ranged from 70 to 100. Tashia, a psychiatric nurse who had been at the hospital for many years, wanted the patient's blood sugar stabilized before moving the patient upstairs. She told Lynn, "No, we're not taking her yet."

"You're a nurse. You can treat the blood sugar just like we can. We need her upstairs. She's being admitted for treatment," Lynn protested.

"You don't know what you're doing!" Tashia yelled. "You're incompetent! You're a horrible nurse!"

The nurses station quieted. Tashia, who was nearing retirement, was known to be a bully, but this was different. She was yelling at Lynn in front of other nurses and patients on stretchers in the hallway, including the patient in question. From their rooms encircling the nurses station, ER patients peered through the curtains at the spectacle.

Lynn raised her voice right back. "Don't you dare call me names!"

Tashia got into Lynn's face, her finger within poking distance of Lynn's eyes. "You want to hear name-calling? Fine! Everyone thinks you're a skank!" Lara hadn't heard that before. Lynn was a petite, beautiful black woman. Lynn didn't say anything. She walked away.

When Lara finished her charting, she caught up with Lynn in the hallway. Rose was already there, patting Lynn on the back. Lara asked if she was okay.

"Yeah," Lynn said. "I felt like if I came back at her, I'd be yelling at an old woman. She's an angry, bitter woman."

Still, Lara could see that she was shaken by Tashia's outburst. This was Lara's only complaint about South General: A small but unavoidable group of the nurses was verbally abusive. While at other hospitals, the bullying could be more covert or passive-aggressive, at South General, hostilities were blatant. "There's some serious attitude here. Maybe it's from years of having grown up in this rough area," Lara observed. "People put up an angry, defensive wall. It's difficult to break down that attitude with each individual coworker."

Despite racial tensions, Lara, one of the few white nurses at the hospital, hadn't landed in anyone's crosshairs. Evidently someone had noticed that Lara seemed to get along with everyone, because in November, the ER director selected her as one of fifteen people to join a new hospital-wide committee. A healthcare management company had developed the Relationship-Based Care program with the goal of improving staff members' attitudes toward each other so that they could work better as a team. South General had just signed up.

The committee's mission was compassionate and holistic. The mandatory three-day RBC conference emphasized the message, "If you take care of yourself, you'll be a better person, better mom, better wife, better coworker, better nurse. When your coworkers are looking out for each other, it will become a more therapeutic environment," Lara said, excited to help. The instructors asked the groups to brainstorm what they could do to improve relationships in their hospitals.

Lara's committee, consisting of six ER staff members and six nurses from other floors, decided that their first short-term goal would be to set up crisis intervention help for staff. Hospital professionals grappled with traumas and tragedies in different ways. Lara suspected that another South General nurse was turning to narcotics to cope. Fatima was a 28-year-old night-shift ER nurse. A tech recently had told Lara that just before shift change, he had seen Fatima roll a needlebox cart into a storage closet. *That's a good idea!* Lara couldn't help thinking, understanding immediately that Fatima was desperate enough for partially used vials of narcotics that she would stick her hand into a box full of used needles in a hospital that treated many patients with HIV and tuberculosis.

The tech had followed Fatima into the closet and turned on the light to see Fatima's hand in the needlebox. "What are you doing?" he asked.

Fatima immediately withdrew her hand. "Uh, the box was full, so I'm putting it away," she said.

"So why's your hand in there?"

Fatima mumbled an unintelligible excuse and the tech had let her go.

During Lara's next shift, she was heading toward an RBC meeting when she saw Fatima in the hall. Lara recognized the signs: Fatima was pale, sweaty, and sluggish. Her face had a greenish sheen. *Oh my God, you are dope sick*, Lara thought. She played dumb. "Hey, Fatima, isn't your shift over?"

"I got called into the office. When people don't like you around here, they make stuff up about you. So I'm here to tell my side of the story," Fatima replied.

She probably doesn't even see it, just like I didn't, Lara thought. She wanted to help Fatima, to tell her that she could still turn herself around without losing her nursing license. But she wasn't sure how to convey that she knew about her habit. Lara worried that Fatima could accuse her of slander and get her fired. Fatima was barely an acquaintance; they passed each other in the hallway only occasionally during shift change.

Lara decided to ask her Thursday night group what to do. For years, her group of eight women—all friends from NA—met once a week to check in with each other. They could tell Lara how to handle the situation.

But at the network's next meeting, Lara didn't have a chance to discuss Fatima. The bulk of the dinner was spent consoling a woman whose father had died, so Lara didn't mention some recent disappointments in her own life. She had learned that she wouldn't be able to volunteer occasionally as her kids' school nurse after all. School nurse volunteers were required to take a CPR course run by the county, but the course was offered only once per semester and Lara wasn't able to attend that day. The county wouldn't allow Lara to work in the school even though she was a CPR-certified nurse who cared for critical patients regularly.

Also, Lara's marriage was deteriorating. John was openly flirting with other women and gambling again but denying that he had a problem. Sometimes Lara thought about leaving him, but she didn't know how her family would manage. Even though he still wasn't working, Lara couldn't fathom being a single mom on a nurse's salary without having

John around for childcare. "If the kids say, 'Can I join T-ball' or 'Can we go to the movies,' I don't want to be in a place where I can't give them that basic childhood stuff," she said. She soldiered on.

JULIETTE   PINES MEMORIAL, November

Juliette was in the doctors' back office, joking around with Clark Preston. The doctors' office was a relatively large room with five computers spread across a U-shaped desk. It wasn't unusual to see doctors flirting with the cute nurses back there. Juliette, who had good working relationships with most of the doctors, ventured into the office when she had questions about patients or to hang out with Clark, who liked the same sports teams and TV shows she did. Clark usually had a funny video or photos of his dogs to show her.

On Juliette's way out of the office, she saw Dr. Fontaine and red-haired Nancy—the nurse-dating womanizer and his former girlfriend—sitting across from each other in close quarters. Nancy, who was on the phone, was pointedly looking down so that the doctor wasn't in her sight line. She wouldn't meet Juliette's eyes, either.

It was a shame that Juliette couldn't forget that Dr. Fontaine had dated three nurses behind Nancy's back. He was otherwise a charming and skilled practitioner. She shook her head and went to the nurses station, where she was charge nurse for the shift. After checking the boards, she went to triage to help out.

When a patient came in with abdominal pain, Juliette flagged Lucy, the tech assigned to triage, in the hallway. Lucy was a lazy tech who got away with dodging her responsibilities because she occasionally babysat for a few of the supervisors. Once, when Lucy had called in sick, her Facebook page revealed photos of herself at a festival.

"Please put an IV in this patient. He has abdominal pain," Juliette said, gesturing to the 55-year-old patient in a wheelchair. The man was vomiting into an emesis basin.

Lucy blinked at her. "Is the patient going to go to the waiting room?" she asked in her thick Dominican accent.

"Yes, but not for long. He'll be within eyesight of triage. He's vomiting, so we have to give him Zofran, and then he'll go to a room as soon as it's ready."

Lucy shrugged. "I can't put an IV in him because he's not going straight back to a room." She turned to walk away.

"Lucy, the patient needs your help now! He'll go back to a room within five minutes, but I have to assist with another patient," Juliette said.

"No, I can't do it."

"You can!" Juliette insisted. "You can put an IV in him because he desperately needs it."

Lucy ignored her, as if she didn't understand; she seemed to have selective comprehension of the English language. She did this frequently to Juliette, even though techs were supposed to follow charge nurses' instructions.

Juliette exploded, upset about Lucy's treatment of the patient. "Oh, will someone just say it to her in a language she understands?" She regretted the words as she said them.

Gabriel, the secretary, whirled around in his chair and stared at Juliette. Lucy stomped out to triage. Erica, the senior charge nurse, hurried after Lucy to calm her down. "Bad move. That was the wrong thing to say," Gabriel said.

"I know, I'm sorry. It was so wrong," Juliette said. "I messed up. Should I go out there now?"

"No, just leave it alone."

For the rest of the day, Lucy ignored Juliette even more blatantly than usual. "Where'd the patient go?" Juliette asked. "What room is that patient in?" Lucy wouldn't look at her. If Lucy had a question, she asked another nurse, even though Juliette was charge.

The next day, Juliette went to Priscilla's office to tell her what happened.

"She's already been in here and she was crying," Priscilla said.

"Oh, give me a break," Juliette sighed. "Lucy was insubordinate before this escalated. Could the three of us please meet?"

"Sure," Priscilla said. She never arranged the meeting.

Juliette bought an apology card and a box of chocolates from the gift shop. When she tried to apologize, Lucy refused to accept them.

"I don't need a card," Lucy said.

"I'm trying to say I'm sorry," Juliette said, genuinely trying to make amends.

"What you did was wrong."

"Yes it was. I'm trying to apologize," Juliette repeated, still conciliatory.

Lucy stood up and walked away. Juliette left the card and the chocolates on her computer.

Weeks later, Juliette shared this scenario during a continuing education workshop. She felt awful about her mistake, but she worried that Lucy's refusal to interact would affect patient care. "Lucy hasn't spoken to me since," she said.

"What Lucy was doing, before the incident and after you apologized, is a form of bullying that is common in nursing today," the facilitator said. "Ignoring is a form of bullying because you're blocking that person out. It doesn't matter if you don't like somebody. That's fine. You don't have to. But you need to be cordial to and communicate with that person at work."

Juliette felt helpless, but Priscilla wouldn't do anything about it. Priscilla was too afraid of confrontation to act like a manager and diffuse the situation. In Priscilla's realm, bullies and slackers went unpunished, and staffers who did go beyond the call of duty weren't recognized. Priscilla didn't reprimand Juliette; in fact, she told Juliette that she had been right about the patient and encouraged Juliette to be charge nurse more often.

Shortly after that incident, Erica, the senior charge nurse Juliette genuinely admired, resigned from the ER to take an administrative position at another medical center. "I'm so tired of the bullshit at this hospital," she told Juliette. Assignments and rule enforcement were too subjective, she said, and the gossipy atmosphere was poisonous.

"You should apply for my job, Juliette," Erica said. "You do a good job when you're charge."

Some of the nurses thought Juliette would apply for Erica's position, but Juliette didn't want it. The job was too stressful. Besides, Juliette didn't care about prestige or hierarchy; she preferred to help patients as a bedside nurse. Rumors spread that Charlene was lobbying for the position to be renamed "head charge nurse" to emphasize that Charlene, as nurse supervisor, had seniority. Juliette had heard that Bethany, a talented nurse relatively new to Pines, was applying. Juliette liked Bethany. If Bethany was sitting at the nurses station and saw another nurse walk by, she would automatically ask, "Do you need help with anything?" Bethany was a thorough nurse, as well. Juliette had passed by patient rooms multiple times and seen Bethany conducting a careful full head-to-toe assessment. Juliette associated Bethany with the clique, but she was upbeat and nice to Juliette.

One day, Juliette checked Facebook while sitting at the nurses station. "Let's take the kids on the ferry this weekend!" a clique member had posted on several nurses' walls.

"That clique is so mean," she muttered.

"Don't feel badly, Juliette." Juliette looked up. She hadn't noticed Bethany sitting nearby.

"When I started working here, I had never, ever seen cliques like the nurses in this ER," Bethany said. "I was amazed."

Because Bethany lived in the same neighborhood as the others, and because she was the most beautiful person in the ER, Juliette had assumed that the clique had embraced her.

"Aren't you in it?" Juliette asked.

"Not at all," Bethany replied. She had heard other nurses talking about her behind her back. "It feels like no one is on my side," she said. "I don't have work friends, so I just go home after work and that's it."

Last month, several members of the clique were standing around the nurses station talking about a party. Bethany couldn't believe they unabashedly discussed the event in front of her. "So," she said, "are you inviting anyone else?"

"Oh, no," Anastasia answered. "It's a thirtysomething party." Bethany was 29.

"I see it all the time," Bethany said now. "They'll make their plans and purposefully discuss them in front of me, while excluding me."

Juliette felt a rush of camaraderie. "Same with me! I have a seven-year-old daughter and you'd think they'd include me in the kids' group playdates, but they don't," she said. "I can't believe they exclude you, too."

Juliette thought about this conversation for days. At least they seemed to like her better than Charlene, who still believed she was a part of the group. One nurse had admitted to Juliette that she was nice to Charlene only so that she would get good evaluations.

Juliette didn't go out of her way to help Charlene anymore. On a busy day when Charlene was supervising the unit, Juliette deliberately focused on assisting other nurses instead. Charlene's power-tripping, disrespectful treatment had worn Juliette down to the point of vindictive inaction. "On a day when the ER was crazy, I enjoyed watching her run around and be completely scattered," Juliette admitted to a friend. "I didn't triage more ambulances when I could have. There was a patient she could've moved out of my zone into the psych pod. That would have given her another bed. She didn't catch on to it and I didn't volunteer the advice. It's not to the point where any patients would suffer; I would never do that. But she has destroyed any sense of loyalty I would have had to anybody else."

It was common at Pines for nurses to plainly avoid helping coworkers they didn't like. For example, when an ambulance arrived, usually one nurse would triage and others would help the assigned nurse move the patient to the bed, get him on the heart monitor, take vitals, and start an IV. But if the assigned nurse was disliked or lazy, nobody would help her unless the patient was in danger.

During Juliette's evaluation, Priscilla told her that on the scale of 1 to 3, Juliette had scored several 2s and a few 3s, averaging about 2.6. "You're doing an excellent job. I'm very happy with you," Priscilla said. "You showed a lot of growth over the year, you help out your team members, you're always available. You anticipate patients' needs, you talk to the doctors about what's needed, and you advocate for patients. The only thing is, you have to be on time more often."

Juliette left Priscilla's office pleased. She was also relieved that she had listened to Lara. Since her conversation with Lara, Juliette had had a dozen opportunities to take Dilaudid from the ER. It was amazing how many nurses "turn a blind eye when you say, 'I'm going to waste this with you,'" Juliette said. But she didn't do it. If her migraine was bad enough to require narcotics and Tim wasn't home, she would take a cab to the ER. She had promised Lara she wouldn't take anything from the hospital, and she would stay true to her word.

SAM   CITYCENTER MEDICAL, November

At 11:00 p.m., nursing home attendants brought an elderly woman into the ER because she wasn't eating. When Sam checked the woman's vitals, she realized that the woman wasn't eating because her pulse was thirty-five beats per minute (normal range is between sixty and eighty). Also, the woman was breathing too rapidly, wasn't moving one side of her body, and most likely had a urinary tract infection. By now, Sam was experienced enough that she could tell when a patient had a UTI because "they just have that smell."

Sam started an IV, drew labs, and, forty-five minutes later, took the woman to get a CT scan. The scan showed that the woman had internal head bleeding. William came in to check on Sam. He seemed to know intuitively that she was worried because she'd never treated a patient this sick.

He reviewed the woman's chart. "Okay, Sam, you take care of the meds, I'll document." He helped Sam assist the patient's intubation, put on restraints (in case the woman woke up and tried to rip out the tube), and titrate (adjust the dose of the patient's medication). He showed Sam new techniques for inserting a Foley catheter, even though, as Sam put it, he was "not a Foley person."

When the ICU was ready, Sam called in report while William emptied the Foley bag and checked the patient's vitals. On the way upstairs, Sam looked at the clock: 1:30. William—the charge nurse, who was not supposed to have any patients—had helped her for nearly two hours. Sam was so grateful that she didn't get annoyed with him when he resumed his usual teasing.

He tugged on her ponytail. "So how are things going with Dr. Spiros? When are you going to see him?"

"Geez, why is this such a big deal to you?" Sam said.

"Oh, well, you know, I look out for my people," William replied.

The next night, when Sam arrived at the restaurant first, she had second thoughts while waiting for Dr. Spiros. She wasn't nervous because he was older; she had dated older men. She was nervous because he was a doctor. At her hospital. *Why are we doing this?* she thought. *How did this whole thing happen, anyway?* Sam knew women who became nurses specifically because they wanted to marry a rich doctor. Sam was not one of them. Actually, she felt "a little weird being that stereotypical nurse going out with a doctor."

She spotted him as soon as he walked in, wearing dark chinos and a collared crimson shirt, and saw that other women in the room noticed him, too. *He looks good,* Sam thought, and then, *Oh my gosh, that's Dr. Spiros right there. I mean, Dimitri.*

The date started off slowly. As they awkwardly talked about work and family, Sam narrated in her head. *And now I'm going to ask you a question, and you're going to answer, and then you're going to ask me a very similar question.* They found their groove by the middle of dinner, at least enough so that Sam was convinced that Dr. Spiros was charming after all. They found that they both were fervent football fans and were able to banter about their rival teams. "It's rare to find a woman who's into football," he said.

At the end of the night, Dr. Spiros smiled warmly. "Well, hey, let's get together again." They set a second date for two weeks later. Then he initiated Potential Hug Sequence. Sam couldn't tell if there would be an attempt at a kiss or whether the hug would be one-armed or two, so she leaned in gracelessly and they ended up patting each other on the back. Instead of saying something to diffuse the awkwardness, Sam shrugged and walked toward her apartment, thinking, *Yep, just let the awkwardness keep rolling because I'm awkward like that.*

Sam didn't think there was chemistry. She was surprised he wanted to see her again. The evening had been fun enough, although they didn't seem to mesh. But what could she do? As she told a friend, "I'm not good at letting people down gently. I can be efficient with a sledgehammer, but how could I do that to a doctor I work with?" At least dating a doctor, if that's what was happening here, made her job even more interesting.

The following night, Sam realized she wouldn't have time for "interesting." When she arrived at Citycenter, 105 patients were already on the board, meaning each nurse had double the maximum patient load. The

ER didn't even have enough equipment for the staff to properly do their jobs; there were only ten bags of saline in the entire department. Sam was the only nurse in Zone 3 because the other assigned nurse had not come in. Zone 2 also had only one nurse. Sam wondered whether her absent coworkers were the latest nurses to quit under Victoria's reign. *If I can make it here, I make it anywhere*, Sam thought.

For the first hours of her shift, Sam raced among her nine patients while, as a tech on her way in told the staff, Victoria (the ER director) and the nurse educator were across the street eating dinner. Both Victoria and the nurse educator had been longtime nurses who easily could have helped out on the floor.

Two of Sam's patients were seriously ill but had been mistriaged; they should have been assigned to Zone 1. One of them had diabetic ketoacidosis, or DKA, a difficult condition for a nurse to handle alone. Sam was supposed to give the patient at least five liters of saline and monitor his insulin drip by doing hourly finger sticks. She managed to draw his blood only approximately every ninety minutes, and even so, that was because his room was easily accessible, across from the nurses station. He should have received one-to-one care.

Because of those two patients, Sam couldn't visit her other patients for three hours. She didn't have time to go to the bathroom for eleven hours. She was so tired that she caught her foot in the cords of a portable vitals machine and face-planted directly in front of the nurses station. The charge nurse immediately quipped, "Oh no, we can't lose another nurse!"

Midshift, an ER resident made a miscalculation and ordered Sam to turn off the patient's insulin drip. When the DKA patient's ICU doctor came downstairs, he was furious. "Why has he gotten only two liters of fluid? Why is the insulin turned off? Why haven't you taken a finger stick in ninety-six minutes?!" he yelled, gesturing to the empty saline bags still attached to the man's IV.

"I'm sorry but I have seven other patients right now," Sam said. She was still the only nurse in the entire zone. "I wanted to rip this guy's head off!" she said later. "What did he think I was doing, sitting around eating Twizzlers and painting my nails? I had people in the back holding room with chest pain and shortness of breath who I hadn't seen for hours. I had to make sure they were still breathing."

The ER resident and senior resident heard the commotion and dashed into the room. They tried to explain that the ER was overcrowded and that the nurses were short-staffed. "It doesn't matter! This is an ICU patient!" the doctor yelled. "He needs one-to-one care!"

Sam slipped out of the room to attend to her other patients while the residents calmed the doctor down.

The next night, Sam was assigned to Zone 1. As busy as it was, she was thrilled at the chance to work with tough patients. The charge nurses usually assigned her to Zone 3, where Sam didn't feel she was learning as much as she could. Again, nurse numbers were down. An anesthesiologist she worked with was so taken aback by the unreasonable number of patients in the ER that he kept muttering, "This is so unsafe. Someone is going to die; this is so unsafe."

An IT guy, who was in the building to assist with the transition to a new computer system, caught Sam in the hallway. "Um, I think that nurse needs help." He pointed to a patient room.

Sam walked into the room to see a frantic young nurse even less experienced than Sam working alone on a complicated patient. Triage had sent back a patient with a heart rate of 150 beats per minute without an EKG. The patient was a train wreck: He'd had a seizure, couldn't follow commands, and was jaundiced. Sam helped the nurse get a rectal temperature of 102, then went to find the ER doctor.

Sam found Dr. Spiros outside another patient's room. "Hey, can you order some Tylenol for Mr. Rhodes?" A fever could cause a high heart rate.

"I don't think he can swallow anything," Dr. Spiros replied.

Sam gave him a "don't be dense" look. "No shit, Sherlock. I want it rectally."

Dr. Spiros laughed and gave her the order.

William, the charge nurse that night, saw them laughing together and followed Sam to her next patient room. He typed the patient's information into an EKG while Sam connected the leads. "So how was your date with Spiros?" he asked her.

"It was fine. No big deal. We just hung out."

"What did you wear?"

"Jeans. A sweater. Boots. Why?"

William shrugged. "It makes a difference. Do you like him?"

"I don't know. It's too early to tell," she said, dodging.

William looked at her for a long inscrutable moment before leaving to check on other patients.

At the eleven o'clock shift change, Grace, an older nurse, tried to transition her patient to another nurse. The younger nurse refused because she was overwhelmed. Grace explained the situation to Sam.

"Are you kidding me? Everyone's overwhelmed!" Sam said. Sam had been overwhelmed plenty of times since her first day, but she kept her head down, focused on her sickest patients, and never once refused to take another. Sam took Grace's patient without reservation. Grace had been working at least eight hours longer than Sam, and had every right to hand off her patients and go home. If Sam didn't take the patient, he would be assigned to the inexperienced nurse with Mr. Rhodes, the sickest patient in the ER. Sam's patient total was now at ten, the most of any nurse. "We have to work as a team," Sam said. "On bad nights like this, teamwork is even more important than usual."

Sam believed that nursing schools should instill the value of teamwork, but that hadn't been her experience. The phrase "nurses eat their young" was, to Sam, "the understatement of the century." While some of her nursing instructors had been friendly and helpful, many of her clinical instructors were not.

Early on in her schooling, when Sam hadn't emptied a patient's Foley, an instructor yelled at her about it in front of the other students and nurses. "You're screwing up! How could you not empty the Foley bag? That's gross!" the nurse yelled at Sam, her tone nastier than her words.

"Well, no, I didn't empty the Foley. I didn't know I was supposed to. We're only a month into clinicals," Sam had managed to say before dissolving into tears.

That instructor made other students cry and once screamed at a pregnant student so loudly that the woman left class early with chest pains. Sam stuck with the program. Other aspiring nurses did not.

MOLLY   November

SOUTH GENERAL HOSPITAL

Molly was assigned to a patient who had developed a 104-degree postoperative fever after a minor surgical procedure. Molly introduced herself, then started an IV to deliver fluids and medicines. An hour later, when she checked on the patient, the woman was feeling better. In a tired, crackly voice, she said, "Thank you, Molly."

Molly couldn't believe it. In ten years, no patient had taken the time to thank her by name. That small gesture made Molly feel important, "not in the world, but to that patient," she said.

As Molly continued to work at South General, it happened again. But, for Molly, while the patients were preferable to Pines', the nurses were not. The racial divide was pronounced: The white nurses worked together and the black nurses worked together. Except for Lara, whom the black nurses seemed to accept, South General nurses rarely crossed that line.

As much as Molly liked South General, her commute was ninety minutes each way, which meant her workday totaled fifteen hours. Knowing that South General was not the ideal hospital she sought, she decided to drop the hospital from her agency rotation and pick up more shifts at Citycenter and Academy.

CITYCENTER MEDICAL

One afternoon, a foreign-born woman came into the ER with abdominal pains and breast tenderness. Women of childbearing age with abdominal complaints automatically got a pregnancy test. Some of the women had no idea they could be pregnant. Others came to the ER because they would rather Medicaid pay hundreds of dollars for a hospital visit than spend $10 themselves for a home pregnancy test. Molly took the urine sample to the lab room and placed four drops onto a pregnancy test kit.

After Molly's second post-IUI pregnancy test had been negative, she had kept her chin up. But when a third IUI was again unsuccessful, she started to get discouraged. Her follicles weren't responding well to the fertility medication. The IUIs, lab tests, and drugs already had whittled most of her insurance coverage. If Molly's next IUI was unsuccessful, her doctor had told her they would have to move on to IVF, an even more expensive process that she would have to pay for entirely out of pocket.

Molly had never been the sort of person to "What if?" but even she wasn't immune to these creeping doubts. What if the next IUI didn't work? What if her money ran out? And, worse, what if she couldn't get pregnant at all?

When Molly returned to the patient's room, she asked the woman if she could discuss the test in front of her husband. The woman nodded.

"The results were positive. Y'all are pregnant," Molly said.

The couple immediately burst into joyful tears and hugged, ecstatic. "We have been trying for a while," the woman said through misty eyes. "I have lost a baby in the past."

Molly wiped her eyes and, smiling, left the room. She couldn't decide whether her tears were "sweet tears, happy tears, or jealous tears." Whichever they were, Molly couldn't remember ever feeling that way before.

ACADEMY HOSPITAL

In late November, Molly wore Thanksgiving scrubs for an Academy shift. "Oh, would you look at that," Molly overheard the baby nurses titter, hyperaware that she didn't bother to follow their trends. Molly didn't mind the comments; the young nurses probably considered her cheerful animal-printed scrubs the equivalent of, in her words, "the grandma sweater with the embroidered flowers." The Academy girls wouldn't be caught dead in printed scrubs. But patients often commented on Molly's with a smile.

Nurse divisions were particularly stark at Academy. Academy nurses had a "look," a uniform within the uniform. Most of the nurses were new grads who wore designer scrubs (such as Urbane), North Face zip-up tops, and $120 Dansko nurse clogs. Molly wore her old running shoes for comfort.

The divisions went beyond the clothes, though. The major clique consisted of what Molly called "the cute little trendy girls" who had graduated from Academy's prestigious nursing school. The Academy graduates were talented, prepared nurses who would not leave any coworker in the lurch professionally. But socially, they distanced themselves from nonalumni.

One of Molly's favorite nurses was Claire, who had spent two years as a medical/surgical nurse before coming to the ER. Claire was friendly, helpful, and overweight. She had told Molly quietly that clique members weren't nice to her and made her feel inferior, even though she was more experienced. Two months later, Claire quit. "It makes me sad," Molly said. "She was big, and being a cute nurse at Academy really equals being part of the 'in crowd.' For some nurses, being included like that makes them happier workers and better able to focus on their job, so when they're blatantly left out, their days are much more difficult. The profession has that reputation of older nurses eating their young, but I feel like the younger nurses were eating their fat."

At Pines, Molly did not believe that Juliette's size was the reason the clique excluded her. Juliette was the type of person whom you had to get to know in order to love, and some people didn't look past their first impression. Juliette could say something completely benign, but her tone of voice could make it sound negative, and her blunt mannerisms could seem abrasive. Molly tried to persuade her to leave Pines and work for the agency instead; the agency would hire her back without question. She thought Juliette would be happier outside of Pines' strange social bubble.

Molly had befriended Juliette when they were both new nurses. She came to know her as funny, outgoing, loving, kind, and generous. Juliette had a handful of close friends for whom she would do anything, and she often let them know how much she cared for them. She was much softer than people realized. If Molly were to play armchair psychologist, she would guess that Juliette was the way she was because she had a difficult childhood with an alcoholic mother who chose booze over her daughter. Molly believed Juliette had constructed a tough exterior to protect her feelings but at the same time was desperate for approval. It was a combination that unintentionally could come across as simultaneously harsh and needy.

The traits that nettled Juliette's colleagues were some of the same characteristics that made her an excellent nurse. Juliette was fiercely loyal to her patients, standing up for them no matter the cost. Patients also appreciated that she was straightforward; she told them the real scoop and then did everything in her power to help make them better. It was a mistake to dismiss Juliette without giving her a chance.

Nurse on Nurse

Nurse-to-nurse bullying has been called "a silent epidemic," "professional terrorism," "insidious cannibalism," and "the dirty little secret of nursing." And it is crucial that the public learns about it—and hospitals eradicate it—because it affects patient care.

Workplace bullying can happen in any profession. It may come as more of a surprise from nurses, who are expected to be nurturing, empathetic, and caring. But the numbers are staggering. In the United States, a *Journal of Nursing Management* study found that 75 percent of nurses had been verbally abused by another nurse. It is so pervasive that even the American Nurses Association observed, in literature for its members, "Most of us could probably recount at least one story in which we as nurses encountered or witnessed workplace bullying."

Nurse bullying is a significant problem in many corners of the world, in countries as diverse as England, Japan, Portugal, Finland, Australia, New Zealand, Ireland, Taiwan, Poland, Canada, and, a country with particularly high rates, Turkey. Worldwide, experts have estimated that one in three nurses quits her job because of it, and that bullying—not wages—is the major cause of a global critical nursing shortage. "We are not 'angels in white,'" a Japanese nurse told me.

One of the most sobering statistics comes from Boston Medical Center's director of nursing education and research, Martha Griffin, who found that nurse bullying is responsible for 60 percent of new nurses leaving their first jobs within six months and 20 percent leaving the profession entirely within three years. "It is destroying new nurses," a Kansas nursing instructor told me. "I have five students who graduated less than a year ago who quit the nursing profession because of this behavior. It makes me very sad."

It is tempting to attribute nurses' hostility to their high-stakes work environment. But studies show that more nurses experience bullying from peers than do doctors or other healthcare staff. And nurses are verbally abused more frequently by each other than by patients, patients' families, and physicians.

As distressing as it is for a nurse to be bullied by a physician, disruptive-behavior expert Alan Rosenstein reported that nurses are more upset by nurse-on-nurse "backbiting and unnecessary scrutiny." As one nurse wrote him, "I expect that behavior from the surgeons, *not* the nurses, because I rely on them as my peers."

In 1986, nursing professor Judith Meissner coined the phrase "nurses eat their young" as a call to action for nurses to stop ripping apart inexperienced coworkers. Nearly thirty years later, the practice festers, and while younger nurses may more often be targeted, no nurse is immune. As a Washington State Post-Anesthesia Care Unit nurse said, "There is a culture of treating other nurses like dirt." The mystery is why this behavior continues.

Bullying among nurses goes by several names, including nurse-on-nurse hostility and lateral aggression. Rosenstein noted that nurse bullying is usually less direct than doctor bullying; it is more frequently behind-the-back "undermining, clique formation, and other types of passive-aggressive behaviors." Indeed, a *Research in Nursing & Health* survey found that the most common bullying methods are, as Juliette experienced, "being given an unmanageable workload (71 percent) and being ignored or excluded (58 percent)." Nurse bullies have admitted to other researchers that their most frequent weapon was "to stop talking when others entered the room."

According to Griffin, the five most frequent forms of lateral aggression among nurses, in order of frequency, are: "Nonverbal innuendo (raising of eyebrows, face-making), verbal affront (covert or overt, snide remarks, lack of openness, abrupt responses), undermining activities (turning away, not available), withholding information . . . , [and] sabotage (deliberately setting up a negative situation)."

Several other behaviors fall under the bullying umbrella, including when nurses gossip; ignore; condescend; belittle; humiliate; in-fight; unjustly criticize; fail to support a coworker because of dislike; give the silent treatment; make slurs or jokes about race, religion, appearance, demeanor, gender, or sexual orientation; or exclude a nurse from socializing. Bullying includes giving hints that a coworker should quit his or her job and excessively monitoring a peer's work. Pennsylvania State professor Cheryl Dellasega has written that other common relationally aggressive behaviors include "manipulating or intimidating another nurse into doing something . . ., teasing another nurse about lack of skill or knowledge, running a smear campaign, or otherwise trying to get others to turn against a nurse."

Verbal sexual harassment, unwanted touching, and physical intimidation also feature in the nurse bullying landscape, though less prominently. Canadian researcher Brian McKenna learned about incidents among nurses such as "sexual harassment with the promise of employment for compliance" and "colleagues 'setting up' a nurse to be exposed to sexually inappropriate behavior from patients."

The Workplace Bullying Institute reported that nurses regularly call its help line. Founder Gary Namie has said, "The same people tasked with saving lives of strangers turn on their own if they don't like someone's makeup or the car she drives." Nurses told me of coworkers they call "the Troll" or "Bitch on wheels."

Studies support Molly's observation that nurses "eat their fat;" Finnish researchers found that bullying victims have a higher body mass index than other nurses. But nurses of all shapes and ages shared stories about other nurses making fun of their clothes, gossiping, berating peers until they quit, and purposely withholding information to embarrass them in front of doctors and other nurses. A Virginia ER nurse said that when she was a new graduate, older nurses tried to humiliate her in front of the attending, took credit for her work, told physicians that she didn't know what she was doing, and changed her charting to sabotage her career. A Michigan nurse manager's director forced her to retire because she refused to bully staff like her predecessor did. Bullying behavior happens, the nurse said, "because when there is little support for nurses, they make themselves feel better by making someone else look worse."

"Structural bullying," or unfair or punitive actions by supervisors, is a major problem in the field. A New Zealand study found that more than one-third of nurse respondents believed they were neglected, had learning opportunities blocked, and were given responsibilities for which they were not equipped. Nurses report that charge nurses, nurse managers, and other supervisors can penalize nurses they don't like by giving them undesirable schedules or patient assignments, piling on the workload, or pressuring them not to use their vacation or sick days. A nurse told University of Massachusetts professor Shellie Simons, "During my first pregnancy, because the charge nurse did not like me, I was assigned the most infectious patients: HIV, tuberculosis, and hepatitis."

Some administrators use vague standard descriptors like "core values" to arbitrarily punish nurses. In the Northeast, a nurse was sent home without pay for wearing her hood up during the walk from the parking garage to the hospital, because the dress code for nurses on hospital property (even when they are not on the clock) prohibited hoods, jeans, and flip-flops. "Our hospital uses the term 'professional behavior and attire' to discipline at will, and all it takes is one complaint," said a nurse at that hospital. The hospital's managers demanded that nurses cover tattoos and piercings, "even though they were hired with them. They requested a nurse to alter her hair color because it was dyed an unnatural shade of red." The administrators did not enforce these dress code policies on physicians.

Misunderstanding among specialties
Prejudices and perceived tiers among nurse specialties and degrees contribute to the animosity. A *Hospital Access Management* article reported that "nurses create a kind of hierarchy within their own ranks in which trauma and cardiac critical care nurses, for example, consider themselves the 'cream of the crop.'" Some nurses joke that RN stands for "Real Nurse," which denigrates Licensed Practical Nurses. (LPNs have taken approximately one year's worth of courses; RNs have at least a two-year degree, a three-year diploma, or a four-year bachelor's degree.) Nurses told me about rivalries among specialties, between hospital and rehabilitation nurses, and between hospital nurses and nurses at doctors' offices. A cardiovascular ICU nurse said that because her specialty is often considered the top in the field, when she floats to other units, they give her the worst assignments. A nurse practitioner said that she and her colleagues call ER nurses "trauma jockeys" because they enjoy "blood and gore" and "gossip about the people who come through and the gore they see."

Several nurses said that other units mistakenly believe their specialty is easy. "They think we don't work very hard and that we're not as tough as med/surg or ER nurses," a Maryland postpartum nurse said. In nursing school, one of her clinical instructors, a medical/surgical nurse, told the class that if she were in postpartum, "I would get so bored. I like working hard."

A school nurse in Louisiana told me, "People think I put Band-Aids on all day, but it's not that simple." School nursing is far more complex than the stereotype implies. "I think the public generally believes that school nurses want to take it easy and just do some first aid," said Carolyn Duff, president of the National Association of School Nurses, which estimates that there are approximately 70,000 school nurses in the United States. "What's really true is that nurses who work in schools are highly skilled and highly educated generalists who are responsible for both the children and the adults in their building."

In fact, school nurses may have a larger potential patient load than other nurses. School nursing requires the technical skills to treat chronic disease conditions, as well as the intellectual skills necessary for disaster planning, Duff said. "For students who may not see the school nurse often, planning occurs for them whether their parents know it or not. Take something as simple as immunization compliance: School nurses are accountable for making sure their populations are immunized according to state regulations. They know which students are not immunized and make sure when there are outbreaks, those students are excluded from school for their own protection. They have a constant awareness of each student's particular needs."

A South Carolina trauma nurse confessed that she looks down on floor nurses and nursing home nurses. "I will absolutely admit that I am biased. To me, everything less than critical care is somehow below nursing. I work at the highest level of my degree and scope of practice. Why should someone operating at the bottom also be called a nurse? It's like that sad-but-true joke: 'What do you call the person who graduates from medical school at the bottom of their class?' 'Doctor,'" she said. "Sometimes I almost wish that my RN came with a gold star next to it, because I crave some extra recognition for how hard I work. I am an RN, BSN, CEN, and almost a SANE [Registered Nurse, Bachelor's of Science in Nursing, Certified Emergency Nurse, Sexual Assault Nurse Examiner]. Yet to the doctors and the patients I'm 'just a nurse.'"

Part of the problem may be a lack of understanding among the specialties. For example, when I interviewed floor nurses across the country, I raised Molly's complaint that floor nurses made excuses to avoid taking new patients at shift change. They told me that the reason they prefer not to take new patients then is because the chaotic timing could jeopardize patient safety. When ERs transfer a new patient at shift's end, some floor nurses call it a "dump and run." An Indiana psychiatric nurse said, "We don't like taking patients at shift change because that's the time when everything and everyone are the most disorganized, so the patient won't get the attention he or she deserves. It's not fair to the patient and it's stressful for the staff."

For approximately half an hour, the outgoing floor nurse is so busy giving report that she cannot give a new patient the necessary one-to-one time, which can involve a more complete medical assessment, settling in the patient and family, activating orders, writing admissions paperwork, starting labs, collecting specimens, documenting, setting up the room, making sure the patient is stable, etc. "We don't just take vitals and tuck them in," said an Arizona pediatric oncology nurse. The floor nurse needs to be with the new patients so she can pick up on a potentially life-threatening situation. As a Washington, DC, acute care nurse practitioner said, "It's not safe to leave a patient who was just sitting in the ER alone in a room for that long while I'm speaking with someone else."

Prejudice against minorities

Lateral aggression may be directed toward nurses who look, sound, or act different from the majority of the staff. Researchers have found that nurses have been targets because of their accents or ethnicity, because they are a float or per diem nurse, or because they received a promotion or honor that coworkers think is undeserved.

Gender falls into this category as well. Male nurses said that while their gender helps them with patients and administrators, it puts them at a disadvantage among fellow nurses. A study of Minnesota OR nurses found that male doctors treat male nurses better than female nurses and that they have better camaraderie. "I think I have better relationships with physicians than many female nurses because they know me better. And I stick out. You're not going to remember every interaction you have with a tiny twenty-three-year-old blonde girl named Laura, because there are a dozen of those on my unit. You're going to remember interacting with the random scruffy-faced dude who successfully helped a mother breastfeed for the first time," said an East Coast nurse who is the only murse in a building of hundreds. "This also means that my mistakes are held against me longer and harder. But overall, I think my opinions are trusted more, and I'm viewed as more authoritative, even when I'm not. For the record, I don't think it's fair. I've been given opportunities that much more deserving nurses have been passed over for."

In nursing school, the same murse said that his conspicuousness led instructors to have higher expectations of him than his female classmates. "My successes were highlighted in front of everyone, as were my failures. It's like when the instructors were looking for an example, they picked the person who stood out the most, because I'm a guy," he said. Now, at work among his colleagues, other nurses are more likely to "think I have a stick up my ass when I question anything," and socially, "I usually end up feeling like the little brother, big brother, or comic relief, not part of the actual clan."

The workplace "can be challenging" socially for male nurses, a New York City murse admitted. "I'm not really involved in my colleagues' social functions outside work. Baby showers, wine tastings, bachelorette parties . . . Sounds fun, and while I do consider many coworkers my friends, a lone married man in his early thirties with a bunch of young women at these events would just be awkward." Even when nurses like him don't rely on their coworkers for socializing, nursing is such a team-oriented profession that bonding outside of the hospital can easily affect the working relationships within it.

Cliques

It would be shortsighted to dismiss Juliette's complaints about her coworkers' social exclusivity as trivial or irrelevant. Much of any work-place bullying comes from cliques, which both galvanize and hide the perpetrators. In material about workplace bullying, the American Nurses Association specifically stated, "Misuse of power can also occur when a nurse who, acting as charge nurse, shows favoritism toward friends or those in a personal clique while treating others poorly by assigning them more difficult assignments or by not offering to help. This misuse of power is done without regard for the nurse and the patient, and it exposes the vulnerability of both." It is this sort of treatment that distressed Juliette.

Nurses spend long hours together and are dependent on coworkers both professionally and personally. Many studies have found that nurses have higher job satisfaction when they have positive relationships with colleagues. Of course, benign work relationships can form that leave some nurses feeling devalued or left out. A Louisiana pediatric nurse explained, "Some places have set weekends, so when you work full-time you always work with the same crew. Sometimes if you get switched or request the opposite weekend, it's like you're not a part of the team because you never worked with them, so they don't help you like they help the others."

More trouble comes when a nurse's standing devolves from not quite fitting in to being alienated. A Michigan ICU nurse was tormented by a nurse practitioner who tried to rally other coworkers to "take her down." The nurses tried to sabotage the ICU nurse, refusing to answer her questions and to teach her the electronic health record system. The nurse left the hospital because of this treatment.

A 21-year-old Southern ER nurse described a clique of supervisors as "something straight out of *Mean Girls*. They make each other stronger, like female bullies in high school." Without the pack, these nurses seem socially needy and insecure, but "when they're together, they go around wreaking havoc. While you're running around frantically trying to take care of five patients, they're sitting at the desk reading *People*, and looking at you, laughing, 'Looks like you're having fun over there.'"

Mean girls. Humiliation. Sabotage. Why is there such a strong bullying culture in a profession known for its empathy and compassion, and a profession in which even bullying victims enthusiastically gush about how much they love their job?

Oppression causes in-fighting

In 1909, Dr. Leon Harris told *The New York Times* that nurses were "subjected to a despotic set of rules and regulations which in their stringency and utter lack of justice compare favorably with Siberian prison rules." The head nurses, whom Harris called "tyrants," regularly fired young, pretty nurses in favor of less attractive women, and "abuse their position of power. Like many of their sex, their inclination to be petty and mean and small in their dealings with other women comes out strong."

Harris went on to inform the *Times* that "the abominable outrages practiced on our young women at these institutions in the name of 'hospital discipline'" included hazing young nurses, disgracing them for trivial reasons, micromanaging their lives outside of the hospital, forcing them to work when they were sick, ordering them to do kitchen work or scrub floors if the head nurse didn't like them, and stripping nurses of the two hours of "off time" they were supposed to have during their twelve-hour shifts (a break that will have disappeared a century later). Certainly, nursing has changed since then, but Harris's description illuminates the roots from which nursing grew.

Many people insultingly believe, like Harris, that nurses catfight because it's women's nature to, and the vast majority of nurses are female. Australian researcher Elaine Duffy has observed that people dismiss bullying "with statements like, 'This is typical of bitchy females working together,' implying that such behaviors are typically female." That rationale is far too simplistic, but is related to a more plausible explanation.

In 1970, Brazilian philosopher Paulo Freire theorized that when a dominant group forces its own values and norms upon a less influential group, the oppressed group develops low self-esteem and becomes angry and aggressive as it tries to internalize those standards. As group members are made to feel inferior, they begin to disdain their own culture. Because the oppressed group won't engage in violence against the more powerful dominators, its members turn on each other, dividing and infighting, sabotaging each other. Freire called this conduct "oppressed group behavior."

Some nurse scholars contend that nurses are an oppressed population because of a history of submissiveness to mostly male physicians and administrators. In the early 1900s, doctors controlled nursing school curricula, steering programs to instruct nurses primarily on how to support physicians. Without autonomy or control over their occupation and treated by medical professionals as subordinates, nurses took on the characteristics of an oppressed group. As the Center for American Nurses reported, "The culture of the healthcare setting has been historically populated by images of the nurse as a 'handmaiden' in a patriarchal environment. The balance of power has not been in the nurse's favor. . . . Too often, nurses have acquiesced to a victim mentality that only facilitates a sense of powerlessness."

Browbeaten by doctors, administrators, patients, and patients' families, nurses also came to accept bullying as an inevitable part of the job. "Unfortunately, many nurses have been taught to simply 'grin and bear it,' and as a result of prolonged abuse, nurses have become an oppressed group with nowhere to channel anger but at other nurses," according to St. Joseph's University researchers.

Venting to doctors or administrators could jeopardize nurses' jobs, so they redirect their rage, frustration, or fear against each other, for which there are few repercussions. Interestingly, studies have found that when nurses are empowered at work, bullying occurs less frequently. This correlation supports the idea that when oppressed group members gain influence, they are less likely to lash out at each other.

Stress and burnout lead to bullying

When a healthcare organization does not empower employees—or when it restructures, downsizes, or keeps nurses short-staffed—nurse bullying increases. Studies have found that environments with volatile workloads, degenerating patient health, and increasingly confrontational patients and visitors create "a perfect storm for workplace bullying."

This could tell us that when nurses are overly stressed and under excessive pressure, they become hostile toward the people they most frequently encounter during the workday: other nurses. Indeed, experts say that nurses who are burned out at work "are more likely to vent their frustration by abusing other nurses." What other outlet do they have? In departments where nurses are rarely afforded the time to eat or go to the bathroom, they certainly wouldn't be able to go for a walk or step outside to compose themselves. Stuck in their unit for hours on end, they can be so physically and emotionally worn out that they have little left for themselves, let alone each other. Nurses who are too drained or busy to take the time for self-care are more likely to engage in lateral aggression.

This theory could help to explain why bullying is so rampant among healthcare professionals. Not many workplaces are as tense and simultaneously as emotionally and spiritually draining as a hospital. It is evident how the cycle might perpetuate: Multiple studies have found that bullied nurses have much higher levels of burnout than their peers. If these victims, now burnt out, need an outlet themselves, they might be more likely to engage in the same bullying behavior.

Does hazing make nurses stronger?

There may be a reason why nurse bullying commonly targets young, inexperienced, or newly transitioned nurses. It's arguable that there is a difference between the kinds of workplace bullying that are universal across professions and the type that qualifies as nurses "eating their young."

Nurses told me that colleagues want a new nurse to prove herself before they accept her as part of the team. "There is a sort of test new nurses need to pass to become part of the nursing clique," said a California nurse practitioner. Because of the nature of the job, nurses hold one another accountable to strict standards. "Due to the broad base of knowledge we must have, and many of us being 'Type AAA' perfectionist personalities, we have very high expectations of our peers," a Missouri public health nurse said.

As a result, some nurses are short on patience and stingy about sharing knowledge, in order to toughen up new nurses. "Eating their young" refers to "the fact that a new nurse has to earn the right to work in the unit. No one gets any slack for being new," said a Pennsylvania OR nurse. "You have to jump right in and be able to care for the most difficult patients as if you've been doing it a hundred years. Even when I moved to a new facility and had been doing the same job previously, there was this feeling of being tested to see if I would measure up and fit in."

This philosophy leads some nurses to assign new nurses the most difficult or highest number of patients without assisting them, or to give them a hard time when they don't know what to do. "Nurses put their own on steep learning curves to test their mettle. It's sick and often counterproductive," said a Virginia labor-and-delivery nurse. "Older or very insecure nurses often push the younger ones by giving them too many tasks to complete and not enough support."

But making someone feel worse about her skills is not the same as making her a better nurse. And sometimes the "testing" goes too far. As I interviewed nurses for this book, many stories sounded similar to those of the college girls I interviewed for *Pledged*, a book investigating sororities. Like sorority sisters, nurses told me about overbearing cliques, governance by administrators more focused on money and image than on people and substance, arbitrary standards regarding their looks, and, most relevant to this section, a long tradition of hazing and questionable rites of passage.

Nurses eating their young is a form of hazing, different from other types of workplace bullying both within and outside of the nurse profession. It is as if nurses, like sorority members, have to endure a pledge period during which they must prove themselves worthy of a group that has already admitted them. A Texas nursing school professor referred to nurses eating their young as "sorority initiation." Nurses in other states told me about rituals such as an OR's tradition of initiating new nurses (most often the young, pretty ones) into the department by dunking them into the scrub sink with the water running.

Even American Nurses Association (ANA) literature called nurse bullying "a type of initiation to determine if the new nurse is tough enough to survive in nursing." (The ANA added, "But the problem extends beyond the new nurse to include nurses at all levels as potential victims.") A Florida psychiatric nurse told me, "Older nurses being harsh to newer nurses is almost like a ritual. I think sometimes it's done subconsciously. We can be harsh to new nurses to make them strong for the many challenges they will face in this profession."

When a North Carolina nurse started out in the ER, she said the old guard "punished" her for being young and attractive. If every other nurse had zero patients and she had four, her colleagues would assign her a fifth. "The existing nurses had been there for eons and felt they owned the place. They treated new staff however they pleased. I cried on the drive home every day for my first six months," she said. "I was in the Marine Corps before this, I survived boot camp. [I thought] surely I could take all of the mean, snarky, underhanded hazing. But I wasn't at that hospital longer than a year because of it."

An Idaho murse said he was hazed a few years ago partly because he was a new graduate, but mostly because he is male. "I was treated like an idiot for the first several months. They made snide remarks or didn't value my opinion. Also, as a man, I was expected to act differently in crisis. Starting as a new nurse was terrifying. When someone is actively dying in front of you or having a psychotic episode, it takes some getting used to, regardless of gender," he said. "When I was giving report, it was as if I were being interrogated by the Gestapo. I'd be asked questions I didn't know and treated like an idiot for not knowing the answers. I had to earn every ounce of respect that I got. 'Eating their young' comes from the need to weed out nurses who don't belong, but there must be a better way to go about it. My experience was awful."

Researchers have described how experienced nurses use lateral aggression to keep younger nurses and students in their place. By making the less experienced nurses doubt their ability, they create a perceived hierarchy tiered by seniority. This is not unlike sororities grinding pledges down to rebuild them in the preferred mold. "Here, a select group of senior nurses take any opportunity to tear a nurse down. Entering an ICU, I thought I'd have a great preceptor to teach me everything I'd ever need to know. But I really felt like I was set up for failure," said a cardiovascular nurse who was hazed repeatedly. "New nurses are inevitably going to make mistakes, but senior nurses feed off it and make it worse. I understand that you need to know your stuff, but those nurses are there to teach you."

When an inexperienced coworker was assigned to a case that was out of her depth and she was afraid she couldn't properly serve the patient's needs, she asked her preceptor and the charge nurse for help. "They left her to drown," the cardiovascular nurse said. "She broke down in tears in the middle of morning doctor rounds. Unfortunately, I think this will continue, because when new nurses bring this up as bullying or harassment, it gets pushed aside or sounds like tattling."

Significant numbers of Greek alumni believe their college sorority is more cohesive because they suffered through hazing together; and that because they participated in the hazing tradition, so should every group that follows. Similarly, Boston Medical Center's Martha Griffin has observed, "Tolerance for some forms of nursing practice lateral violence is seen historically in the context of a rite of passage or expressed in the thought 'this is how people were to me, when I was learning.'"

Australian researchers report that nurse bullies "are usually themselves past or current victims and most are convinced that their experiences have strengthened them for their nursing role." Under the guise of teaching younger nurses to be strong, these nurses appear not only to prefer to see new colleagues fail than succeed, but also to help them along in the process of failing. "Why do we tear each other down so much?" a Texas ER nurse wondered. "[They act like] they earned their stripes the hard way, the 'old fashioned way,' so they don't want to make it any easier for the new nurse learning the ropes. It's like the parent saying, 'When I was your age, I got beaten with a log, so you should be thankful when I do it to you.' Right, it was terrible the things you had to go through to get to where you are now. Shouldn't you then want to make it easier for someone else, so they don't have to experience that kind of heartache?"

Much like sorority members, the nurses I interviewed were split on whether nurse hazing is ultimately beneficial or detrimental to the profession. At first, Emma, a Mid-Atlantic surgical nurse, was furious when an older nurse hazed her at the Pyxis by "making me feel stupid, when my main goal was to get my patients their medications as efficiently as possible. [I felt] this sort of hazing was totally unnecessary and counterproductive," Emma said.

Now that she has been on the job for a few years, however, Emma finds herself defending the practice. "Older nurses feel a need to set a high standard and not baby new nurses. Sometimes this comes off as very harsh and unnecessary, but in retrospect, I really appreciate being challenged to be diligent early on, even if it meant being called out on my failings in front of others. This sort of corrective hazing that a few older nurses are known for might not be the most delicate way to help someone see their errors, but it certainly is effective. I was fortunate that the nurses on our unit generally don't 'eat their young' just for the sake of it, but rather to guide and provide the opportunity for new nurses to prove themselves."

In recent years, as workplace bullying generally has become an increasing part of the national dialogue, some nurses worry that supervisors are abandoning a no-nonsense teaching style because new graduates might consider it bullying. "We've coddled these new young nurses. There is way too much hand-holding," said a Virginia Neonatal Intensive Care Unit (NICU) nurse. "If a new nurse screws up or doesn't have her stuff together, she needs to know. We have to hold ourselves and each other accountable for our patients' care. Nurses should eat their young to get rid of the weak. If you can't deal with an older nurse correcting you and watching out for your practice, how are you going to handle resuscitating a dead patient solo, or dealing with an alcoholic sex offender who is making disgusting comments to you?"

Even some younger nurses are willing to let the practice continue if it prepares new graduates by whipping them into shape, like a nursing boot camp. "Nurses take an immense amount of pride in what they know, what they've seen, what they've experienced. And unless you know what they know, seen what they've seen, or experienced what they have (and you won't, especially when you're a new grad and new to a unit), you don't know jack until you prove yourself otherwise. So suck it up, earn your place," said a New York pediatric ICU nurse who graduated two years ago.

A nurse in Lebanon argued that bullying among nurses is "good because it is part of the learning process. It helps you sharpen your communication skills. We learn how to face our bully, act with knowledge, and continue doing what we do best for the sake of the patients." Similarly, the New Zealand study found that a small number of nurse bullying victims viewed the situation positively because it enabled them to stand up for themselves and to "feel stronger." A Washington, DC, pediatric oncology nurse remembered when older nurses drilled her relentlessly about various patients and diseases. "One nurse was so intimidating that I was crying as I tried to give report to the next nurse. But you do certainly learn things quickly that way."

Another similarity to sorority hazing: Nurses eating their young continues because nurses often don't report it. Researchers say that nurses tend to keep quiet because they are afraid of retaliation, they don't think reporting the behavior will penalize the bully or result in change, or the perpetrator is a manager. Like patient assault, lateral aggression has become so ingrained in the culture of the profession that many nurses don't report the behavior because they—both victims and perpetrators—don't realize that it is unacceptable. In one study, when nurses confronted their aggressors, three-quarters were "shocked that the victims felt that way."

Some older nurses said that they don't mean to treat new nurses harshly; their language or tone can reflect the tension of an urgent moment. An Arizona pediatric oncology research nurse tries to give students as many appropriate nursing tasks as possible. One day, however, this nurse's young patient was declining and she needed help from seasoned nurses, residents, and respiratory therapists. As the nurse was attempting to contact the child's parents, a student approached her to ask, "What should I do?" The nurse recalled, "It seems like an innocent enough question, but I had fifteen people I was listening to and giving information to. The last thing I needed was some clingy, high-strung student asking what she should do. I said, 'Stand in the corner. Watch, and don't say a word!' I knew the minute it came out of my mouth that I had just eaten my young. I simply was not nice. But if a student doesn't have the wherewithal to know she's in the midst of a tremendous learning situation just by observing, I certainly don't have the time to explain it to her at that moment."

In Washington State, a day surgery nurse explained that although she enjoys precepting on occasion, "It all depends on where my head is on any given day. I'm very Type A and if I'm in a 'gotta get it done' mode, then mentoring can drive me nuts, because obviously a new employee (especially new grads) takes lots of time getting stuff done that I know I could be doing so much faster. And sometimes I feel I must jump in and do part of the job. That is not good mentoring," she said.

Because so many departments are short-staffed and turnover is frequent, some inexperienced nurses are automatically expected to take on massive responsibility and pressured to work on critical patients whether or not they are ready. A nurse in Singapore said that nurses eat their young because they expect new nurses "to be as skillful as if you were already thirty years into the job. And if you are not up to their standards, you may be given a tongue-lashing, taken off the learning curve, or banished indefinitely to the Siberia of nursing chores to clear bedpans and clean backsides," a repercussion reminiscent of the 1909 *New York Times* article.

When these new nurses get overwhelmed, complain that they have too many assignments, or don't have the experience to handle their tasks properly, older nurses can get frustrated; they might have little sympathy because they are or were in the same boat. "We work hard, come to work on time, prepared, focused, and ready to jump into the trenches," said a twenty-year veteran of a Midwestern NICU. "We have had years of terrible hours, schedules, and holidays—obviously tons of shitty, unfair assignments—and we just did it, trusting that the seasoned nurses had a plan with the assignment choices."

At the same time, if inexperienced nurses are too casual, older nurses might think they don't take their work seriously. The generational divide is severe. In the United States, the average nurse is 47, and many nurses are delaying retirement through their late sixties, according to a 2014 *Health Affairs* study. "The younger nurses have good skills and, with our guidance, demonstrate excellent skills over time. The issue is that they lack respect and can be rude and arrogant. You lose patience with nurses who can't wait their turn, won't shut up and listen, can't stay off their phones, argue with policy, or show their butt-cracks. They whine about their assignments, take chances when asking for help would be safer, take long lunches, interrupt, and bad-mouth other nurses within earshot. They come to work rushed and on the phone, eating, and often not in scrubs; ignore parents of sick children while they are charting; and often surf the Internet," the Midwestern nurse said. "There is a pecking order and a prejudice against the younger nurses because they are hard to work with. When my generation of nurses started, we were so intimidated as new nurses that we came in early, took notes, and focused on the task at hand. We have years of experience and skills that can't be matched."

While "kids-these-days" gripes are predictable and inescapable in any profession, they are louder in nursing because the workforce skews older. Widening the generational divide, nursing degree programs have changed since older nurses began working. Until the late 1970s, nurses attended school in the hospital setting, where they learned both in classes and in the wards, explained Canadian nurse and author Donna Yates-Adelman. "Today, baccalaureate degree nurses graduate with very little hands-on clinical experience and are left to catch up after they graduate," she said.

"This has created a rift between the new graduates and the working nurses (many who are hospital-trained), who see it as having to help finish the new nurses' education."

Indeed, a Florida Atlantic University study revealed that the young nurses most affected by nurses eating their young "were those with university education; they felt they were resented for learning too much theory and not enough practical training." Canadian researchers found that "older, diploma-prepared nurses expressed resentment for new baccalaureate degree graduate nurses. These older nurses would relax at the desk and watch their new colleagues flounder. Young baccalaureate nurses . . . concealed their educational background to prevent ridicule and resistance."

The quandary leaves new nurses feeling stuck. To earn respect from their coworkers, they need the experience gained from what amounts to on-the-job training. But some coworkers aren't necessarily willing to give them that training because they don't respect the new nurses. When a Kansas nurse's colleague grumbled, "I hate nursing students," the nurse said, "I told her, 'This from someone who was once a nursing student.' How quickly we forget where we came from."

Younger nurses say they feel like they can't win: If they are too timid, coworkers push them to toughen them up; if they are too confident, coworkers try to take them down a notch. "In my ER, new nurses are lumped into the same boat: know-it-alls who know nothing who are trying to steal the thunder of the older nurses around them. Which is hysterical," said a Texas nurse who has been at her job for less than a year. "These experienced nurses have years of wisdom they could share to help a younger nurse. But when they do, it's to assert dominance. They hold it over your head: 'Remember that time I saved your ass?' And they use it and use it and use it against you."

No matter the cause, lateral aggression, like doctor–nurse bullying, is a problem that goes beyond hurt feelings. It can be just as psychologically damaging as physical abuse, and the effects can last for years. Nurse victims can suffer from symptoms of depression, anxiety, fear, shame, self-blame, guilt, post-traumatic stress disorder, and eroded self-esteem.

Furthermore, multiple studies have found that bullying can have substantial economic consequences for healthcare institutions. Researchers found that higher rates of workplace bullying are associated with higher rates of nurses quitting or intending to quit. This turnover can cost workplaces between $40,000 and $100,000 per nurse, and the sick days nurses take to cope with or avoid incidents can cost additional hundreds of thousands of dollars.

Nurse bullying also has been proven to increase medical errors and accidents and decrease productivity. Besides the distraction of dealing with the behavior and the effects of the emotional fallout, Griffin observed that "lateral violence stops newly licensed nurses from asking questions, seeking validation of known knowledge, and feeling like they fit in, and stops them from acquiring the tacit knowledge-build necessary in clinical practice." When nurses are afraid to ask questions, they are less likely to be able to provide safe care.

From sorority to sisterhood

Nurses are a sisterhood, a sisterhood that can be empowering, invigorating, edifying, spirit-raising, the stuff of the "secret club" about which a nurse rhapsodized in the introduction to this book. But this sisterhood (males included) could be so much stronger if nurses weren't divided by perceived hostilities, misdirected anger, and vast generational rifts.

Beginning in nursing school, nurses learn to be advocates for patients, but not necessarily to be advocates for each other. As new graduates during a time of vulnerability, some nurses are trampled by the same coworkers they need to support them through their transition to practice. Strong mentors can dramatically help both to change this atmosphere and to help new nurses thrive despite it. A New Jersey nurse practitioner who said it's her "goal to change the attitude of 'nurses eat their young'" advised mentors to "engage in teachable moments, put your ego away, learn something from the mentored, and take pride in the work you do. If you love your work, you will impart that passion to others."

That impression during a nurse's formative years can last for an entire career. Several nurses told me that they chose their specialty because of a particularly impassioned instructor or that they have returned to a cherished mentor for guidance repeatedly throughout their careers. More than a decade after working with her, an Arkansas CRNA is still in contact with a mentor who was "like a big sister to me. She taught me to be a patient advocate, to stand up to doctors, and voice my opinion if I felt like something would affect the patient negatively or if I had an idea that might benefit the patient. She also taught me to say no if asked to do something I wasn't comfortable with. She gave me a confidence in my professional abilities that has allowed me to achieve my ultimate career goal."

The mentor/mentored relationship can benefit both parties. A Washington State PACU nurse precepted two new graduate nurses who remained at her hospital and now work as her peers. "I love the feeling of supporting them and knowing that I provide a safe space for asking questions and sharing stories. And I got a couple of great friends out of it!" the nurse said.

Nurses representing all generations want to strengthen the sisterhood. "We may be fat, old, and wrinkled, but we pitch in and help each other even when it is not our patient. If the youngsters would just lay low and learn instead of being competitive, then they would flourish," said an Ohio NICU nurse. "When something cool is going on, I try and snatch a new nurse to share with her. We have had the occasional nurse who is excited about learning but also cautious. She is easy to tuck under your wing and share everything you know with her, [while] often learning from her newer views at the same time."

Young nurses said they want the same thing. Experienced nurses "are the foundation of hospital care, and their strength and giving nature inspires me to want to learn more and succeed as a nursing student," said a Massachusetts first-year student. "One nurse I work with has a great skill of being able to explain complex body functions in ways students are able to understand. After becoming a nurse, I hope I can be as influential to students as the nurses are to me."

When a nursing team is able to build an ideal sisterhood, the result is glorious. A Florida high-risk OB nurse said that the camaraderie among her nursing team is "unparalleled." At and outside of work, these nurses grew to know and to respect each other. "When we finish our individual nursing assignments, we check on one another to see that everyone has completed their nursing responsibilities and assist them if they haven't. Working holidays is part of the deal, so we plan dinners to celebrate at work since we can't celebrate with our families. Our job creates a place of comfort, happiness, support, and sisterly love. I know I could depend on these nurse sisters for anything I may need. It's just the way it is with nurses."

It is the way it could be.

CHAPTER 5

BURNT TO A CRISP:
How Nurses Cope—and Why Some Crack

"The nurse owes the same duties to self as to others, including the responsibility to preserve integrity and safety, to maintain competence, and to continue personal and professional growth."
 —CODE OF ETHICS FOR NURSES, PROVISION 5

"Compassion fatigue made it so much harder to take care of patients. Here I was, using all of my might to drag myself out of bed and march on, and I'm seeing these people whining over hangnails and really minor problems while I'm holding back tears and contemplating killing myself."
 —A NORTH CAROLINA ER NURSE

"I love the free entertainment that patients provide. People say and do the most ridiculous things, and I've got a front row seat to the absurdity."
 —A COLORADO TRAVEL NURSE

SAM   CITYCENTER MEDICAL, December

On weekend nights, Citycenter's ER regularly saw hordes of boisterous drunken patients brought in by police, EMS, or, occasionally, friends. Many times, the patients demanded to leave, but hospitals were supposed to keep intoxicated patients because they could be a harm to themselves or to others; and many of them were injured but too drunk to know it. The staff was allowed to discharge these patients when they were clinically sober—able to follow commands, walk with a steady gait, and tolerate oral fluids—even if they were not legally sober.

One chilly evening, EMS brought in a patient who was particularly riled up.

"I'm leaving this fucking place!" said the patient, a large man in his twenties.

"No, sir, you can't leave. You're drunk," Sam replied. She stepped to his bed and stood in his way, as nurses were supposed to, to prevent him from walking out.

"I'm not drunk!" He started to sit up.

"Yes, you are drunk. As soon as you sober up, we'll let you leave," Sam said.

"I *am* sober." He swung his legs over the side of the bed.

Sam, composed, stood her ground next to the bed. "Lay back, take a nap. We'll get you some juice if you want."

"I don't want any fucking juice!" the man yelled.

Sam looked him hard in the eyes. "I'm really sorry but you're not leaving. That's the way it's going to go. You can sit down or we can have security help you sit down."

The moment the man's feet touched the floor, William was at Sam's side. "Hey, buddy, you need to listen to what she's saying," William said.

The man eyed William's imposing build and got back in bed.

In the hall, Sam said, "I didn't need your help. I can take care of this myself."

William looked amused. "You needed a little backup."

Sam rolled her eyes and checked on her next patient. Police had arrested a man who told the officers that he needed medical treatment because he had "the shakes" from alcohol withdrawal. (If an arrestee told local police he needed his diabetes or hypertension medications, or even that he'd had abdominal pain for three weeks, the police would bring him in to the ER.) He obviously was looking for an excuse to decrease his time in a jail cell. Sam recognized the patient, a man in his midtwenties who'd come into the ER drunk the week before. As Sam entered the room, Dr. Bernadette Geiger, the compassionate attending with the high voice, joined her. A police officer was sitting in the visitor's chair, bored to be babysitting his perp.

The patient, slouched in the bed, sat up eagerly when he saw Dr. Geiger. "Oh, Doc! You remember me from the last time I was here. You know my problems; you know I need to be admitted. I'm having a really rough go of things."

"No, sir, I'm terribly sorry, I don't remember you," Dr. Geiger said as she conducted a quick exam. "I take care of so many patients every day. I'm sorry, but this is protocol. You seem fine to me." The patient would go straight back to jail.

When Sam and Dr. Geiger left the room, Sam said, "Dr. Geiger, we had him last week!"

Dr. Geiger winked. "Of course I remember him, but he's not going to play any games with me."

Sam grinned, happy to learn a new tactic.

• • •

On their second date, Dr. Spiros cooked dinner for Sam at his apartment. She was already flustered when she arrived late, after getting lost and then spending an embarrassing amount of time attempting to parallel park in front of his building. Inside, she looked around while Dimitri drained ravioli and poured glasses of wine. It still felt strange to call him Dimitri.

Dr. Spiros's apartment was decorated with matching earth-toned accents from the bathroom to the living room. Only the office was unadorned, with minimal furniture. Sam browsed photographs on the mantel to make conversation easier. They had seen each other at work only once since their last date; they had figured out tonight's logistics via text. *I should not be here*, she thought, scolding herself for being unable to gently say no to a second date. *When a guy cooks a girl dinner, he wants to get laid.*

They sat down at a table complete with cloth napkins. She had to give Dr. Spiros credit: He had made the pasta and sauce from scratch. She wasn't sure how to feel, though, when he started talking about his ex-wife. "She didn't like my hours as a resident, and now she's trying to get a hundred grand from me," he said. "I'm not even an attending yet and she's squeezing money out of me." His phone dinged and he looked down at it. "Speak of the devil. An email about the money she wants."

Sam looked down at her plate. *Ohh, this is awkward*, she thought. *Not cool to have the phone at the table, either.* Dimitri changed the topic by talking about his now-defunct relationship with the Citycenter tech. Was nothing private? Would he talk about Sam to coworkers, too?

After dinner, they chatted on the couch. There was a lot to like about Dr. Spiros. He was hot, although that wasn't a priority for Sam. He had plenty of interests outside of medicine, yet could understand, as she said, "what it meant to have an awful, crazy day at the hospital." But their conversations kept veering toward his plans to teach medicine in underdeveloped countries. He was barely a doctor and here he was, ready to share his supposedly vast experience with the world.

"Teaching is great and all, but I'm just trying to not kill people at this point," Sam joked.

Dr. Spiros seemed to be trying to impress her, expounding on his work in the ER and talking about expensive nights on the town. He described his trips to far-flung locales, but Sam had never traveled outside of the continental United States. Sam noticed that he was nestled into the opposite end of the couch. *Does he want me to jump his bones or something?* she wondered. He made no moves, so neither did she. She decided he must have asked her out as a rebound after his relationship with the tech ended. Perhaps he was talking so much about himself because they had little in common besides Citycenter, and she was still so new to the hospital that she didn't know their colleagues well enough to discuss them. She wondered if the great, suave Dr. Spiros was nervous.

After a while, she said it was late and she should go. Dr. Spiros gave her leftovers in a Tupperware container—a cordial, if grandmotherly, gesture. When they said good night, he went in for an awkward pat-on-the-back hug. "Okay, I'll see you later," he said, defeated.

On the drive home, she worried about how they were going to interact at work. The dates had been so awkward—were they even dates?—that she had no clue how to follow up on them. *I need to not date anymore*, she resolved. *I'm going to just put my head down and do my job. Dating can come later in life.*

During Sam's next shift, William caught up to her in the hallway and wrapped a strong arm around her shoulders. The top of her head barely reached his chest. "So? How's my competition?" he asked, cocking his head suggestively.

"I'm not sure. It might be over," she said. She described the end of the date.

"Oh yeah, you guys are done. Definitely," William said.

"Thank you. That's nice," Sam said, sarcastic.

"Well, hey, that means you and I can hang out!" he said, batting her ponytail.

Sam huffed. *What a flirt*. William flirted with everyone. "You have a girlfriend."

He started to say something, but Sam held up her hand and walked away.

The next time Dr. Spiros was on duty, Sam managed to avoid him by interacting only with a resident, which was unpleasant; the resident blatantly looked down on Sam and the other nurses. But Sam realized that although the resident was patronizing, she wasn't intimidated by doctors anymore. Her dates with Dimitri had changed her perspective by dissolving the mystique around physicians. "You go into nursing bright-eyed and bushy-tailed, thinking the doctors know everything. You only see them at work, so you assume they're like robots that go into sleep mode after work," she said. "Getting to know Dimitri taught me that doctors are human, too, and they can be just as weird as you are."

Sam vowed, "I'm just going to go up to them and say excuse me and say what I have to say. They won't bite."

MOLLY   December

ACADEMY HOSPITAL

During a brisk week in December, Molly took two consecutive day shifts: one at Academy followed by one at Citycenter. At Academy, which typically wasn't overwhelmingly busy even during the holiday season, she was surprised at the unusually high numbers of patients. Many of the patients in the Academy ER told her that they had already spent time at Citycenter that morning. After waiting in the Citycenter lobby for an average of three hours, when they finally received a room, nurses told them the doctor wouldn't be able to see them for several more hours. They had come to Academy instead. Molly was mystified. Citycenter wait times were typically long, but not so long that patients were driven to another hospital. She wondered what was going on.

A patient came in with a systolic blood pressure of fifty-eight. Awake and talking, the patient was in her forties and bedbound with multiple sclerosis. Molly focused on getting the patient stabilized and improving her blood pressure. She gave the patient four liters of IV fluid, which did nothing. She administered a blood volume expander. She tried two different medications to increase the blood pressure. None of this was working, yet the patient was still awake and answering questions appropriately. Molly noticed the patient's lactate—a blood lab that could indicate sepsis—was elevated and that she had a high white blood cell count. She did everything she could to raise the woman's systolic pressure.

Finally, the patient's systolic blood pressure reached seventy-one, the highest it had been since her arrival. Molly called the ICU, which sent a resident to write admission orders. "When she gets upstairs, I want her started on Dobutamine," the resident said.

Molly called the ICU nurse. "Make sure y'all have a Dobutamine drip to get started when she gets there."

"No problem," the nurse said.

As soon as a bed assignment was available, Molly began to prepare the patient for transport.

Suddenly, the patient's ICU doctor walked in, followed by a team of four residents lined up like ducklings. Molly inhaled sharply. It was Dr. Bitch. Dr. Baron whipped the curtain aside and strode into the room, followed by the four residents. She headed straight for the patient's monitor, barely glancing at the patient. "Wait. This patient is not stable enough to go to the ICU," she said.

"This is the best she's been in the six hours she's been here," Molly replied.

"She's too unstable for transport," the doctor insisted.

Molly looked at the patient, who was listening to the conversation. One of the first things Molly had learned in nursing school was to treat the patient, not the monitor. The only information Dr. Baron had was the monitor's blood pressure numbers. "Why don't you talk to her?"

The doctor did not. "We can manage this patient. She can't be transported like this."

Molly bit her tongue. The ICU was just two floors up, perhaps a five-minute walk. "The patient has been in this condition—awake, talking, and joking—for six hours," she said.

"I want her started on Dobutamine right now," the doctor announced.

"We don't carry it here, but the patient's ICU nurse is getting it ready and will have it available upstairs," Molly said.

"No. I want it now. Call the pharmacy and have them make it up."

Molly was astounded. "She can be in the ICU before the pharmacy would have a chance to make it."

"I don't want this patient transported now," Dr. Baron proclaimed, and stalked out of the room, leaving her residents behind.

It was 7:15 p.m., past the end of Molly's shift. Once Molly and the residents were in the hallway, out of the patient's earshot, Molly told them, "I do not care for your attending."

"No one does," one of the residents muttered.

Molly made eye contact with each of the four. "This patient has a room and will receive one-to-one care with an ICU nurse trained to manage a patient this sick. The ER is short-staffed tonight because two nurses called out. My priority is this patient, and being managed in the ER is not in this patient's best interest."

The residents stared at her blankly. "We cannot resolve this issue for you because she is our attending," one of them said in a crisp foreign accent.

"What she's doing is not in the patient's best interest. What this patient needs is available in the ICU right now."

"But she's our attending," said another resident.

"Y'all can't give your opinion to someone?" Molly asked, surprised that none of these doctors was advocating for the patient.

No response. Molly said good-bye to the patient and walked out of the room. On her way out, a tech stopped Molly to say, "Thank you so much for sticking up for yourself, because no one ever says a thing to these doctors."

CITYCENTER MEDICAL

The next day, when Molly arrived for her Citycenter shift, the ER was teeming with hospital brass asking staff members about the department. Another nurse filled her in. The Joint Commission had sent surveyors to the ER for a surprise inspection. They were so disgusted by the lack of cleanliness and the nurse-to-patient ratio that they nearly shut down the ER on the spot. When the inspectors swabbed EKG lead wires, they found several different strains of bacteria. They gave the hospital forty-five days to fix the ER or TJC would close it. Citycenter ER administrators were frantically trying to set the department straight.

The mood among the nurses had lifted instantly. Until now, Citycenter nurses had believed they were stuck with their lot—that because their supervisor was part of the problem, they had nobody to approach for help. Even the patient load seemed more bearable because of the hope that TJC's intervention would make the ER safer for patients and staff.

Molly's favorite news was the charge nurse's response to the inspection. Some charge nurses were given cue cards to follow so they could cover up some of the most blatant violations between the time inspectors registered at the front desk and reached the ER. Nurses were supposed to rush to move drinks from the nurses station, lock IV carts, relocate patient stretchers that blocked doors, secure oxygen tanks, clean rooms, and so on.

Citycenter's charge nurse that day was Renée, the longtime veteran. When TJC checked in with the administration, a hospital official rushed to Renée in desperation and said, "TJC is in the building and heading here. Get the staff together and do what you can."

To Molly's delight, Renée answered, "No. I want them to see what this place is really about."

LARA   SOUTH GENERAL HOSPITAL, December

A few weeks after Fatima's meeting with administrators, Lara finally told her Thursday night NA group about her coworker. The women said that it was important to get to know Fatima better before mentioning the drugs because she had to trust Lara to allow her to help. Lara didn't work night shifts, but she tried to make small talk the few times she passed by Fatima in the hall. "I don't know her well enough to be like, 'Hey, there's a big suspicion about you,'" Lara said to the group. "I still have to ease into being her friend." One woman suggested anonymously sticking an NA pamphlet in Fatima's mailbox, but Lara worried she'd get paranoid.

Nothing had come of Fatima's meeting, as far as Lara knew. Administrators couldn't fire a nurse without a concrete case. Lara had noticed that Fatima was arriving early and staying late, another tactic Lara had used. She often entered other nurses' patient rooms, clearly, Lara thought, looking to score leftover vials.

Working extra hours wasn't necessarily a red flag to someone who hadn't been in Lara's shoes. Some nurses worked 3:00 p.m. to 7:00 a.m., a full sixteen hours. Recently, Lara had spoken with a nurse who had worked twenty consecutive hours. "You can work twenty hours? That's safe? How is that even legal?" Lara had asked him.

"I don't know, but here I am. It happens all the time," he replied.

Lara continued to devote herself to her Relationship-Based Care committee work. December could be an especially tough month for nurses because they had to deal with their patients' anxiety on top of their own holiday stress. The committee was encouraging people to make a conscious effort to be nicer to each other, with posters in the staff bathroom and reminders during meetings. They turned "RBC" into a mild reminder for coworkers to calm down. Rather than telling a nurse she was acting like a jerk, staffers would joke, "Hey, check yourself, that's not very RBC of you." Since the formation of the committee, there had been no fights on Lara's shifts. The committee hoped the more empathetic atmosphere would improve employee relationships and the ambience for patients. As Lara said, "What if you brought your kid into the hospital and you saw nurses calling each other skanks?"

Lara also suggested that the department have huddles at every change of shift, so the day's entire team could touch base about who would be working where and whether they needed more assistance. Lara explained, "The huddle is about how we can work well as a team. If you're in triage and you do blood work for the nurse in the back, that's going to take a load off her. A lot of people weren't happy because some trauma nurses sit and do nothing when there aren't any traumas. That's one of the main things: If your area isn't very busy and you have the time, there's most likely someone who needs help, so what can you do to help them?"

Lara led the ER's first huddle. "Okay, team, today's going to be a good day," she said. "We have ten nurses working today. Rose is charge. Rachel's doing trauma. Peter is in triage . . ." She listed each staffer's assignments, including the cleaning crew she had invited to the huddle because they were part of the team, too. This way, everyone knew they were accountable for their area, and also the entire group knew where the weaker or new nurses were, and could help them accordingly.

"Anyone got anything going on today? Willa, how are your knees?" Lara asked a nurse in her sixties.

"They feel rough today, baby," Willa said.

"Okay, everyone, we gotta look out for Willa. If you see her pushing a stretcher, go help her. She should not be pushing a stretcher today," Lara said. "Guys, remember there's no 'I' in team. We're all in this together!" She punched a fist in the air, intentionally cheesy. The group laughed and scattered to their zones.

The nurse manager told Lara that the huddles were the most helpful and positive meetings the department had ever had. Hopefully, once the huddles became routine, administrators would join them.

Lara's next idea was to set up a specific room for post-trauma crisis intervention. The committee was still working on developing ways to help the staffers after something devastating happened, as with a recent case in which a 12-year-old died from a bullet wound. "People die on our shift, sometimes several people in one day, and then we just go back to work. Imagine if you just did CPR on a kid and it didn't work. Then you deal with coworkers who are being rough on each other, and patients are angry because they're waiting. And there's no downtime," Lara explained. "You can only hear a mother scream after coming to see her dead child once and you will be affected by it. That scream, I can't even begin to describe it. The secretary answering the phone, security, janitors, every-one—they're hearing this incredible anguish and are expected to be unaffected by it."

At the start of a committee meeting, Lara presented her idea. "I was thinking we should have a debriefing room, a place where we can gather our thoughts after something awful happens. Everyone from the nurses who worked on the patient to the janitor who mopped the blood off the floor could take five minutes to think, talk, or pray." Lara thought this strategy could ease the tensions that were typically high for hours after a tragedy.

"That's a great idea," said a tech. "We need a place to go and sit for a minute."

"Which room should we use?" Lara asked.

"We could use part of the lunchroom," said a unit secretary.

"Then we'd be focusing on eating instead of catching our breath," a floor nurse said.

"Why don't we use this room right here?" asked another nurse. "It's only used for meetings sometimes anyway."

The group became animated as they came up with low-cost ways to make the room more serene. "We could put in one of those little waterfall-on-the-rocks things!"

"And a white noise machine with peaceful sounds."

"I have the perfect picture I can bring in to put on the wall."

"I could bring in some lavender, that's a therapeutic smell."

"Ooh, I have a cool plant I can donate."

Lara was so excited that once the committee settled on colors for the room, she volunteered to purchase the paint out of her own pocket.

• • •

Two weeks before Christmas, Lara went to her mother's house one last time to finish clearing it out before it went on the market. She posted on Twitter that she was having a sad day. In the middle of the night, Lara opened her laptop and scrolled through dozens of replies about her mother and the house, which had been the neighborhood hangout. The uplifting messages made her smile.

Then she read the next post on her Twitter feed: John had tweeted to a woman with a half-naked photo, one of those porn star models that hundreds of men posted to daily, "Alabama, you're so hot. I want to put this picture on my truck."

Lara knew that John had cheated on her in the past, she knew about his gambling addiction, she knew about his sex addiction. But to post something like this where all of their friends and family members could see it, right after Lara's tweet about mourning her last day at her childhood home? No. Lara was done. People had told her that the last straw before a divorce often was relatively insignificant compared to past transgressions. She understood that now.

Lara turned on the light in the bedroom. "Hey, John, when you tweet to another female, like your friend Alabama, everybody sees it," she said. "So now everyone we know is looking at your conversation with the porn star."

John jumped out of bed, looking panicked. He ran to his computer and started deleting tweets. Lara took a deep breath and whispered a quick, quiet prayer: "Please give me the strength to do this."

"John, I cannot do this anymore," she said, her voice steady. "I'm going to move out. You have health insurance. Get help for this sexual addiction. You need to make an appointment."

"Stop playing this bullshit game," he said.

Lara had thought for sure that he would beg her to stay, but he didn't. "I'm not going to your family's holiday party tomorrow," she said.

He didn't believe her. The next morning, he loaded the car while Lara finished feeding the kids breakfast. "Just get your suitcase and come on," he said.

"I'm not going," she said.

"Get your goddamn suitcase. You know you're going to go."

"No, I'm not," she said.

He looked momentarily surprised, then began to usher the kids out the door. Lara kissed her children good-bye and told them that she had to go to work. As soon as the door shut behind them, Lara burst into tears. She was proud of herself for finally standing up to him, but wondered, still, whether she was giving up too soon.

Why Nurses Crack

After twenty years of working as a cardiac nurse in Washington State, Elena Uhls became so stressed that she sank into a major depression. The combination of the unit director increasing her patient load to twelve at a time, the nurse manager asking her to perform tech duties on top of her own, and patients and techs treating her disrespectfully had broken her spirit to the point where she grew suicidal. "I was crisp," she said, using nurse slang for "burnt out." "I felt worthless. I made errors, forgot things." She considered switching careers, but she couldn't imagine herself in any other job. "I was so paralyzed. I knew it was possible that I'd accidentally kill somebody if I didn't take time off. Every day as I drove home, I slowly plotted my death. Depression is painful; suicide felt like the only way out."

Once she found a helpful doctor and took antidepressants, Uhls recovered her basic mental health, but she isn't the same nurse she used to be. A traveler, she floats among hospitals, avoiding the workplace where "every day was a nightmare." She said, "I know in my heart I'm not that loving nurse I once was. If I can make a difference, I try, but what can I do in a few hours? I [used to] try to be their coach, their cheerleader, their educator, whatever it took, but not now. I still care, but not with the same light heart. It's more businesslike. Maybe it's better that way."

We rely on nurses to be our healers, our heroes, to comfort us, to soothe our hurts and salve our psyches. But how often do we pause to wonder who takes care of the nurses?

Nationwide, nurses' top health and safety concern is the effects of stress and overwork, according to the ANA Nursing World Health and Safety Survey. More nurses are worried about this issue now than in 2001, when the average shift length was shorter and patient loads were lighter. Their second biggest concern is that they will suffer a disabling musculoskeletal injury because of their constant heavy lifting; throughout an eight-hour shift, a nurse lifts an average of approximately 1.8 tons.

Injuries are a major stressor for nurses, who must lift and move patients in addition to working on their feet most of the day. The number of nurses reporting work injuries has increased in the last decade. The ANA found that "Nearly all nurses still indicate that they have worked despite experiencing musculoskeletal pain, including eight in ten who say it is a frequent occurrence." Other common nurse injuries include needle sticks, strains, sprains, bruises, cuts, head injuries, broken bones, or dislocated joints. A Virginia women's health nurse added, "Many nurses have bladder issues by age fifty. 'We don't pee so you *can*!' How's that for a women's health nurse motto?"

A number of nurses interviewed for this book reported feeling over-worked, overwhelmed, and underappreciated for several reasons. For twelve to fourteen hours at a time, they must demonstrate physical and emotional stamina, alert intelligence, and mental composure, even if they are berated by patients or bullied by doctors and other coworkers. Many healthcare employers don't engage nurses in decision making, although nurses are at the forefront of patient care. Nurses are under pressure to work quickly and correctly, taking sometimes contradictory orders from professionals who will blame them if something goes wrong. They are stressed because, an Oregon nurse manager said, they are responsible "not only for the patient but also the family, the team of support specialists, hospitalists, physical therapy, occupational therapy, social work, hospice if needed, meals, medications, teaching, spiritual support, keeping the patient clean and comfortable and documenting, documenting, documenting."

Nurses must constantly face traumas, tragedies, and patients who will die on their watch, no matter what they do. A New York City pediatric ICU nurse recalled, "The other day, one of my coworkers said, 'I'm taking care of a brain-dead baby today and I just can't take it.' When there's no hope left, that's when it gets really sad." Nurses are expected to care for the dying, to save the degenerating, and to minister to all manner of injury. And they are expected to do it without breaking their composure. "Some nurses are exposed to repeated horror on a regular basis, things that a regular Joe couldn't handle," said a Virginia NICU nurse. "The worst thing you could ever imagine seeing, we see at work. My hospital doesn't have anything in place to help. If you can't deal with it, you leave."

While doctors and other hospital personnel are also exposed to death and suffering, nurses may be more susceptible to the lasting emotional impact. Nurses spend the most time with patients individually and have a hand in every level of their care. "Nurses are not only 'first responders,' but are also 'sustained responders,'" author and clinical nurse specialist Deborah Boyle has observed. "Nurses become part of a mosaic of caring within a family framework that may be fraught with anticipatory loss, tension, disbelief, and physical disfigurement. In the acute care setting they are responsible 24/7 for the patient's care and the family's response to the illness trajectory. Often, they cannot leave the situation after bad news is shared or a death has occurred. It is this extended time and the placement of the nurse at the center of the interchange that makes nursing's role unique."

Nurses can also become emotionally attached to their patients, some of whom die in front of them. "The patients become part of our family. It's a whirlwind relationship because you meet someone, and the next thing you know, you're looking at their naked body and listening to their innermost anxieties. In return, you listen, try to help, and share parts of your own life," said a Maryland hematology nurse. "If they die, it's very hard; you have lost someone you became close to very quickly, someone you were cheering to beat the odds. As a nurse, you can't dwell on your loss. You have other patients who need you. One might think that you would build a tough exterior that doesn't let the hurt in, but to truly be effective, you can't. You share your grief with work friends because people at home can't understand the connection that you share with patients."

For all of these reasons, nurses are the hospital employees most likely to develop work-related psychological disorders. Eighty-seven percent of surveyed nurses at one university hospital exhibited symptoms of anxiety, depression, PTSD, or what researchers call burnout syndrome. Nurses have relatively high rates of suicide, depression, and anxiety relating to job stress. University of Kentucky researchers found that 35 percent of surveyed nurses are mild to moderately depressed, compared to 12 percent of the general population and 12 percent of emergency medicine residents. Occupational reasons for this depression include not enough time to provide emotional support to patients or to complete their nursing tasks, too much time spent on non-nursing tasks like clerical work, and not enough staff for proper patient care, all of which could be alleviated if hospitals increased nurse staffing.

Nurses' schedules can leave them little time to recuperate from arduous patient care. They might stress about missing family birthdays, recitals, sports games, and holidays. They are not necessarily paid commensurate to their sacrifices. Nurses told me about sleepless nights during which they were so worried about patients that they called the unit to check on them, and days off that they spent doing something for a patient instead of for their family. And it is difficult to explain the letdowns of the job to people who aren't nurses. "People don't know how hard it is to compartmentalize your life when you have a bad day at work, like when a patient dies or declines, and then you have to come home and act like nothing is wrong," a Maryland OR nurse said. "Your husband and children have a difficult time understanding and it's impossible to explain. They don't teach that in nurses' training."

Workplace stressors are affecting nurses' mental health across the world. In Quebec, where the local nursing union has asked the government to end sixteen-hour shifts because understaffed nurses are "overworked and exhausted," five nurses killed themselves in an eighteen-month span. At least one of them left a suicide note in which she blamed her hospital's working conditions. When the woman's sister-in-law contacted the hospital, she was allegedly told, "She's not the first to commit suicide and she won't be the last."

In 2013, the U.K.'s Royal College of Nursing announced that 82 percent of nurses go to work while sick because they worry that understaffing would harm patient care. Reporting that stressed nurses are "forced to choose between the health of patients and their own," the RCN revealed that staff shortages and increased workloads caused more than half of surveyed nurses to become ill. In a separate report, South African nurses conveyed similar issues, in addition to poor security, lack of government support, and unhygienic hospitals.

Burnout, compassion fatigue, and PTSD

Experts estimate that approximately 30 percent of nurses are burnt out, which has been defined as a "loss of caring." Burnout symptoms include irritability, difficulty concentrating, low energy, and sustained thoughts of quitting. Many nurses also experience a related but lesser known condition that is often confused with burnout. "Compassion fatigue," also called secondary traumatic stress disorder, can occur when empathetic nurses unconsciously absorb their patients' traumatic stress. They experience the traumas emotionally, sometimes mirroring the patients' anxiety. As they pour their energy and compassion into caring for their patients, many of whom do not improve, they fail to care properly for themselves and/or their own families. The resulting sense of helplessness has been called "a combination of physical, emotional, and spiritual depletion" and "a state of psychic exhaustion."

This can happen to nurses who treat children the same age as their own or to nurses who have nothing in common with their patients. A St. Louis oncology nurse quoted Holocaust survivor and psychiatrist Viktor Frankl to States News Service in 2012: "'What is to give light must endure burning.' I think people who care for others understand. Caregiving is painful."

The ANA lists compassion fatigue symptoms including anxiety, depression, disrupted sleep, memory problems, fatigue, headaches, upset stomach, chest pain, and poor concentration. Nurses suffering from compassion fatigue might be less able to feel empathy toward patients or their families and more likely to abuse drugs or alcohol; they might avoid or dread working with certain patients.

Distinguishing characteristics of burnout versus compassion fatigue vary by the expert, but there seems to be a general consensus that burnout is caused by stress related to the job (understaffing, lack of support) while compassion fatigue is caused by stress related to the patients (connections with patients or families, caring for the suffering or dying). Burnout can lead to emotional exhaustion, but compassion fatigue causes heavy-heartedness. Michigan nurse and staff educator Shari Simpson explained at an Association of Pediatric Hematology/Oncology Nurses annual conference, "Compassion fatigue does not mean one is no longer capable of feeling compassion. It's the feeling of compassion weigh[ing] so heavily on you that the way you experience life is affected."

Both conditions, author Deborah Boyle wrote, "are associated with a sense of depletion within the nurse, a 'running on empty' feeling." And nurses can experience burnout and compassion fatigue at the same time. A trauma nurse in North Carolina was hit by this double whammy. "Doctors are demanding, patients are demanding, management is demanding. If the doctor orders a wrong medication, and the nurse gives it to the patient, whose fault is it? It's your fault for giving it. If a drunk patient gets out of bed and falls, it's your fault for not being there to stop him, but the doctor won't give you an order for restraints. Everything in hospital healthcare comes down to the nurse. Every second of every shift, you are giving, doing, running, caring—it's draining," she said.

For this nurse, the combination of compassion fatigue and burnout contributed to a depression that bordered on suicidal. "I have had days where I would have rather crashed my car than go into work. I was getting sucked dry. The neediness of everyone! It's like a never-ending rendition of 'If you give a mouse a cookie' and as nurses we don't like to fail. It's not allowed," she said. "As a nurse I am completely in tune with my patients, their needs, and the needs of their family. I really can lose track of myself. If it comes down to helping a patient to the bathroom or being able to empty my own bladder after eight hours, it's going to be the patient every time. It's not totally healthy. But I can't imagine doing anything else."

On a particularly bad day, she arrived at a preshift meeting in which supervisors scolded the nurses. "What I heard was, 'Customer service is really lacking in the Emergency Department. It doesn't matter what's going on in your personal life. We don't care. It is always all about the patients,'" she remembered. "And this whole time, I had been thinking of killing myself. In my head, I kept putting a gun in my mouth and pulling the trigger; it was like I was watching a movie over and over again." Eventually, the nurse confided in a psychiatric resident and her husband, who helped her to pull through. Today she is a stable, healthy nurse who continues to love her work.

Employees in any helping profession can be afflicted with compassion fatigue, including social workers, counselors, chaplains, and humane workers. But nurses are particularly vulnerable, Boyle wrote, because "they often enter the lives of others at very critical junctures and become partners, rather than observers, in patients' healthcare journeys. Acute care nurses in particular often develop empathic engagement with patients and families. This, coupled with their experience of cumulative grief, positions them at the epicenter of an environment often characterized by sadness and loss." Simpson calculated that if an inpatient nurse sees an average of even just four patients during a twelve-hour shift, in twenty years she will care for more than 11,000 patients and families. A clinic nurse who sees ten patients per shift will care for nearly 43,000 patients. Those numbers require an extraordinary amount of compassion.

It is possible that the nurses who care the most might bear the highest risk. Researchers report that some types of personalities are more susceptible to stress and compassion fatigue, such as people who are overly conscientious, perfectionistic, and self-giving. And nurses are already highly empathizing people. "We are programmed to be able to do it all; we give our life and soul to the profession," said a Florida psychiatric nurse. "Sometimes, if you feel you can't help an individual, you feel you have failed."

Compassion fatigue may have increased in recent years because of the demands of managed care. Because doctors and nurses have more time pressures to see more patients and complete more paperwork, they have less time to enjoy, for example, "the connection that many family physicians shared with their patients, [which] was replenishing, which helped them cope with the stressors of practicing medicine," Indiana University School of Medicine researchers observed.

Nurses are also vulnerable to post-traumatic stress syndrome (PTSD), a psychiatric disorder experienced by 8 to 10 percent of the general public. University of Colorado researchers found that 22 percent of surveyed nurses exhibited PTSD symptoms. All of them had observed a traumatic event such as a patient death, massive bleeding, open surgical wounds, or trauma-related injuries, or they had performed futile care on critically or terminally ill patients. Other events that could lead to PTSD include helping with end-of-life care; handling postmortem care; dealing with combative patients; taking verbal abuse from patients, family members, doctors, or other staff members; performing CPR; experiencing stress because of unsafe nurse-patient ratios; and failing to save specific patients.

ICU nurses are subjected to many of these events on a daily basis. An Emory University study discovered that ICU nurses experience PTSD at a rate similar to female Vietnam veterans. Among ICU nurses, 24 to 29 percent exhibited PTSD symptoms, compared to 14 percent of general nurses. (Outpatient nurses are less likely to develop PTSD than inpatient nurses.)

A PACU nurse in Washington State said she suffered from PTSD for several months after caring for a coding post–heart attack critical care patient who died on her shift. The hospital offered no resources to help her cope. "There was nothing available to me. I still cry thinking about the situation and how I was supposed to give 150 percent to this patient who was basically already dead," she said. This trauma came on top of the usual nurse stresses. "Often, I feel it's an impossible job. [Some of us] go home feeling we were unable to give the care we wanted because we were so overworked by patient numbers, acuity, and needing to be everything to everyone: nurse, friend, coworker, empathetic listener, computer specialist."

Second victim syndrome

In 2010, Kimberly Hiatt, a veteran pediatric critical care nurse at Seattle Children's Hospital, accidentally gave an eight-month-old critically ill infant 1.4 grams of calcium chloride instead of the correct 140-milligram dose. The infant died days after the mistake. Hiatt was fired, even though it was not clear that the miscalculation directly caused the death of the infant, who had heart problems. A ten-fold overdose of calcium chloride, which is given to support circulation and prevent heart and neurological problems from low blood calcium, would not necessarily be fatal.

Hiatt, who told staff about her error as soon as she realized it, officially reported it herself. "I messed up," she wrote on the hospital's electronic feedback system. "I've been giving CaCl for years. I was talking to someone while drawing it up. Miscalculated in my head the correct mls according to the mg/ml. First med error in 25 yrs. of working here. I am simply sick about it. Will be more careful in the future."

Hiatt reportedly was stunned that the hospital fired her for making one significant medical mistake in her entire career. Administrators had given her glowing reviews; two weeks before the incident, her evaluation awarded her a 4 out of 5 and called her a "leading performer."

To keep her nursing license, the state nursing board required Hiatt to pay a fine and agree to a four-year probationary period during which she would be supervised when dispensing medication. But Hiatt had difficulty finding a new job, even though she aced an advanced cardiac life support certification exam, qualifying her for a flight nurse position. Seven months after her mistake, depressed and isolated, Hiatt, at age 50, committed suicide.

Hiatt apparently suffered from "second victim syndrome." According to the Institute for Safe Medication Practices, "Second victims suffer a medical emergency equivalent to post-traumatic stress disorder. The instant patient harm occurs, the involved practitioner also becomes a patient of the organization [because he/she needs medical help]—a patient who will often be neglected." A 2011 survey found that surgeons who thought they made a medical error were more than three times as likely to have considered suicide as those who did not.

Humans are going to make mistakes. Washington University researchers found that 92 percent of doctors surveyed had perpetrated a near miss or actual mistake and 57 percent confessed to a serious error. Retired anesthesiologist F. Norman Hamilton wrote in a *Seattle Times* letter to the editor following Hiatt's death, "If we fire every person in medicine who makes an error, we will soon have no providers. We all make errors. It is only by the grace of God that most of them do not result in great harm or death."

While second victims usually require immediate emotional support, healthcare organizations largely don't help employees through "the deeply personal, social, spiritual, and professional crisis," the ISMP reported. "Although the first victims of medical errors are the patients who are harmed and their families, the second victims are the caregivers and staff who sustain complex psychological harm when they have been involved in errors that harm patients while caring for them. . . . But, too often, we remain silent and abandon the second victims of errors—our wounded healers—in their time of greatest need."

That's what Seattle Children's administrators did to Hiatt. Instead of easing her out of second victim syndrome, they arguably threw her under the bus, appearing to blame her for the fatality. Paradoxically, then-hospital CEO Tom Hansen wrote an internal memo in which he said, "Of course, we will also support our staff members during this difficult time." Hansen went on to write, "It is important to me that all staff and faculty feel it is safe to report when mistakes are made, and that everyone is confident that we recognize the difference between an honest mistake and reckless behavior."

In direct contradiction, Seattle Children's fired the staff member who seemed to need a great deal of support, damaging the career of a nurse who apparently thought it was safe to report that she made an honest mistake. After Hiatt's case hit the news, a Washington State Nurses Association survey found that half of nurse respondents believed "their mistakes are held against them." Even more worrisome, a third said they would hesitate to report an error or patient safety concern because they were "afraid of retaliation or being disciplined" and more than a quarter would hesitate to report those concerns because they were afraid they would lose their job.

Following the incident, the hospital changed policies, including instating a rule that only pharmacists and anesthesiologists could prepare doses of calcium chloride in nonemergencies. Also of note: In 2003 and 2009, Seattle Children's staff allegedly had made two other fatal medication errors. After the 2009 death, Seattle Children's medical director Dr. David Fisher said in a statement, "This was not the fault of any one individual." It appears the hospital's problem was much larger than the single nurse it pushed forward as the scapegoat when her error occurred in 2010.

Instead of firing a nurse who reportedly had made a single notable error in a quarter-century of service, the hospital could have tapped her to help devise a system that would have caught her error in time, thereby both improving the hospital and allowing Hiatt to contribute to her own healing process. Firing her helped no one. As University of Missouri Health Care patient safety director Susan Scott told msnbc.com, "If my mom got an insulin overdose from a nurse in a hospital, I would want that nurse to give her that insulin tomorrow." That nurse would probably be the least likely to make that mistake again.

What hospitals aren't doing

Hospitals aren't adequately addressing nurses' work-related health issues, but are they legally liable for causing them? In 2013, Ohio nurse Beth Jasper, a 38-year-old mother of two, died in a car accident while driving home from a twelve-hour shift. Her widower filed a wrongful death lawsuit against Jewish Hospital, claiming that administrators knew that Jasper was "worked to death." Jim Jasper alleged that the understaffed hospital regularly forced nurses to take extra shifts and go without breaks. The case was dismissed because the judge determined that the hospital could not be responsible for a death that occurred after work hours.

Certainly, hospitals aren't doing enough to prevent these problems. In Massachusetts, when a newborn died minutes after an emergency caesarean section, a veteran nurse told *The Boston Globe* that she "came very close to losing it psychologically" because of grief, but hospital administrators did not want her to see an independent psychologist in case he could be called to testify in a malpractice lawsuit. (The *Globe* article gave no indication that the death was attributable to human error.) "The hospital is more worried about lawsuits than they are about the effects the incident has on the staff," the nurse told the *Globe*. How can nurses best address the health of their patients when they are expected to shove their own health issues under the rug?

Lara's debriefing room idea is an effective low-cost solution. As a hospice nurse told me, at times nurses need to go somewhere to "have a little cry." Other small concessions that hospitals could provide are opportunities for nurses to eat, take a break or a short walk, and check in with loved ones outside of work. Nurses also could use easy access to support groups and trained counselors. Some nurses said that even when their hospitals hold debriefing sessions, administrators refuse to offer coverage for nurses who want to attend. They neglect staff members who truly might need these sessions to understand, reflect on, and share feelings about what they have seen.

So many of these problems could be solved by hiring more nurses, which would reduce patient load and nurse mistakes, give nurses more time to do their jobs well, decrease stress, and provide coverage. An analysis by health economists found that, by a conservative estimate, hospitals can recoup more than 99 percent of an average nurse's salary (70 percent of salary plus benefits) from reduced medical costs and improved productivity alone. It should be stated that staffing for hospitals is not a zero-sum game: "Registered nurses are a revenue center rather than a cost center," said ANA senior policy fellow Peter McMenamin. A strong nursing staff can generate revenue for hospitals not only in improved productivity but also in retaining top physicians.

In the time it takes for hospitals to make this happen, however, nurses themselves could do a better job of focusing on self-care. Nurses sacrifice their own health to attend to ours. They are so accustomed to working nonstop to take care of other people that they often forget to nurture themselves. It isn't uncommon for nurses to donate blood or bone marrow to specific patients. "People will just about kill themselves to give care to others without taking care of themselves," Canadian health services officer Norma Wood has said. "It can get into a martyr situation where patients matter more than we do." Researchers recommend that nurses take self-care measures, including changing work assignments or shifts, taking time off or reducing overtime hours, getting involved in a project of interest, and focusing on work-life balance.

It can also be helpful for nurses to talk about their feelings. "I believe most nurses don't seek counseling or support outside of friends and families. We need to do a better job of permitting ourselves to seek support," a longtime Michigan nursing school professor said.

Some hospitals do have programs, counselors, chaplains, on-call coping liaisons, or debriefing sessions. Barnes-Jewish Hospital in St. Louis recently launched a successful program to help staff cope with these issues. The hospital offers a compassion fatigue course, stress-reduction workshops, support groups, meditation, and discussions about difficult cases. Three-quarters of the staff members who have taken the formal class have been nurses, said Patricia Potter, director of research for patient-care services at Barnes-Jewish. Particularly in the medical ICU, where the head nurse has championed the program, nurses have seen a noticeable difference in their relationships with each other and their ability to communicate effectively as a team. Program graduates "tell me that they are recognizing more when they feel stress, and that the skills we've taught them have been very helpful to reduce the perception of that stress," Potter said.

Many nurses have shared that, with experience, they have learned to view patients medically rather than emotionally, and to separate their work experiences from the rest of their lives. They learn how they react to various situations and they develop coping mechanisms to prepare themselves accordingly. University of Akron professors found that registered nurses younger than 30 are more likely to burn out, experience "significantly higher rates of the most intense levels of frustration, anger, and irritation" than older nurses, and are less likely to find ways to cope with these emotions. As a result, the researchers suggested that experienced nurses could serve as emotional mentors to younger nurses to help them navigate the profession's demands.

A young Maryland medical/surgical nurse said that a nursing school mentor was instrumental in preparing her for the emotional side of nursing. "She let me know it's all right to let things affect you and that doesn't make you any less of a nurse. She taught me how to handle bad days. She was very open with me about her own experiences starting out and how they shaped her, which I draw on a lot now," the nurse said. "Mostly, she demonstrated how to stay calm in intense and emotionally charged situations, and let me know that nursing is not always as ideal as people make it out to be and everyone feels that at some point or another."

Why it's worth investing in nurses' mental health

"The greatest common risk to patients is the understaffing of nurses," Minnesota ER doctor Gary Brandeland, who has written about medical mistakes, told *The New York Times*. "A nurse may make a critical mistake, and a patient might die. She has to live with the error, but the real culprit, the root cause often is that she or he was understaffed and overworked and a mistake was made. The hospital doesn't pay for it on a personal level. They just get a new nurse."

In times of budget cuts and healthcare changes, hospitals may be reluctant to alleviate understaffing and/or to provide resources to help nurses deal with burnout, compassion fatigue, PTSD, second victim syndrome, and other assaults on their mental health. But administrators must openly acknowledge that their nurses' health is worth the investment. Burnout and compassion fatigue have been linked to decreased productivity, more sick days, and increased turnover among nurses, which are correlated with higher patient mortality rates, lower patient satisfaction, and compromised patient care. Nurses suffering from these issues are more prone to make mistakes. The ISMP has reported that fatigue alone can cause reduced accuracy, inability to deal with the unexpected, slower recall, and reduced hand-eye coordination, all of which could greatly impact patient care.

Researchers have also found that nurse burnout is linked to hospital-acquired infections, which kill approximately 100,000 patients a year. The researchers theorized that burnt-out nurses might be less vigilant about washing hands (and reminding visitors and other clinicians to do so) and other infection control procedures. They calculated that in hospitals that reduced nurse burnout by 30 percent, the number of urinary and surgical site infections dropped by 6,239, which saved $68 million a year. Washing hands matters: When the Michigan Health and Hospital Association implemented a checklist to remind staff to clean their hands and keep the field sterile, within three months the median rate of infection in central line catheters had fallen to zero.

It would also behoove administrators to decrease staff turnover, and not only because hospitals must expend resources to train and hire new employees. Inadequate nursing staffing has been called a national emergency. When nurses resign from a hospital, they create a cycle in which the remaining nurses are left short-staffed and more stressed. A Drexel University study found that when nurse turnover rates increase, so do the odds of nurse injury and patients' risk for pulmonary embolism/deep vein thrombosis.

Meanwhile, it is up to nurses to bolster each other, and to appreciate when hospitals get the system right. Nurses at a midwestern NICU rely on a particularly effective chaplain and each other's strong support. After a tragedy, the team discusses the case to talk about the plan of care and what could have been done differently. They often follow up with parents whose children died in the hospital.

"One of the worst parts of coping with traumas and tragedies is when the family is present," said a pediatric ICU nurse in New York. Parents might watch CPR breaking their child's ribs, alarming bedside procedures, the monitor numbers dropping, or their children in an altered mental state. "Believe me, it's shocking what we do to these children; the brutality of a [cardiac] arrest can be very intense. We are trained to be the eye in the storm, to stay calm. But in the periphery of the storm, that's where some of the worst damage can be done; parents suffer PTSD, they have nightmares. So do we, though."

Recently, as the New York nurse gave compressions to a baby in cardiac arrest, the child's parents were on their knees sobbing and praying in the corner of the room. After the team had lost the pulse twice more, a doctor escorted the parents out of the room so they would not be present for emergency surgery. "The surgeon got there and the baby's chest was opened at the bedside so he could do manual heart massage and his fellow could rewire the pacer wires. The child ended up being fine. That is the miracle of medicine," the nurse said. "This baby left three weeks later in his parents' arms with a Superman cape tied around his little neck. No residual neurological damage, no cracked ribs. Nothing. That's what you have to remind yourself of the next time a kid codes and things don't go so well."

In the University of Akron study on burnout, 99.9 percent of the nurses surveyed nevertheless reported feeling happiness or pride during the previous week at work. "Sure, there can be an overall feeling of being burnt out at work, but things happen that give you that sense of

worth, pride, and happiness," a Kansas ER nurse told me. "I've been completely beaten down after three twelve-hour shifts in a row, then gotten
a compliment from a patient that turned my feelings around. Helping
a particularly sick patient can be physically and emotionally draining,
especially when you're feeling burned out, but if the patient opens their
eyes and gives you a smile, or you get a sincere hug from the wife, that can
make it all seem worthwhile."

This fortitude is part of what makes nurses so incredible, and is one of
many reasons that should convince administrators to consider nurses valuable contributors rather than replaceable employees. "I work where kids
die," an Arizona pediatric oncology nurse said. "What words can be used
to describe that? If I allowed myself to, I would cry every day. Instead, I
try to focus on the time that that sweet little life was a part of mine. I try
to keep things as fun as possible for the child. Kids who are dying know
they are dying. If I can elicit one little chuckle from them, then I've had a
really blessed day."

Nurses know to take solace and joy in the moments they are able
to comfort a patient. Among the tragedies, miracles shine—wondrous
flashes, whether flickers of hope or impossible resurrections—in which
nurses played a part. These triumphs add up, and experienced nurses
learn to clasp them close, to draw on them when they need a lift above
the darkness. Instead of dwelling on lives lost, nurses can hold fast to
remembrances of those they have rescued. Perhaps that's also how Seattle
Children's should have considered Kimberly Hiatt. As Georgia nurse
Brittney Wilson, who runs The Nerdy Nurse blog, said, "She made
a mistake . . . but how many lives over those twenty-seven years did
she save?"

JULIETTE   PINES MEMORIAL, January

The ER was still overcrowded. Pines already had closed to ambulances
twice the week before and turned the ER's minor care room into a
medical surgery unit. For this particular holiday season, out of twenty-
three rooms in the ER, eighteen were occupied by "boarders," patients

who had been admitted to a hospital floor that didn't have a bed ready. How could a hospital run an ER with only five rooms? As far as the nurses knew, eighteen boarders was a record.

Some nurses surmised that the patient overload was a result of some of Westnorth's new policies and agendas; understaffing led to less frequent bed turnover and longer ER waits. Others guessed that because of the recession, more people had lost their health insurance, causing them to come to the ER instead of a doctor's office. Sometimes, too, Juliette wondered if life spans were increasing. It seemed like fewer people were dying, and fewer patients had Do Not Resuscitate orders. "There are so many old people we shouldn't be doing all these interventions on to keep them alive. Just let them be," Juliette said.

Juliette had a 90-year-old patient who was nonresponsive, shaking, and exhibiting a sodium level of 171 milliequivalents per liter (normal range is 135 to 145), which indicated severe dehydration and/or kidney disease. Juliette readied herself for end-of-life comfort care.

Dr. Preston found Juliette at the nurses station. "Her daughter wants her treated," he said.

"But she has an active DNR," Juliette said.

Dr. Preston shrugged. "It's not worth the cost of what the lawsuit would be to go against the family."

Juliette's jaw clenched. This was absurd and she was comfortable enough with Dr. Preston to tell him so. "Clark, you're telling me, if I'm ninety and I have a DNR and I'm dying, but my daughter or husband says, 'I want you to do everything you can to save her,' that you would go ahead and try to save me?"

"Yes, we would. That's what Pines wants us to do," said the doctor as he scribbled orders for an IV, antibiotics, a catheter, and blood draws. "Pines wants us to go with the family's wishes if the person isn't awake or able to say anything."

Juliette had seen this before at Pines. If the family was present and wanted the hospital to override the DNR, the staff would first try to convince the family that the patient's wishes were clear. If the family insisted that the doctor keep the patient alive, he would usually do that.

"What is the purpose of having a DNR if we ignore it?" Juliette asked.

"Juliette," Dr. Preston said, patting her on the back as he left the room, "take off your cape."

This year, Juliette was scheduled as the charge nurse on Christmas Eve and New Year's Day. Because Molly wasn't flying home for the holidays, she had graciously volunteered to work eight hours of Juliette's twelve-hour Christmas shift so that Juliette could spend most of the day with her family.

On New Year's Day, when Juliette arrived for her shift as charge nurse, the waiting room was packed with drunks. This was the worst holiday to work because ERs were beset by hordes of intoxicated patients. There was a three-hour wait for patients to be seen. The trauma doctor was busy with the unusually high number of traumas that had come in overnight, including three teens whose car had crashed into a tree and a man whose wife had run over him on purpose. The charge nurse wasn't supposed to have any patients at all, but every other nurse had several boarders already. Juliette assigned herself eleven patients.

She was glad to see that Ruby was on duty. A fifteen-year Pines veteran with wild curly black hair, Ruby was a recently divorced nurse who was prone to making off-color comments. She rubbed some colleagues the wrong way, but she had always been friendly to Juliette. On the few occasions when they worked shifts together, Juliette was quick to assist Ruby when she needed it and Ruby would reciprocate. It was helpful for nurses to have a partner like that.

Juliette was also relieved that Dr. Lee was the day's trauma doctor. A small bespectacled Asian man, Dr. Lee was a favorite of the nurses. He was one of the rare Pines physicians who said "please" and "thank you" to them. He was patient, generous about sharing information with nurses, and receptive to nurses' input. And another rarity: He was quick to respond when a nurse paged him.

Juliette moved as many intoxicated patients as possible into the hallway to clear the rooms. Even Dr. Preston stopped Juliette to whisper, "What are we going to do? We have no room for any new patients."

"We just keep trying to move people out as best we can," Juliette said.

At 11:00 a.m., Carla, a young nurse and a new member of the clique, approached Juliette. "Room Two is angry from waiting and may just go."

"Fine, let her," Juliette said. She stopped by the room. The patient, who had driven her Audi into a stop sign and had minor lacerations, was pacing and hollering, "I have to get *out* of here. I have to *go*."

"You have to wait for the trauma doctor to give you discharge instructions," Carla said.

"I want my clothes."

"Your clothes were cut off of you at the scene because you crashed your car," Juliette said. "The paramedics came to help you and you were put on a backboard." The woman's blood alcohol level was two times the legal limit.

"I want my fucking clothes!" she yelled. "I want my belongings!"

It was standard procedure for staff to cut clothes off of trauma patients for quick and easy access, if paramedics hadn't already done so. "You wouldn't believe how many people get upset because their clothes are cut off when we're trying to save their life," Juliette later explained. "If we can save an item because you're awake and alert, we will, but if we can't, we can't. And the medics are prone to cutting things off right away."

Juliette moved on to another room, expecting the woman to leave as soon as her discharge instructions came through.

The medic phone rang. "Pines, can you take two Priority One traumas?" Priority 1 meant a patient would die without imminent intervention.

Juliette gestured to the secretary. "Call Dr. Lee and find out if we can take them."

"Stand by," Juliette told the medics.

The secretary hung up the phone. "If it's okay with you, he can do it, he says."

"We'll take them," Juliette said to the medics. "Can you give me report?"

Juliette assessed her staffing. Her single trauma nurse was already overwhelmed and Juliette would need another. She assigned both of her techs to the incoming Priority 1 patients. She asked Ruby, who was in the center of the ER, to give report to her on her four patients so that Ruby could leave them to assist the trauma nurse. From that zone, Juliette could handle Ruby's patients—mostly drunks—as well as her own and still observe enough of the ER to handle charge nurse duties.

Juliette moved a drunken dreadlocked man from Room 4 to the hallway, near a buxom 21-year-old who had vomited all over her low-cut minidress. When Dr. Preston walked by her, he shook his head to the nurses and murmured wistfully, "She was somebody's New Year's Eve dream date until she started puking on herself."

The Priority 1s were an elderly couple who had been hit by a car. When the medics wheeled the couple in, Juliette assigned herself the patients. She was able to get the woman into the OR right away to treat abdominal bleeding, and the man into the OR within two hours for head bleeding. Juliette was glad she had accepted the traumas because they both needed immediate treatment. She later found out that both people survived.

After the couple moved upstairs, Juliette made her rounds. She could hear the Audi driver in Room 2 cursing at Carla. "You fucking bitch, I told you I want to talk to the doctor!"

Carla, looking stressed, exited the room. "What do you want me to do?" she asked Juliette.

"Just get her out of here. Discharge her."

The woman was still yelling, between snippets of a conversation she was having on her room phone. Now she was refusing to leave. "I paid for this room!" the woman screeched. "I'm not leaving!"

Juliette picked up a hall phone and dialed 911. "I've got a verbally abusive, threatening patient I want out," she told Dispatch. She returned to the patient. "Ma'am, you're going to have to leave."

The phone still at her ear, the woman paced in her blue paper scrubs. "I don't have to leave, you fucking bitch."

"You've been discharged. You have your things," Juliette said.

"Whoever cut my clothes off is going to pay for them."

"Fine. But I have a sick patient I need to put in this bed. You can wait in the hallway."

"I'm not waiting in the hallway." The woman resumed her phone conversation. "Can you believe these people?"

Juliette stretched a new sheet over the bed, then reached over and unplugged the phone from the wall. "I've told you: You need. To leave. The room." She took the woman's purse from the stretcher and handed it to her so she could clean the stretcher.

"Don't you touch my shit!" the woman yelled. Juliette calmly headed to the room's hand-sanitizing dispenser.

At that moment, the police arrived and ushered the patient out of the room while Juliette explained the situation to the officers. Immediately, the woman's demeanor changed. In a saccharine voice, the woman said to Juliette, "I need some discharge instructions and you better have some backup for those things you're saying about me."

"Backup?" Juliette hooted. "I don't need backup. It's all written in your chart."

Dr. Lee approached the patient. "I'm sorry it took so long. You are discharged. There's nothing wrong," he told her.

"Well, I need something for my pain," she said.

Aha, Juliette thought. *A drug-seeker. That's why she demanded to leave, but then refused to. She just wanted a prescription.*

Dr. Lee wrote her a prescription for Tylenol-codeine #3. The woman looked at the paper. "I'm allergic to that," she said.

"Is it written in your chart?" Juliette said. She leafed through the chart. "Hmm, it doesn't say here that you're allergic to Tylenol number three."

The woman glanced nervously at the police officers. "Never mind, I'll just take it," she mumbled.

The story in the ER for the rest of the day was how Juliette had heroically unplugged the phone on the patient. Afterward, three nurses told her that she had been a wonderful charge nurse. "You made New Year's run smoother than usual, Juliette!" Ruby exclaimed. "It was so much less frantic. Great job!"

MOLLY   January

ACADEMY HOSPITAL

Molly's fertility doctor was offering her one last IUI cycle, her fifth. She would give herself shots for ten to twelve days, then have IUIs on two consecutive days. The protocol change meant that she had a clinic appointment on a morning she was scheduled to work at Academy. She hated to inconvenience Academy supervisors; Academy was the easiest money she made.

But the ER director assured her that the staff loved working with her and would try to accommodate her appointments. "You are an asset to our department," the director said, and assigned Molly a 3:00 p.m. to 3:00 a.m. shift. She told Molly how much the managers appreciated that she was a hard worker, self-sufficient, and always willing to help other nurses.

A 25-year-old named Jan, a petite Hispanic nurse who had graduated from Academy's nursing school, was one of the most grateful nurses at Academy. Like many of the baby nurses in the Academy clique, Jan would come to Molly with her questions rather than admit to the other baby nurses that there was something she didn't know. Molly was happy to help nurses who wanted to learn from her. "I like teaching," she explained. "I try to say stuff in a nice way so they don't feel stupid. So many times in nursing school I was made to feel stupid, and I don't want to do the same to other new nurses."

In the early evening, Molly happened to see Jan standing in the supply closet looking confused.

"Do you need something?" Molly asked.

"What do I need to do a chest tube? They're doing one STAT and I need to get back in there."

Molly had drained chest tubes, which were used for patients with a collapsed lung, more times than she could count. The chest tube was inserted through the ribs to help the lung reinflate. "Okay, we need the chest tray for the doctor," she said. Jan pulled the tray from a shelf. "We need the collection chamber for the blood or air coming out of the patient. We need some sutures. And then we need the sterile gowns and supplies for the doctor."

After Jan collected the items, Molly followed her to the patient's room, where a doctor was prepping the sterile field—cleaning the patient's chest and opening supplies on a table covered in sterile drapes. The patient, a college student, was crying. A collapsed lung was painful and made it difficult to breathe. Like many young, thin males his age, the student had coughed and suddenly had shortness of breath. A chest X-ray had revealed the problem.

"Open up the collection chamber. You need to add water into the funnel," Molly told Jan quietly so the patient wouldn't realize that his nurse wasn't experienced with the procedure. "The tubing needs to be attached to the suction. Good. Now we'll wait for the doctor to insert the tube and then we attach the chest tube to the suction."

After the successful procedure, Molly told Jan she had done well. Away from the patient, she told Jan a story. "Something to remember with chest tubes is if the doctor makes the hole too big in the chest, then air can escape into the rest of the body. Once I helped a doctor put a chest tube in a guy who was intubated. Well, every time the respiratory therapist squeezed the ambu bag, the patient's balls would inflate!"

Jan started laughing. Molly continued, "The chest tube had just gone in, so they're bagging him real fast and no one is noticing this but me. They started out normal testicle size but they were very large grapefruits by the time I figured out what was going on. The guy was naked and the air is tracking from around the chest tube hole through his lungs and into his groin. I had to say, 'You know, his balls are blowing up every time you bag him.' So they called in a cardiothoracic surgeon and had to suture the air leak shut."

"I'm glad you didn't tell me that beforehand," Jan laughed. "Thanks for your help. I totally understand chest tubes now."

Midshift, a 16-year-old girl was brought by ambulance to the ER from a school dance, where she had gotten drunk, thrown up, and passed out in the bathroom. When her father arrived, he screamed at her. Then the girl changed her story.

"Dad, I think when I was passed out, someone raped me," the girl sniffled.

Her father immediately redirected his anger. He demanded that the nurses call the police and start an investigation. Everyone in the room except her parents knew the girl was lying.

Teen patients commonly said anything they could think of to avoid dealing with their parents' reactions. Molly had treated dozens of teenaged girls who made up the same story, and not one of them had been sexually assaulted, creating what Molly referred to as "a 'girl who cried wolf' mentality." Most patients didn't realize that if police officers seriously considered somebody to be a sexual assault victim, they brought the patient to a hospital with a sexual assault nurse examiner (SANE) on staff, which Academy did not have at present. The patient wouldn't come through triage or sit in the waiting room; the staff would usher her straight back to a private room for the SANE's evaluation, a policy that Molly called "a very hush-hush process hidden in the ER." Therefore, ER nurses knew that if EMS or the police brought a patient through triage, they did not believe the individual had been sexually assaulted.

When the father went into the hallway to call the police himself, Molly turned to the girl. "If you really were raped, we will do everything we can to help you," she said. "If it's not true, we have a big problem: Someone will get arrested, go to jail, and possibly serve time just so you can get out of trouble for drinking. Now tell me, what's worse: being grounded for something you did or someone going to jail for something he didn't do?"

The girl looked down. When her parents came back into the room, she muttered, "Maybe that didn't happen. I don't remember."

On another occasion, the daughter of a local VIP got drunk at a school dance and passed out. A friend's parents brought her to the ER. When the girl's father arrived, he yelled so loudly that Molly closed the door to the patient's room for a while. Soon after Molly opened the door again, the girl had an epiphany.

"Daddy, Daddy! Jesus is talking to me!" she shouted. "He's showing me what I did wrong! Daddy! Kneel beside the bed with me and let's pray! Dear God! Thank you for giving us your son to take away our sins! Thank you for showing me what I did today was wrong!"

The father fell for it. He knelt next to the bed with his daughter. "Praise God! Praise Jesus!"

"Daddy! We need to go to church when we leave here and let everyone know that alcohol isn't the way. Jesus is the only way!"

Her father shook his head, feeling it. "Amen! Praise Jesus!"

"Daddy! I want to speak in front of the congregation and let them know that Jesus is good! Alcohol is not good! Daddy, this will never happen again!"

"Amen, baby. I love you."

And the yelling was done. The Academy ER had a sticker sheet of glittery Oscar statues that were reserved for patients who put on Oscar-worthy acts. The nurses would stick one on a patient's chart so that everyone who treated the patient knew what to expect. Some staffers didn't like Oscar because it gave the practitioners preconceived notions. But Molly thought it was funny and a stress reliever.

Molly had to give credit to this resourceful teen. As a nod to her performance, Molly stuck Oscar onto the girl's chart.

CITYCENTER MEDICAL

One afternoon, medics brought in a woman who had attempted suicide by turning on a barbecue grill in her bedroom and inhaling the gas. It looked like she would survive. As Molly documented at the nurses station, a pregnant nurse walked by and sniffed. "Ta'quisha, you get grilled hot dogs for lunch?" she asked loudly. Ta'quisha, a tech, told the nurse about the attempted suicide; she was smelling the fumes off the patient.

"Now I'm hungry!" the nurse said.

At the end of the day, an ambulance brought in a 60-year-old man who had been found slumped over at his desk at work. The man twitched and his eyes rolled toward the back of his head. The staff at the nurses station was busy watching the attending doctor question the EMT to determine whether the patient had suffered from a stroke or a seizure.

"Is anyone watching him?" Molly asked, jumping up to help. "Does he have a line?"

After the patient was intubated and sedated, Molly brought him into radiology for a CT scan. The neurology team crowded into the viewing room, excited to see what had gone wrong in the man's brain. As the scan materialized on the monitor, a voice behind Molly shouted, "I win!" She turned to see the neurology resident making the victory sign. "It's not a stroke, it's a seizure!" he said happily. "Who else had seizure?"

Many hospital staff members got through the day by relying on a morbid sense of humor. Molly had come to know the funnier doctors well enough that they joked with her frequently. It was impossible not to laugh at some of the patients, too, like the guy who came in with his penis stuck in a metal washer (it was a large washer). Or the middle-aged man who decided to experiment with his garden bounty one night when his wife was out of town. Unfortunately, he couldn't then remove the cucumber from his anus. In the hospital, he was moved from the ER to the OR because, the small-fingered doctor told her nurses, "I wasn't able to get it and it's sideways now." Molly noted, "There's a multibillion dollar sex toy industry that's discreet and online. Why do people use common household produce?"

Staff played games to make the day more fun, including Guess the Blood Alcohol Level pools. Some of the nurses kept a running list of the most amusing patient names to come into the ER. One doctor tried to crack up his nurses by writing ridiculous discharge papers, such as: "Dear Homeless Guy, I am disappointed that you are both drunk and smelly. That won't get you any pussy." This doctor also liked to joke with Molly about how to break fatality news to family members: "Raise your hand if your loved one is still alive. . . . Not so fast, you two!"

Making Fun of Patients: The Truth Behind Dark Humor, Double Entendres, and the Butt Box

Humor and pranks might seem crass in an emotional environment where people are coping with or fighting illness, trauma, tragedies, or death. But that's exactly why nurses depend on them.

Researchers have found, historically, that healthcare professionals use humor with their patients and each other in all but three circumstances: around uncooperative patients, with patients who are upset, and when interacting with dying patients' loved ones. Plenty of studies have shown that humor can help patients; in addition to spontaneous banter, many doctors (such as oncologists) use prepared jokes about their treatments. Studies also reveal that nurses use humor with patients more frequently than doctors do.

What's less well known is that behind the scenes, doctors' and nurses' humor among colleagues is different—and darker than might seem appropriate to an outsider.

At the milder end of the spectrum, nurses try to lighten the mood by staging pranks on each other or unsuspecting doctors. Some nurses like to crouch in an empty room, turn on the call light, and when the summoned nurse enters, jump out to scare the bejeezus out of her. In one hospital, a nurse hid under a sheet on a gurney that two nurses were told to transport to the morgue. On the way, the hidden nurse groaned and then began to sit up, sending her coworkers shrieking down the hallway.

A California nurse has sprayed Mucomyst (an inhaled substance that treats breathing problems) into the top gloves in the supply box so that the next taker would have sticky, smelly hands. Nurses have awakened night shift colleagues with a sternal rub, an uncomfortable method to test for unconsciousness by firmly fist-rubbing midsternum. An Illinois nurse remarked, "I am not the only nurse I know who has farted in a sedated patient's room and blamed it on the patient when someone walked in." Nurses are not above leaving fake poop in bedpans for unsuspecting staffers (including on the front seat of an ambulance). A unit in Oklahoma has a pranking tradition that sends new nurses on a scavenger hunt for a "window that opens" on a floor where no such window exists.

When a young Southern nurse asked an older nurse how to warm a bag of blood before administering it to a patient, the older nurse joked that she should microwave it. The gullible nurse's resulting explosion resembled a crime scene.

During a Virginia nurse's first week in the ER, a physician exited a patient room holding up a large splotch of brown mush on a gloved finger. The doctor asked the nurse, "Hey, do you think this looks like it has blood in it? I can't decide." The nurse recalled, "Horrified that he's walking over to the nurses station with shit on his finger, I stutter and tell him I don't see anything. He looks perplexed. He then proceeds to lick the sample off his finger. 'It doesn't taste bloody,' he says. It was chocolate pudding. I'd been punk'd." Juvenile, yes, but a common hospital prank.

A doctor at Pines Memorial set up new students by teaming with a nurse like Molly to hand him a urine specimen cup full of apple juice. When teaching the med students how to diagnose, he'd drink the juice and say, "It tastes infected." Molly joked that someday she was going to hand him a cup of urine without telling him.

Nurses say that urologists tend to have a lewd sense of humor and a strong affinity for penis jokes ("Urology department—can you hold?"). Operating room nurses proudly boast that their unit has the bawdiest sense of humor in the hospital. "We get very naughty; we blame it on the fact that we wear what look like pajamas all the time. Just about everything that comes out of our mouths is a double entendre that probably borders on harassment, but that's how we get through the days," said a Pennsylvania OR nurse.

When the Pennsylvania nurse pokes her head beneath surgical drapes to check a patient or flush a catheter, her male colleagues make slurping blow-job sounds. If the surgeons turn the lights off to better view the monitor, they announce they do their "best work in the dark." As the nurses help them fasten their surgical gowns, the doctors quip, "Tie me up like you mean it."

Much of the time, hospital humor is harmless because nobody is offended. But when the patient isn't unconscious or family members are within earshot, doctors' and nurses' jokes can be misinterpreted. A Texas nurse remembered a case when a patient stopped breathing; staff hustled his brother from the room so that they could work the code. The patient died. Afterward, the brother furiously reported the nurses and doctors to hospital administrators because he saw them joking with each other as they tried to save his sibling's life.

What were they thinking? And what could have been so funny during such a traumatic time? Few outsiders are aware of doctors' and nurses' reliance on "gallows humor," a phrase popularized by Sigmund Freud in reference to a story about a man joking as he goes to the gallows to die. Also known as dark humor or black humor, gallows humor is a morbid way to joke about, or in the face of, tragedy or death. Gallows humor describes, for example, when a doctor calls out a patient's long list of extensive injuries to a nurse and then adds, "and he's got a stubbed toe, too." Or when nurses call a coworker "Grim Reaper" because, through no fault of his own, three of his ER patients die in one night.

When patients are dying, some doctors and nurses say they are "circling the drain," "headed to the ECU (the Eternal Care Unit)," or "approaching room temperature." A nurse team calls motorcyclists who don't wear helmets "donor-cycles." Some staff refer to the geriatric ward as "the departure lounge." Gunshot wound? "Acute lead poisoning." Patient death? "Celestial transfer." That's gallows humor.

One of the best true-life examples of gallows humor occurred a few decades ago. In the middle of the night at a hospital in an unsafe neighborhood, three ER residents were waiting for their pizza delivery when a gunshot victim was rushed inside: It was the delivery boy, who had been walking toward the building when a mugger shot him.

The doctors tried to save the victim, but had to call his time of death after forty minutes of resuscitation efforts. "The young doctors shuffled into the temporarily empty waiting area. They sat in silence. Then David said what all three were thinking. 'What happened to our pizza?'" recounted bioethicist Katie Watson in a 2011 Hastings Center Report. "Joe found their pizza box where the delivery boy dropped it before he ran from his attackers [and] set it on the table." The hungry doctors stared at the box. Then one of them asked, "How much you think we ought to tip him?"

Many nurses told me that gallows humor is common and necessary. A survey of New England paramedics found that nearly 90 percent used it; in fact, gallows humor was by far the respondents' most frequent coping mechanism, much more so than talking with coworkers (37 percent), spending time with family and friends (35 percent), and exercising (30 percent).

Gallows humor is not the same as derogatory humor, in which doctors and nurses appear to make fun of specific patients. But many healthcare providers use that, too, to similar effect. In 2014, a Virginia patient who left his cell phone audio-recording during a colonoscopy allegedly recorded his doctors making fun of him while he was under anesthesia. The doctors reportedly said a teaching physician "would eat [the patient] for lunch" and joked about a hypothetical situation regarding firing a gun up a rectum. The patient sued the doctors for defamation and sought more than $5 million in damages.

Despite its propensity to be juvenile or offensive, derogatory humor is a coping mechanism. Staff members at hospitals across the country make fun of patients' names; a Virginia doctor tapes his favorites to his locker. In a Maryland ER, a travel nurse said that "Status Dramaticus" is nurse code for patients with low acuity but high drama, and a "Positive Suitcase Sign" is "when a patient expects to be admitted for a bullshit complaint and brings along a giant suitcase like they're checking into the Hilton."

In North Carolina, whenever a psychiatric patient who often hit people emerged from his room, techs hummed the *Jaws* theme. A study of humor in a psychiatric unit quoted a doctor announcing at the beginning of a meeting, "Let's run an efficient meeting today; only one joke per patient."

Certain groups of patients are targeted more than others, including obese people, particularly in the OR and obstetrics–gynecology departments. In a gynecological surgery case, for example, doctors and nurses played "the pannus game," in which they wagered on the weight of the pannus (the flap of fat on the lower stomach) they were removing. Many healthcare workers trade anecdotes about the items they find or expect to find stuck in the folds of patients' fat. A medical student told researchers, "There's lots of stories about larger older women who when you lift up their fat, you see Oreo cookies, a remote . . . [all] hospital urban legends."

The patients whom hospital workers are most likely to make fun of are people "whose illnesses and health problems were perceived to be 'brought on' by their own behaviors, which 'inhibited' doctors' abilities to take care of them," Northeast Ohio Medical University researchers said, such as excessive smokers, drinkers, or drug users; people who engage in criminal behavior; reckless or drunk drivers; and people who practice unsafe sex.

Other categories include "difficult" patients (who are demanding, aggressive, etc.) and patients who are sexually attractive. A medical student told the Ohio researchers about cases "when the patient is out and people will come in and remark about her knockers being fabulous." Another student assisted doctors who rated the penis size of their patients, and said, "'Don't look at this guy' or 'Look at this guy because he will make us all look good.'" However inappropriate it is to comment on an anesthetized patient's genitalia, the doctors were more likely doing it to lighten the mood for the staff than to pick on that specific patient.

Healthcare professionals are careful to say that they usually make fun of situations and symptoms, not the patients themselves. A medical student explained to the researchers, "There's nothing potentially funny about a sinus infection or earache. They're not amusing. But . . . if somebody comes in with an object lodged in their anus, that's entertaining."

It's so entertaining that some ERs keep an orifice box (also known as "the butt box") into which nurses can plunk the objects that enter the hospital in patients' orifices. Some of the items that patients have stuck into their rectums include: glass perfume bottles, a steak knife (inserted point-first), a six-inch bolt, soda-can tabs, bugs, animals, a broken candle jar, and an entire apple. After Indiana nurses pulled a G.I. Joe out of a man's rectum, they hung the real unfortunate hero by his neck in the nurses station as a prank. When a California patient said he had swallowed "something," nurses played a game of "name that object"; the "something" turned out to be a pipe, a padlock with a key, a screw, two bobby pins, and an unidentifiable object that may have been a battery. Nurses in a Virginia ER had a hard time keeping straight faces when a patient arrived with a vibrator buzzing loudly so far up his rectum that surgery was required to remove it. In hospitals that don't keep a butt box, some nurses surreptitiously take cell phone pictures of amusing X-rays.

Doctors, medical students, nurses, and techs who participate in derogatory humor generally do so in meetings, in the hall, or in group or private conversations. The nurses I interviewed said that gallows humor is more common than derogatory humor, which one doctor has distinguished as "the difference between whistling as you go through the graveyard and kicking over the gravestones."

Why participate in either? Experts say that humor helps medical professionals distance themselves from the anger, grief, stress, and frustration that are inevitable in their jobs. Nurses depend on gallows humor so that they are not overwhelmed by anxiety and sadness. "Sometimes when something happens that is so awful that you want to cry, instead you use black humor to keep from crying," said a Texas nurse practitioner. "They're not really 'jokes.' Mostly it's just trying to relieve the tension."

A Mid-Atlantic travel nurse uses gallows humor to "find the bright side" in tough circumstances. "In a massive trauma, I'll take note of the cheery toenail polish color of a patient, or remark that they picked a great day to wear clean underwear for the car accident," she said. A Canadian nurse remembered a recent code during which the doctor in charge did an impression of another doctor "who was known to freak out during codes. He said, 'Oh my God, somebody help this man!' It brought some levity to the code, had all the nurses laughing, and got everyone relaxed a bit during a very stressful event. The patient survived and the code was not affected at all by the joke."

Gallows humor is a way both to disconnect from a horrific situation and to connect with the other health team members who are together facing that situation. Humor has been shown to improve doctors' and nurses' morale and working relationships. It allows them to express their feelings more easily and to say things that otherwise could be difficult to say. It's also a bonding tool; as researchers have observed, "having a common sense of humor is like sharing a secret code."

Should gallows and derogatory humor have a place in the hospital setting? "How does it feel to be a patient in a room who just got diagnosed with recurrent ovarian cancer and to hear laughter down the hallway?" Massachusetts General Hospital oncologist Richard Penson wondered in a journal article. Referring to patients who overheard a staff member using derogatory humor that they angrily assumed was about them, a psychiatrist described "the stray bullet effect—it's not directed at them but they perceive it [to be]." Other doctors worry that derogatory humor, like the Oscar for dramatic patients, can cause staff members to develop preconceived, negative notions about a patient or type of patient.

But the benefits to staff and ultimately to patients may outweigh occasional wounded feelings. One would hope that doctors and nurses would be permitted to take whatever nondestructive steps they need to be able to provide the best possible care. Bioethicist Katie Watson observed, "Critics of backstage gallows humor who are admirably concerned with empathy for patients sometimes seem curiously devoid of empathy for physicians. Medicine is an odd profession, in which we ask ordinary people to act as if feces and vomit do not smell, unusual bodies are not at all remarkable, and death is not frightening."

Researchers have said that when medical students use derogatory slang about patients, they are deflecting their feelings of anger or disgust away from the patients who frustrate them because they don't take care of themselves and, therefore, waste the hospital's resources. It is, California researchers concluded, "a safety valve for 'letting off steam.'"

Many nurses described these types of humor as defense mechanisms, as an innate reflex. "It's depressing when you're dealing with people hurting mentally, so much that a lot of them want to die. The only way to deal with this is to make extremely inappropriate jokes," an Indiana psychiatric nurse said. "An example would be joking about ridiculously poor suicide attempts, which sounds terribly insensitive. The other day we got a patient who 'attempted suicide' by taking a few of this med, a few of that, a couple sprays of Raid, and a shot of bleach. Like, really? Is that the best you can do? Of course, we already know the answer (a cry for help), but sometimes it's the inappropriate jokes that make the job a little easier to handle."

The public would find nurses' frequent use of gallows humor "scandalous," said a Texas travel nurse. "Laypeople would think I'm the most awful human being in the world if they could hear my mouth during a Code Blue or Priority 1 trauma. It's a by-product of being placed in situations where death is common and unimaginable horrors are just another day at work. Gallows humor helps to deal with some of the horrible things we see in a way that bonds us together as a team against the bad stuff. We have to take care of these dying, abused, neglected, sick patients and then turn right around and take care of the minor things without missing a beat," she said. "Bad things happen, and I can't stop it. All I can do is try to support my patients to the best of my ability. Keeping that in mind helps me sleep at night. In the midst of those traumas and tragedies, I compartmentalize: I allow a part of myself to mourn and feel sad, while the majority of my attention is focused on the task at hand. I'm trying to save a life and that is my primary goal, but sometimes the stress of doing that task builds and needs a release. We use gallows humor to relieve that stress."

Joking, even during codes, can empower healthcare workers, provide a fresh perspective, create a sense of control, and locate joy or playfulness in a devastating moment. This is important because nurses must get through the traumas intact so they can be fresh and focused for the next patient and the next. They have to concentrate intensely in critical situations one minute, and then let go so they can immediately move on. Gallows humor helps to ease that transition and to leave work thoughts in the workplace. "Nurses need to blow off the adrenaline pent up after patient care. It's better to dress up those feelings behind laughter than carry that burden home with you," said a Washington State hospice nurse.

A Canadian study found that nursing school educators who used humor experienced less emotional exhaustion and higher levels of personal accomplishment than other educators. In fact, experts specifically recommend that healthcare professionals utilize gallows humor as a survival tactic and to combat burnout. Nurse and humorist Karyn Buxman encourages nurses to find humor in their work: "Start a collection of humorous comments, events, or charting notes, keeping in mind that patient confidentiality is paramount."

Gallows humor in hospitals has not been heavily researched, but the existing literature mostly supports using it. "When is behind-the-scenes gallows humor okay, and when should it cause concern?" Katie Watson, the bioethicist, asked. "To answer, I would first want to think about who is harmed by the joking." Ultimately, in cases such as the pizza-tipping joke, she concluded, "To me, the butt of the doctors' tip joke is not the patient. It's death. The residents fought death with all they had, and death won." And that's why the joke is okay.

Humor is a way for nurses to find dawn in the darkness, to self-empower, and to unite with each other, determined and defiant. Above all, humor is a way to locate hope amid hardship, which is exactly what patients need nurses to do.

CHAPTER 6

THE STEPFORD NURSE:
How Hospitals Game the System
for Patient "Satisfaction"

"The nurse promotes, advocates for, and strives to protect the health, safety, and rights of the patient."
—*Code of Ethics for Nurses*, Provision 3

"Hospitals tend to focus on what they get sued for. Hospitals used to have COWs: computers on wheels. A while ago, a nurse said, 'What's up with the COW in Two?' Well, the patient in Room Two knew she was in Room Two and filed a lawsuit and won. So now hospitals call them WOWs: workstations on wheels."
—a Washington, DC, ER nurse

LARA   SOUTH GENERAL HOSPITAL, February

The first few weeks of Lara's separation from her husband were terrifying, while she tried to figure out whether she could support herself and two small children on her own. She couldn't afford the mortgage on the house, which broke her heart because she and John had built their home, and her brother lived next door. She let John stay in the house because she didn't want their children to have to adjust to two new homes. He was sure his gambling could cover the costs.

At first, Lara waited for John to apologize and agree to get treatment. Even as she moved her things out of the house, she thought he would realize that he needed her and he needed help. He watched the children while she worked and attended NA meetings, but when they exchanged them, he showed no signs of wanting to reconcile. In response to people who asked him why Lara left, John said, "She's jealous about something I wrote on Twitter," trivializing his years of issues down to one tweet.

As much as it hurt, John's delight at being single helped Lara move past her initial doubt about her decision to leave him. It was more difficult for her to get over being sad, lonely, and scared. How would she pay the bills by herself and have enough time for her children? How would she resist the temptation to turn to narcotics?

Eventually, Lara's realtor found a small rental house within her budget and near the kids' school. Several NA friends helped her move, and a girlfriend gave her two U-Hauls worth of free furniture. The men she knew in NA offered her handyman assistance. Many of the women called to say they had gone through something similar, offering consolation and strength.

Still, Lara was unsettled most of the time. She tried to stay busy, because when she wasn't, she either dwelled on her anger or cried. She was able to pull herself together only when she was at work or with Sebastian and Lindsey. It helped to focus on getting them through their homework or finding activities to do together on weekends.

Lara had seen a lawyer to begin divorce proceedings, but she didn't like when the lawyer said, "We're going to get him." Instead, she went to a mediator, who worked things out amicably.

Now Lara's main worry was how to afford her rent. Luckily, South General had been accommodating. The first time she called to ask whether there were any openings on the schedule to increase her hours and her paycheck, the ER director said there were not. "Do you need to just come in to work, though?" the director asked, and created a spot for Lara anyway. She allowed Lara a nontraditional schedule: two twelve-hour shifts plus her children's school hours. Lara dropped the kids off at school, arrived at the hospital by 11:00 a.m., worked for four hours, and left to make the forty-five-minute drive to pick them up.

Lara pulled this shift every weekday in addition to the twelve-hour night shifts. John was happy to watch the kids because he believed the babysitting got him out of paying child support. Lara knew her children were fine with John; for all of his shortcomings, he was a decent father. But it killed her to spend so much time away from them. Every NA meeting she attended was another hour that she could have spent with Sebastian and Lindsey.

At South General, Rose, the ER's kindest nurse, connected Lara with Holly, a skilled, businesslike African American nurse whom Lara liked but had not gotten to know well. Holly, it turned out, had just divorced a cheating husband whose behavior was eerily similar to John's; the women joked that but for the racial difference, their husbands could have been the same man. Every shift they shared, Lara and Holly made a point of checking in on each other, exchanging quick hugs and comparing stories. It was a relief for Lara to hang out with someone who understood her situation.

Several other nurses were so supportive that Lara felt as if she had a sisterhood looking out for her at work. To her knowledge, no one had complained that the nurse manager let her come to work whenever she wanted. Once, Lara was crying in a bathroom stall when she overheard the charge nurse say, "Lara's here but don't give her anything stressful. Just keep her busy." Lara smiled, warmed because, despite some poor choices she'd made in life, she had chosen a career that was flexible enough to accommodate a single mom and that attracted the kind of women who protected each other.

One day Fatima approached her at shift change. "I heard you were having a hard time with your separation," Fatima said. "I hope it goes better than mine did." She told Lara about the fighting and drama that had plagued her own marriage and subsequent divorce. She mentioned that her ex-husband had been an alcoholic, a fact Lara filed away for future reference. Sometime when they were alone, she could talk to Fatima about her own family's battles with alcoholism to segue into a discussion about addiction.

Lara was glad that Fatima felt comfortable enough to approach her. She couldn't mention the drugs because they were in the middle of the ER, but she wanted to. She wanted to say that she knew why Fatima always wore long sleeves in the heated ER (track marks), and that she knew why Fatima's hands were red and puffy (frequently shooting into a vein impeded blood flow). Perhaps after a few more conversations they would be friendly enough that Lara could raise the issue.

She sensed that time was running out.

JULIETTE   PINES MEMORIAL, February

On a relatively slow afternoon, Juliette was documenting at the nurses station. While she relished the adrenaline rush of busy workdays in the ER, she also treasured the occasional quiet spell that allowed her to chat with her coworkers or in the back office with Clark Preston.

Molly had been trying to convince Juliette to leave Pines because the clique bothered her so much. "Why don't you work agency? There's no reason not to," Molly had told her. "You can work anywhere you want, you don't have to do holidays or weekends, and the pay is higher."

Juliette had resisted because the devil she knew was better than the devil she didn't. She had anxiety about putting herself in new work situations. And while the clique overshadowed her job, she was still able to find positive connections with patients and some of her coworkers.

Ruby, the recently divorced nurse, stopped by the nurses station to say hello. "So what's the deal with him?" she asked, pointing to a good-looking murse who was an incorrigible flirt. "I know he's young for me, but what's the deal?"

"If my daughter were in her twenties, I would not let her date him," Juliette replied. "He cheats on his girlfriend every six months."

"I gotta get laid. My little toy isn't doing it for me anymore," Ruby said.

Juliette was both surprised and pleased by the confession. She liked Ruby and respected her as a nurse, but they had not spent time together outside of work. How refreshing it was to gab with a coworker about something personal. "I know someone who's more than willing," she said. On a scrap of paper, she scribbled the name of the womanizer whose dalliances with several nurses had caused his secretary girlfriend to have a panic attack. She handed it to Ruby.

"Hmm, Dr. Fontaine. Isn't he a little short? Cute, though," Ruby said.

"He's always down here. But apparently he's been around the block a number of times."

"Well, I'd just have to wrap his thing up twice then," Ruby said, pondering the piece of paper.

Juliette cracked up. "Are you going to triage? I'll walk you there."

The women walked past the waiting area and stopped abruptly. Erin, a likeable young nurse, was heading toward the back wall with a large pair of forceps. "Uh, what are you doing, Erin?" Juliette asked.

"I have to get some candy out of the vending machine," Erin said.

"Why, does a diabetic patient need some sugar?" Juliette joked, and followed her.

Two techs were kneeling in front of the machine. A dozen snacks were caught between the glass and the shelves. In front of an audience of patients and families in the waiting room, Erin tried using the forceps to reach the bags. No dice.

A few minutes later, Gabriel, the secretary, came over, rolling up his sleeves to reach inside the machine. "I can do it!" he announced. He couldn't do it.

A murse brought a splint instrument that he had manipulated into the shape of a hook. The techs tried to grab the candy with the hook. "What if I get a lacerated finger?" one of them asked.

"That's workman's comp!" Juliette answered. The group laughed.

Soon, Dr. Preston came by. "Come on, Dr. Preston, you can do it!" someone shouted.

Ruby elbowed Juliette. "I bet those fingers can do anything."

The staff and the patients watched as Dr. Preston reached his exceptionally long arm far into the machine and jarred loose a bag of Doritos. Finally, the chips and sweets tumbled from the machine. A cheer went up from the waiting room. Dr. Preston bowed and left.

Back at the nurses station, Juliette saw Dr. Fontaine flirting with a nurse. Ruby sidled by and bent toward Juliette's ear. "Really?" Ruby whispered. Juliette grinned, raised her eyebrows, and nodded.

When Juliette got home that evening, she was still on a high from a fun day at work. As usual, she stripped off her dirty scrubs in her garage so as not to bring the germs into her house, painstakingly washed her hands and arms up to her shoulders, and pecked Tim on the cheek. She found 7-year-old Michelle on the couch.

She hugged her daughter tightly in greeting, but Michelle didn't smile. "Mommy, do you work tomorrow?" she asked.

"Yes, honey. It's Tuesday."

Michelle's shoulders slumped. "It seems like you never have a day off. I want you home in the mornings to help me get ready. I wish you could work just in the afternoons."

Juliette's cheerfulness dissipated beneath her guilt. If she took shorter shifts, she'd lose not only wages but also opportunities to bond with her coworkers, as she had today. She decided then and there to apply for a clinical ladder promotion.

In the past, nurses who wanted to advance their career could study for extra degrees or apply for jobs in management. Juliette had no interest in applying for Erica's vacant senior charge nurse position, or for any other administrative role, because she preferred to care directly for patients rather than supervise her peers.

Juliette loved bedside nursing because she cherished the direct interactions with patients. "I love being around them, being able to make all types of patients feel better," she explained. "I love the moments of connection with the patient and with the family."

Clinical ladders offered nurses like Juliette opportunities for a raise and recognition without having to leave the bedside. While the stages could vary by the hospital, Pines' ladder offered four rungs of recognition: clinician level 1 (entry level), clinician level 2 (proficient), clinician level 3 (advanced), and clinical level 4 (expert). Each level required research, initiative, and a demonstrated level of clinical knowledge and advanced practice work. Juliette had reached advanced clinician level 3 a while ago. She didn't have too much left to do to finish her application for clinical 4. She resolved to complete the requisite research project (which she had started and set aside last year) to reach the top level as a validation of her skills and a rationalization for keeping a demanding job that took time away from her daughter.

To achieve a clinical ladder promotion, nurses had to be in good standing at the hospital. Pines had a policy prohibiting nurses who made one patient identification error from applying for any type of promotion that year. Two mistakes in a twelve-month period and the nurse would be fired. Juliette knew she hadn't made any notable mistakes, but she wanted to make sure she qualified before she put in the work.

"There's nothing specific that I know of," Priscilla told her. As the nursing director, she would have heard if Juliette had committed an infraction or received complaints about her work. "But you have six tardies and you need to watch it."

"I will, I'll be careful. But I'm okay to apply?" Juliette asked.

"Absolutely."

Juliette punched a fist into the air. She was so exuberant that she went to tell Charlene. "Charlene, guess what! I'm applying for clinical four and I'm going to make a really strong effort."

"I'm not sure you can," Charlene said. "I've got everyone's tardies and stay-lates printed out. I'm highlighting all of them. It's a pet project of mine." Charlene didn't want nurses to stay later than their shift because she didn't want to pay them unnecessary overtime. She smiled. "So we'll see."

Juliette deflated.

SAM CITYCENTER MEDICAL, February

Everyone at Citycenter was talking about the surprise inspection. The nurses were ecstatic and relieved that The Joint Commission had stepped in. One nurse told Sam that during an interview, she had admitted to the TJC investigator that she was uncomfortable sharing what she really wanted to say. The investigator held up a thick stack of papers to indicate how many others had spoken freely and replied, "You have nothing to worry about."

The day after the inspection, Victoria sent a mass email to say she was transferring to another department to pursue other opportunities. A nursing administrator would take over as interim ER director. Victoria's words didn't fool the nurses. Everyone knew the real reason she had been transferred. A nurse who was friendly with Sam included her in a Facebook message to several coworkers that said only, "Ding dong, the witch is dead."

Once Victoria left, the changes came quickly. The hospital immediately hired more than a dozen new nurses and instituted a bonus policy for nurses who worked extra shifts. The ER now would have mandatory daily checklists that monitored code carts and supplies. Maintenance workers deep-cleaned every room, waxed the floors, and painted the walls. Reportedly during the inspection, one of the surveyors had asked to see a room considered to be clean. A nurse led him to an empty room that was ready to receive an incoming ambulance patient. The surveyor saw blood splattered on the wall, empty bags hanging from IV poles, used blood culture bottles, capped IV needles on the floor, and trash on the counter. When administrators later dispatched multiple housekeepers to that room, it took ten hours to clean it to infection control standards.

Sam was pleasantly surprised by the interim ER director, who seemed willing to listen to the staff. On her first day, she changed Sam's status to "weekend alternative": For $10 more per hour, Sam would work weekends plus one weeknight per week, with one weekend off per month. She had been trying to get weekend alternative for ages, because, she rationalized, "if I'm going to be working in hell I'd at least have a regular schedule doing it." Her previous discussions with HR and her supervisors had gone nowhere. The new director made it happen in one day.

The director quickly gained respect from the ER staff because she was willing to do whatever was necessary to help the department. She came in on weekends and cleaned stretchers. She put on scrubs and transported patients. "She is terrific," Sam said. "It's great to have someone in an authority position supporting us like she does. It makes a tremendous difference."

Sam was sitting at the nurses station with William when Dr. Spiros stopped five feet away from them to talk to another nurse. William waggled his eyebrows toward Dr. Spiros, whose back was turned, then mouthed at Sam, "Your boyfriend's here."

Sam's gray eyes narrowed behind her glasses. Angrily blushing, she whispered, "You can be done with the comments and the looks because there's nothing going on."

By now, Sam could discuss patient care with Dr. Spiros, but she still felt too awkward to say anything more to him than was professionally necessary. It was weird enough that she knew what he looked like when he wasn't in scrubs and that she had been inside his home, let alone that they'd had an almost-but-didn't relationship. At work, rather than waver between calling him Dr. Spiros or Dimitri, she tried not to use his name at all.

Sam didn't mind being single, though it would have been helpful to have an extra ally in the hospital. She could admit to herself that she had a crush on William, but knowing he had a girlfriend, she would never act on her feelings. She was content to appreciate their growing friendship. Despite his teasing, Sam enjoyed working with William, and not only because he was an excellent, sure-handed nurse. He respected her and he made her feel appreciated. Sometimes he called her hospital cell phone just to say hi or to ask if she needed help.

One night, the charge nurse was doling out assignments and put William on Zone 1. In front of the staff, she asked him who he wanted to work with that night.

"Sam," he said.

As Sam smiled to herself, proud and touched that William had chosen her out of all of the other nurses, she looked up and saw CeeCee glaring at her.

It was obvious that CeeCee assumed that she and William were close. Certainly, he was nice to her. CeeCee was always badgering him with social requests: "William, let's do a group bike trip!" "William, come on the ferry with us this weekend!" Sam knew that William was warm to everybody. He had told Sam that he joined the young nurses' social outings so that they would continue to feel comfortable seeking his help at work. He didn't want them to think that because he was often the charge nurse, he was unapproachable.

Sam remembered when, as a nursing student, nearly everyone her senior seemed unapproachable to her. That had changed as she had gained experience treating patients and become accustomed to her colleagues. Without a doubt, William had played a major role in her growth, as a teacher and as a friend. He felt like a safety net, especially, as Sam put it, "when the place is so unsafe that I could lose my license."

Now Sam was growing more confident day by day. She had a good general sense of the ER, knowing where the sick patients were even if they weren't hers. She had learned how to get other people to work more efficiently with her; for example, if she needed lab results urgently, instead of inputting a lab request into the computer, she wrote it on a paper lab form, brought it down to the lab herself, and said, "We've done these labs. I need you to run them, please."

One night medics brought in a 58-year-old trauma patient who had driven his car into a tree. He was awake and alert, though he didn't remember the accident. While two residents examined the patient, Sam, as the recording nurse, stood in the back of the room taking notes. Shirley, the ER nurse practitioner, stood next to her.

As Sam watched the heart monitor, she noticed that the patient was having several premature ventricular contractions, extra heartbeats that disrupt the regular heart rhythm. While some PVCs are normal, the patient had many more than the average person. The patient's nurse was busy drawing blood and the residents were engrossed in their assessment.

"Hey, Shirley, our buddy here is throwing a lot of PVCs," Sam told the NP.

Shirley watched the monitor. "You're absolutely right," she said, then addressed the other nurse. "Let's add magnesium levels to the labs and get a cardiology consult."

The next night, Shirley approached her at the nurses station. "Sam, nice catch last night. The trauma patient turned out to be a cardio patient." She explained that the cardiology team believed the man had had a heart attack or another massive cardiac event that had stopped his heart from functioning efficiently. The force of the air bag hitting his chest had probably restarted his heart, albeit at an irregular rhythm. The man had received a pacemaker that morning.

"Sam, you have good situation awareness and a good sense of what's going on with your patients," Shirley said. "I think you'd be a fantastic NP."

Sam's confidence soared.

MOLLY   March

ACADEMY HOSPITAL

Molly's first patient of the morning was an unemployed, heavily tattooed gang member with a cocaine habit. He had a small bowel obstruction because he had been shot in the stomach a decade ago. Molly tried not to judge her patients. (She'd had several tattooed dudes come in and say, "I hate needles." You just never knew.) Recently at Citycenter, Molly had treated a trauma patient who had been shot three times and killed the other guy. Molly was creeped out by the man, but pleased with her ability to treat a murderer by separating the man's crime from the medical treatment he needed.

When Molly entered the room, the gang member was telling Maxine, a medical student, that he was in severe pain. "Can y'all please talk to the surgery resident and get an order for pain medication?" Molly asked the student.

"Okay," Maxine said. "I already ordered a Foley."

"I'm not putting a Foley in a patient who is able to urinate on his own," Molly said. She explained to Maxine that Foley catheters commonly caused hospital-acquired infections. If a patient developed an infection in the hospital, Medicare and Medicaid could refuse to pay for the visit. Hospitals had strict policies about which patients could get a Foley. Patients able to walk to the bathroom, like this man, were not supposed to have one.

"But we need to accurately measure urine output," Maxine argued.

Molly held up a plastic urinal jug. "This has very accurate markings for measurement. The way we measure urine output in patients with Foleys is to empty the urine into the same urinal the patient would use to pee in, anyway. So I'm not putting the Foley in."

The patient watched the back-and-forth with interest.

"But the resident wants it." Maxine looked confused: If a doctor said it, it must be gospel.

"It's not going to happen. Just because a surgery resident said it doesn't change the policy," Molly replied.

An hour later, the patient still hadn't received pain medication. By now, he was technically no longer an ER patient; he was an ICU patient boarding in the ER because no ICU beds were available. His orders would come from the admitting team of ICU doctors rather than the ER. Although Molly was slammed with other work, as usual, she wanted to make sure that the patient was looked after. He was in obvious pain, but boarder patients were often the last patients the attendings would visit.

Molly found the ER doctor in the hall. As she was about to ask Dr. Ward for the meds, Maxine came out of the patient's room, held up her hand, and said, "We're taking care of it."

"You told me that an hour ago and he still has no orders," Molly said.

"I texted the surgery resident and she said she'd take care of it," Maxine replied.

"When?"

Maxine paused. "I'm not sure."

"That's why I'm asking the ER doctor. He's been in severe pain and vomiting since he came in here."

Maxine tilted her chin condescendingly. "Don't you think you should let *us* take care of it?"

"I've given you an hour to take care of it."

Dr. Ward finally chimed in. "Imagine that's your dad in the room. Would you sit there for an hour with him in severe pain and just wait around for someone to do something? How about you text *that* to your resident?"

Maxine looked sheepish. "Yes, sir."

Five minutes later, the surgery resident was in the room. Molly followed her in and asked for the order, which the resident wrote immediately.

When the room emptied, the patient turned to Molly. "You're the best nurse I ever had. Thanks for looking out for me."

Molly considered patient advocacy the most important role for a nurse. She was surprised at how often she had to push hard for patients because doctors weren't doing the right thing. She spent a great deal of time hounding doctors for pain medications for cancer patients and elderly patients. When Pines had offered to ban Daryl, Molly's assaulter, from the hospital, Molly had declined because he could be a patient someday: "If he had a legit medical reason to seek treatment, I didn't want his options limited."

Similarly, she wanted to ensure that her patient was cared for as an ailing human being, not as a gang member. "I felt for this guy," she said. "I'm sure he had received substandard care in his life because of his appearance and past. I treated him the way I'd like to be treated. To him, that was the best nursing care he'd ever had. That made me happy, but at the same time, it's pretty sad."

PINES MEMORIAL

One day in late March, Molly took a shift at Pines on a day she knew the hospital could use the help. Because she was already established in the ER as a talented nurse with a strong work ethic, the ER office manager gave her hours whenever she wanted them.

Two hours into her morning, she decided to take a urine pregnancy test. It was more than two weeks after her IUI and she couldn't let her hopes teeter for another day. She took a test and specimen cup from the lab room and went to the staff bathroom. With a pipette, she drew a few drops of urine from the cup and dripped it onto the test. Then she waited. *Please.*

This cycle had been Molly's last chance to get treatment covered by insurance. After more than eight months of fertility tests, treatments, and appointments, besides wanting to conceive a baby, she yearned to be finished with the uncertainty in her life and back on track to work reliably for her employers. While the stakes increased with every cycle, these results seemed a great deal more important than the others. If the IUI didn't work, she would have to undergo IVF, which would cost nearly $25,000 out of pocket for only a 30 percent chance of success. Molly and Trey would have to charge it on their credit cards.

Molly consulted her watch. Three minutes had passed. She looked at the pregnancy test. No color change. Negative. Molly stared sadly at it. Her stomach dropped.

But Molly had to return to work; there were no breaks at Pines. Nurses had no room for their own personal struggles in the hospital. She tried to brush off her emotions. *Oh well, at least I'll earn lots of credit card points toward cash back,* she told herself. *And now I need to get back to my patients.* She trashed the pregnancy test and returned to the ER.

That afternoon, Bethany—the nurse whom Juliette had assumed was part of the clique—sought Molly out to talk. Priscilla had given the senior charge nurse title to three of the four nurses who had applied for the job that Erica had vacated. (Charlene had complained about this, but made sure to tell everyone, "They'll all be equal, but I'll still be over them.") Bethany was the only rejected applicant. When Bethany asked Priscilla about it, Priscilla said she had heard the only reason Bethany applied was to prevent Juliette from getting the job.

"That's not true at all. Why would I do that?" Bethany told Molly.

"Juliette didn't even apply," Molly said. "She didn't want a new job; she's working really hard for clinical level four."

"Right," Bethany continued, "and then Priscilla said, 'Between you and me, I would never hire Juliette for that position.' A manager should never talk to employees about other employees!"

Molly was floored. Priscilla gave Juliette the impression that she loved her. Juliette was a hardworking nurse who always tried to do right by her patients, and she was assembling a strong portfolio for her clinical ladder application. "If she feels this way about Juliette, she should tell her, and her performance evaluations should reflect it," Molly said. She struggled with whether to tell Juliette because she knew it would hurt her feelings. But Juliette needed to know that the private information she shared with Priscilla might not be remaining confidential.

Staff politics were only one of many reasons that Molly was glad she had left Pines. Pines had the best educated and best insured patients that Molly had seen; they were probably among the smartest and wealthiest in the area. They were also the most demanding patients Molly had ever met.

Recently, the Westnorth Corporation announced to staff that care should be tailored to the patient surveys that were administered randomly after discharge. Thanks to the Affordable Care Act (also known as "Obamacare"), hospitals took their patient satisfaction surveys very seriously because their scores affected the amount of federal money they received. Since Westnorth had taken over the hospital, patient satisfaction scores had dropped. Administrators now were scripting nurses' discussions with patients and ordering them to use memorized key words in what the hospital called "guided conversations." For example, the survey asked, "Did your nurse educate you on your condition?" Patients tended to answer no, despite receiving discharge instructions about their diagnosis and treatment. Therefore, Westnorth now instructed nurses to say, specifically, "I am going to educate you on your diagnosis."

At Pines, the patients could be difficult to please. "You can come in with appendicitis and we fix you but your room was cold, so you're pissed off and give us a poor rating," Molly said. "I don't care whether the patients are 'satisfied.' I care that they get the treatment they need." A patient once found Molly in a room performing CPR and yelled, "I ASKED YOU FOR A PILLOW FIFTEEN MINUTES AGO!" During CPR!

Too often, Pines patients demanded specific procedures, after speaking with doctor friends or searching for ideas on the Internet. If the patient's orders didn't match the doctor's orders, the patient might leave the hospital dissatisfied, even if he was cured, simply because he didn't receive the treatment he demanded.

One of the worst patients Molly could remember was an annoying woman who pressed her nurse's call light every few minutes. "I'm cold," she'd say, so Molly would cover her with a blanket. Molly would just be sitting down at the nurses station when the woman rang again. "I want some water." Molly brought her the water. Five minutes later: "I don't like it with ice." Molly brought her water without ice. Another few minutes, then: "It's too warm. I want one piece of ice."

Thinking the woman should have to "work a little harder" to contact her nurse, Molly moved the call light out of reach. The woman called her on the room phone, asking for another blanket. Molly complied. Three minutes later, the patient rang her again. Molly was wise enough to know that some patients were difficult because they were lonely and scared. But she had four other patients just as lonely and scared as this woman, who was taking up way too much of her time. Nurses flipped coins to avoid patients like her.

Those were the kinds of people who answered the patient satisfaction surveys. Not the man to whom Molly gave her own meal because he missed putting in his dinner order and hadn't eaten all day. Not the little old lady who had taken her first-ever airplane flight, fallen at the airport, and needed a CT scan that messed up her intricately braided cornrows. She'd had her hair done because she was meeting her great-granddaughter for the first time. Molly spent 45 minutes rebraiding the woman's hair into its updo. As an out-of-town resident, the grateful woman wouldn't receive a survey. Instead, Molly got in trouble with the charge nurse for braiding hair.

And no one would hear from the 30-year-old man who was dying of AIDS. He had been estranged from his family, and had just reconciled with his mother when his condition deteriorated. While Molly was triaging him, he begged his mother, "Please don't leave me. I don't want to die alone." Soon afterward, he became unresponsive.

At 2:00 a.m., the patient was admitted to a medical floor for end-of-life care. When Molly wheeled him upstairs, his mother turned to her in tears. "I can't stay here and watch my child die."

"I understand this is very painful, but he specifically said he didn't want to die alone," Molly said.

When Molly left the man's room to return to the ER, the mother left, too. At 7:00 a.m., when Molly's shift ended, she called the floor to ask if the man was still alive. "Yes, but barely," came the answer.

"Is anyone with him?" Molly asked.

"No. His mother never came back."

Molly had just finished an exhausting twelve-hour night shift, but she wanted to honor the man's last wish. She clocked out, took her things to his room, and sat next to him, holding his hand for two hours until he passed away.

"Of course," Molly said later, "since he was an admitted patient—and dead—he couldn't be polled about his hospital experience."

Patient Satisfaction, Tricking Patients,
and the Stepford Nurse

When Department of Health and Human Services administrators decided to base 30 percent of hospitals' Medicare reimbursement on patient satisfaction survey scores, they likely figured that transparency and accountability would improve healthcare. Centers for Medicare & Medicaid Services (CMS) officials wrote in the Federal Register, rather reasonably, "Delivery of high-quality, patient-centered care requires us to carefully consider the patient's experience in the hospital inpatient setting." They probably had no idea that their methods could end up indirectly harming patients.

Beginning in October 2012, the Affordable Care Act implemented a policy withholding 1 percent of total Medicare reimbursements—approximately $850 million—from hospitals (that percentage will double in 2017). Each year, only hospitals with high patient satisfaction scores and a measure of certain basic care standards will earn that money back, and the top performers will receive bonus money from the pool. Private health insurance companies, such as Blue Cross Blue Shield of Massachusetts, are reportedly following the lead of what the government calls the Hospital Value-Based Purchasing Program.

Patient satisfaction surveys have their place. But the potential cost of the subjective scores are leading hospitals to steer focus away from patient health, messing with the highest stakes possible: people's lives.

The questions and the problem

The vast majority of the thirty-two-question survey, known as HCAHPS (Hospital Consumer Assessment of Healthcare Providers and Systems) addresses nursing care. For example, in a section about nurses, the survey asks, "During this hospital stay, after you pressed the call button, how often did you get help as soon as you wanted it?" There is no similar question regarding speed of doctors' or other staff members' response times.

This question is misleading because it doesn't specify whether the help was medically necessary. Patients have complained on the survey, which in previous incarnations included comments sections, about everything from "My roommate was dying all night and his breathing was very noisy" to "The hospital doesn't have Splenda." A nurse at the New Jersey hospital lacking Splenda said, "This somehow became the fault of the nurse and ended up being placed in her personnel file." An Oregon critical care nurse had to argue with a patient who believed he was being mistreated because he didn't get enough pastrami on his sandwich (he had recently had quadruple bypass surgery). "Many patients have unrealistic expectations for their care and their outcomes," the nurse said.

What's more, Medicare calculates scores by tallying only the percentage of patients who rank a hospital a 9 or 10 out of 10 and/or who select "Always" in response to the specific questions. Not "Usually." Not "Sometimes." Not an average rating. "Always." This is a lazy calculation that dismisses a tremendous amount of data. Technically, if a nurse rushes promptly to a patient's bedside for every request—colder water, warmer blanket, lower shades—except one, then the hospital could lose credit for the question.

Medicare awards bonuses (out of the money withheld from hospitals) to the top-performing hospitals nationwide. Pitting hospitals against each other, the equivalent of grading on a curve, does not necessarily compare like with like. Already, results show that Washington, DC, and New York patients are less likely than other patients to give their hospital a top score. Several experts have pointed out that Midwestern patients complain less than crankier counterparts in the Northeast and California, where hospitals traditionally receive lower ratings.

Who gets the survey? Hospitals either call or mail the questions randomly to discharged adults, which theoretically could include drug-seeking patients who leave the hospital irate if the staff won't give them prescriptions. Once, a patient who was in the hospital for chest pain asked Molly to take out her pessary (a small vaginal device), clean it, and reinsert it, not ER duties. When Molly told her she didn't know how to remove it, the woman shouted, "I'm supposed to get it cleaned once a month and I'm a month overdue! It needs to be done *now!*" as if it were Molly's fault she had skipped a doctor's appointment. The hospital didn't do it, risking poor scores because the staff rightly refused to meet the woman's absurd demand. Another man complained to the hospital's patient liaison because when the ER staff saved his father's life, they lost his $8 undershirt. "Those are the people who get called for the survey," Molly said.

While hopefully there aren't many unreasonable patients who would avenge unwarranted anger on the survey, they do exist. The survey questions and methodology, however, don't necessarily elicit an accurate portrayal of care quality. The survey doesn't ask whether the hospital resolved or improved the patient's medical issue, which one would hope would be the primary determinant of a patient's satisfaction with the experience.

A national study revealed that patients who reported being most satisfied with their doctors actually had higher healthcare and prescription costs and were more likely to be hospitalized than patients who were not as satisfied. Worse, the most satisfied patients were significantly more likely to die in the next four years.

UC Davis professor Joshua Fenton, who conducted the study, said these results could reflect that doctors who are reimbursed according to patient satisfaction scores may be less inclined to talk patients out of treatments they request or to raise concerns about smoking, substance abuse, or mental health issues. By attempting to satisfy patients, healthcare providers unintentionally might not be looking out for their best interests. As the *New York Times* nurse columnist Theresa Brown observed, "Focusing on what patients want—a certain test, a specific drug—may mean they get less of what they actually need. In other words, evaluating hospital care in terms of its ability to offer positive experiences could easily put pressure on the system to do things it can't, at the expense of what it should."

The surprise

Hospitals, too, can offer poor care and still get high patient satisfaction ratings, and an alarming number of them do. In my research for this book, I examined Medicare's provider data for thousands of hospitals—the data on every hospital in the country that the agency makes publicly available. I found the hospitals that perform worse than the national average in three or more categories measuring patient outcome. These are hospitals, in other words, where a higher number of patients than average will die, be unexpectedly readmitted to the hospital, or suffer serious complications. And yet two-thirds of those poorly performing hospitals scored higher than the national average on the key HCAHPS question; their patients reported that "YES, they would definitely recommend the hospital."

As a Missouri clinical instructor said, "Patients can be very satisfied and dead an hour later. Sometimes hearing bad news is not going to result in a satisfied patient, yet the patient could be a well-informed, prepared patient."

How far will a hospital go to satisfy a patient? In 2012, when the white father of a newborn baby at Hurley Medical Center in Michigan requested that no black nurses care for his child, the hospital complied. Tonya Battle, a neonatal intensive care nurse for twenty-five years, was reassigned to another patient. Battle sued the board of hospital managers and a nurse manager for discrimination. Hurley settled, paying Battle $110,000 and two other black nurses $41,250 each.

Surely, many patients are both honest and savvy enough to perceive and report the quality of their treatment accurately. But patient opinions and emphases vary widely. A 2012 study found that 61 percent of patients at hospitals with low scores on heart failure process measures (whether certain highly recommended treatments are provided to patients) said they would recommend the hospital to family and friends. Furthermore, about 40 percent of the worst-performing hospitals that treat heart failure reached the top half of patient satisfaction ratings, and 40 percent of the best-performing hospitals were in the bottom half. It is clear that the standard national surveys, developed by the Agency for Healthcare Research and Quality at the request of CMS, don't provide patients the opportunity to appropriately evaluate their care.

Notably, the survey never indicates to patients that hospital funding is tied to its results. The survey's recommended sample cover letter to patients states vaguely that the survey "is part of an ongoing national effort to understand how patients view their hospital experience." That's a major understatement. If patients knew how important the survey was, they might be more conscientious about completing it.

Gaming the system
Much like universities try to influence the *U.S. News & World Report* Best Colleges rankings by gaming the system and misrepresenting the data, many hospitals are doing whatever they can to beguile patients into giving them higher ratings. Recently, hospitals have rushed to purchase

extra amenities such as valet parking, live music, custom-order room-service meals, and flat-screen televisions. Some are offering VIP lounges to patients in their "loyalty programs."

The University of Toledo Medical Center spent approximately $50 million to renovate its hospital entry area, make all rooms private, change food and valet service vendors, and hire an executive chef. In Michigan, Beaumont Hospital spent $500,000 to install room service and a new menu including made-to-order omelets. As a Michigan consultant said, "One bad meal can mean a bad patient satisfaction score." It's probable that private rooms could give patients more rest, and tastier food could tempt patients into better nutrition. But some of that money, as at any hospital, could have been used to hire additional nurses, which would improve patient health more directly.

Because almost every question on the survey involves nurses, some hospitals are forcing them to undergo unnecessary nonmedical training and spend extra time on superfluous steps. Perhaps hospitals' most egregious way of skewing care to the survey is the widespread practice of scripting nurses' patient interactions. Some administrators are ordering nurses to use particular phrases and to gush effusively to patients about both their hospital and their fellow nurses, and then evaluating them on how well they comply.

An entire industry has sprouted, encouraging hospitals to waste precious dollars on expensive consultants claiming to boost satisfaction scores. Posters hang in break rooms even in some of the most prestigious hospitals in the country, displaying key words to remind nurses of the specific jargon they must use with patients. Some hospitals have ordered nurses to keep cue cards in their pockets, or, at several Massachusetts hospitals, to wear laminated cards around their necks that remind them to end each interaction with the words: "Is there anything else I can do for you before I leave? I have the time while I am here in your room." And across the country, administrators are telling nurses to use a patient's name at least three times per shift.

One of the most common scripted interactions is the AIDET, developed by Studer Group, a company that works with more than 800 healthcare organizations worldwide and refers to its services as "coaching." AIDET stands for Acknowledge, Introduce, Duration, Expectation, Thank. Some managers are telling nurses that they must demonstrate "AIDET competency" or they will have to undergo "remediation" or an "improvement plan." They are assessed by "AIDET auditors." Of course, patients can appreciate some of the AIDET information. It's helpful to know how long a wait will be or what a procedure entails. Certain nurses could use the reminder that their patients don't know and wish to know what is going on. But good nurses explain those things to patients anyway, and the best nurses explain them in ways most suited to each individual patient. Evaluating—and penalizing—nurses based on how well they stick to a formulaic script implies that nurses need a blueprint for basic human interaction.

More disturbing, several health systems are now using patient satisfaction scores (likely from hospitals' individual surveys) as a factor in calculating nurses' and doctors' pay or annual bonuses. These health systems are ignoring the possibility that health providers, like hospitals, could have fantastic patient satisfaction scores yet higher numbers of dead patients, or the opposite.

While role-playing can be an effective teaching tool, some hospitals have gone too far, auditioning and hiring trained actors to perform patient roles in playacting sessions for nurses to rehearse these scripts, including call-backs. That's right: Hospitals are spending valuable resources to audition and hire professional actors.

If scripting sounds like teaching to the test, that's because it is. HCPro, a healthcare consulting company, offers a tip sheet entitled "Quick Ways to Improve Patient Satisfaction Scores." The company calls the survey "an open-book test" and suggests that nurses "'remind' patients and/or their families of the 'right' answers."

It's safe to say that the Centers for Medicare & Medicaid Services, the federal agency that utilizes the surveys, does not approve of these tactics. Survey guidelines specifically state, "Hospitals must not use HCAHPS wording and/or response categories in their communication with patients." But what did CMS expect? That's like college admissions officers telling high school seniors they shouldn't get help with their applications. No hospital wants to be the only kid taking a curved test on his own, when other students use tutors who already know both the questions and the answers.

In Massachusetts, a medical/surgical nurse told *The Boston Globe* that the scripting made her feel like a "Stepford nurse," and wondered whether patients would notice that their nurses used identical phrasing. She's right to be concerned. Great nurses are warm, funny, personal, or genuine. It can be hard for nurses, who are not actors, to appear heartfelt and compassionate when they all recite the same script.

At Indiana University Health, a ten-page laminated guide instructs staff to use precise phrases and manipulative strategies. Employees cannot answer patients with "You're welcome" or "No problem"; they are told to say, "It's my pleasure!" They are directed to use strategies including "fogging" agitated patients by telling them, "You're probably right"; "verbal softeners," which replace "That never happens" with "It's possible" or "It's unlikely," and, an interesting strategy for customer service: "Nod and hum." The guide even recommends specific nodding and humming sounds: "Mmmm hum, hmmm?" and "Uh-huh."

Uh-huh. These scripts and strategies assume nurses are unintelligent, lazy, or lacking people skills. Consultants further demoralize nurses when they are condescending and out of touch. Rebecca Hendren, an HCPro administrator, wrote the following in an industry newsletter: "If you haven't found a way to drive home the importance of patient experience to direct-care nurses, find it now. You know how much reimbursement is at stake, but the rank and file caregivers still don't get it. I've written before that the term 'patient experience' has a way of annoying bedside caregivers. 'We're not Disney World' is a common refrain; people don't want to be in the hospital. 'I'm here to save patients' lives, not entertain them' is another common complaint."

Oh, they get it. Make no mistake that nurses "get" the finances that hang in the balance. But they also understand that ultimately, the way that both Medicare and hospitals are interpreting patient experience has less to do with patient health than with the image of the hospital.

The assumption that the "rank and file caregivers"—a patronizing term to begin with—fail to grasp the importance of the patient relationship undermines the nursing profession. "In our staff meetings, we've had to practice role-playing and scripting to make sure the buzzwords in the patient satisfaction survey are covered," a Washington, DC, nurse told me. "Rather than addressing the nurses being spread too thin to provide care that is good enough, they assume the nurses aren't coddling the patients adequately enough."

What annoys nurses is that the concept of "patient experience" has morphed patients into customers and nurses into "rank and file" automatons. Some hospital job postings advertise that they are looking for nurses with "good customer service skills" as their first qualification. University of Toledo Medical Center evaluates staff members on "customer satisfaction." Even the AIDET audit forms explicitly refer to patients as customers.

By treating patients like customers, as nurse Amy Bozeman pointed out in a *Scrubs* magazine article, hospitals succumb to the ingrained cultural notion that the customer is always right. "Now we are told as nurses that our *patients* are *customers*, and that we need to provide excellent service so they will maintain loyalty to our hospitals," Bozeman wrote. "The patient is NOT always right. They just don't have the knowledge and training." Some hospitals have hired "customer service representatives," but empowering these nonmedical employees to pander to patients' whims can backfire. Comfort is not always the same thing as healthcare. As Bozeman suggested, when representatives give warm blankets to feverish patients or complimentary milk shakes to patients who are not supposed to eat, and nurses take them away, patients are not going to give high marks to the nurses.

The hospital image

Recently, at a hospital that switched its meal service to microwaved meals, food service administrators openly attributed low patient scores to nurses' failure to present and describe the food adequately. It is both noteworthy and unsurprising that the hospital's response was to tell the nurses to "make the food sound better" rather than to actually make the food better. This applies to scripting, too: It does not improve healthcare, but makes it sound better.

The University of Toledo Medical Center (UTMC) launched an entire program based on patient satisfaction. iCARE University mandates patient satisfaction course work and training for every university student and employee. "Service Excellence Officer" Ioan Duca told a publication sponsored by Press Ganey, a company that administers the surveys for hospitals, "I am really focused on creating a church-like environment here. We want a total cultural transformation. I want that Disney-like experience, the Ritz Carlton experience, the Texas A&M experience. I want that kind of true belief."

"Belief" is the pivotal word here. Those laminated cards that collar Massachusetts nurses include the phrase "I have the time" not because the nurses necessarily have the time, but because, consultants told *The Boston Globe*, "patients are more satisfied with their care when they believe nurses made time for them."

UTMC is a good example of how an emphasis on patient satisfaction does not make for better care. Remember, this is the hospital that also spent $50 million on superficial changes (such as changing valet service vendors) and evaluates staff on "customer satisfaction." At the time of this writing, according to government data on hospitals' rates of readmissions, complications, and deaths, UTMC appears to be among the worst performers in the state, if not the country. UTMC has higher than average rates of serious blood clots after surgery, accidental cuts and tears from medical treatment, collapsed lungs due to medical treatment, complications for hip/knee replacement patients, and, more generally, "serious complications." In addition, UTMC made headlines in 2013 when, during a transplant operation, hospital staff threw away a perfect-match kidney that a patient was donating to his sister. Instead of focusing so intently on "satisfaction," UTMC should have spent those millions of dollars on improving its actual healthcare.

Many hospitals seem to be highly focused on pixie-dusted sleight of hand because they believe they can trick patients into thinking they got better care. The emphasis on these trappings can ultimately cost hospitals money and patients their health, because the smoke and mirrors serve to distract patients from the real problem, which CMS does not address: Patient surveys won't drastically and directly improve healthcare—but hiring more nurses, and treating them well, can accomplish just that.

Nurse satisfaction

It turns out that nurses are the key to patient satisfaction scores, but not in the way that these hospitals have interpreted. When hospitals do hire enough nurses and treat them well, patient satisfaction scores intrinsically rise. A study comparing patient satisfaction scores with surveys of almost 100,000 nurses showed that a better nurse work environment raised scores on every HCAHPS question. Furthermore, the patient-nurse ratio also impacted patient satisfaction scores. The percentage of patients who would "definitely recommend" a hospital decreased with each additional patient per nurse.

There are a few things that good work environments for nurses have in common: favorable patient-nurse ratios, positive nurse-doctor relations, nurses who are involved in hospital decisions, and task-focused managerial support. University of Pennsylvania researchers have found that better nurse work environments lead to improved patient health, too, in the U.S. and in countries as varied as Australia, Canada, China, Germany, Iceland, Japan, New Zealand, South Korea, Switzerland, Thailand, and in the United Kingdom. The researchers observed, "Increased attention to improving work environments might be associated with substantial gains in stabilizing the global nurse workforce while also improving quality of hospital care throughout the world."

When hospitals improve nurse working conditions, rather than tricking patients into believing they're getting better care, they actually provide it. Higher staffing of registered nurses has been linked to fewer patient deaths and improved quality of health, according to a study by influential nursing professor Linda Aiken, the director of the University of Pennsylvania's Center for Health Outcomes and Policy Research. For every 100 surgical patients who die in hospitals where nurses are assigned four patients, 131 would die when they are assigned eight. When a hospital hires more nurses, failure-to-rescue rates drop. Patients are less likely to die or to get readmitted to the hospital. Their hospital stay is shorter and their likelihood of being the victim of a fatigue-related error is lower. Even in Neonatal Intensive Care Units, where medical issues could be disastrous for hospitals' most vulnerable patients, the fewer the nurses, the higher the infection rates.

Hospitals and healthcare systems view nurses as one of the largest budget expenditures. However, by investing in nurses and treating them so well they want to stay, hospitals could earn millions in Medicare bonuses, avoid costs associated with employee turnover, and save money on healthcare expenses (with lower expenditures per patient, including shorter stays, less pharmaceutical use, and fewer tests).

And they would save lives. A Center for Health Outcomes and Policy Research presentation reported that in poor working environments for nurses, patient falls with injuries are 90 percent more likely to occur frequently (once a month, or more often), medication errors are 73 percent more likely to occur frequently, and hospital-acquired infections are 55 percent more likely to occur frequently than in good working environments. In good working environments for nurses, patients are 19 percent less likely to die after common surgical procedures. The presenters concluded that if all U.S. hospitals improved their nurses' working conditions to the levels of the top quarter of hospitals, more than 40,000 lives would be saved every year.

The trade-off seems like a no-brainer. Would you rather be bribed during your hospital stay with made-to-order omelets or would you rather be, for example, not dead?

Even Studer Group, the survey "coach," admitted that nurse communication is "the single most critical composite on the HCAHPS survey." (Indeed, one of the most effective ways to improve patient satisfaction scores, hospitals are finding, is to have nurses check in with patients every hour.) But Studer Group, which calls nurse communication "The Most Bang for Your Buck," is thinking backward. Nurses are more likely to communicate well in hospitals that give them the time, energy, and morale to do so rather than in workplaces that spend those bucks on a script.

If hospitals really want more bang for their buck, then instead of splurging on gourmet meals for patients (who don't select hospitals for the food), they could manage even just one covered meal break per shift for nurses; hospitals say they do this, but many don't. They could let their nurses park at work for free rather than hire a fancier valet service for patients. They could quit trying to cheat both patients and nurses by diverting funds to superfluous perks instead of investing in staffing, and, therefore, in patient care and well-being.

And if CMS truly wants "to promote higher quality and more efficient healthcare," as the Federal Register stated, it likely would meet that goal and have more accurate ratings in the process if it based reimbursement on surveys not only of patient satisfaction but also of nurse satisfaction. A simple measure of hospitals that would reflect healthcare quality, patient satisfaction, and nurse satisfaction could be to rank hospital departments by their nurse-to-patient ratios.

Instead, hospitals are responding to the current surveys and weighting system by focusing on smiles over substance, hiring actors instead of nurses, and catering to patients' wishes rather than their needs. Then again, perhaps it's no wonder that companies are airbrushing healthcare with a "Disney-like experience," a glossy veneer. One of the leading consulting companies now advising hospitals on "building a culture of healthcare excellence" is, oddly enough, the Walt Disney Company.

CHAPTER 7

THE CODE OF SILENCE:
Painkillers, Gossip, and Other Temptations

"I will abstain from whatever is deleterious and mischievous, and will not take or knowingly administer any harmful drug."

—THE FLORENCE NIGHTINGALE PLEDGE (A NURSES' ADAPTATION OF THE HIPPOCRATIC OATH)

"It's insanely easy to steal medications. There have been plenty of times where I've emptied my scrub pockets at home and found ketamine, Dilaudid, morphine, and Ativan."

—A TEXAS ER NURSE

LARA   SOUTH GENERAL HOSPITAL, April

Lara stood silently at the bed of a 9-year-old girl who had died of internal injuries sustained in a car accident. The car had crashed because the girl's parents had been fighting in the front seat. In his rage, the father had swerved the steering wheel. Now the father, uninjured, was in the hallway yelling at the trauma team, "You killed my daughter!" The mother was being treated for shock.

Lara could not bring herself to leave the dead girl's bedside. From the outside, it didn't appear as if anything was wrong with the girl. She looked like a doll. She looked like she was sleeping peacefully. She could have been friends with Lara's daughter. For the first time in her nursing career, Lara wept openly at the hospital, despite the bustle in the corridor, the other needy patients, and the footsteps that tapped into the room behind her.

An arm wrapped around her waist. Lara looked up. Brianne, a long-time ER nurse, embraced her. An elementary school nurse on her off days, Brianne was crying, too. Nurses mostly didn't afford themselves the time to cry; they forced themselves to go on with their day. Lara believed that South General nurses were more "honest" about their emotions than nurses at other hospitals where she had worked. Lara felt they were "more real, more vulnerable, they let themselves feel the moment with colleagues and patients' families. We let them know that we're sad along with them." Lara had seen South General nurses get on their knees with grief-stricken family members to pray with them.

From then on, Lara asked to work with Brianne whenever she had the chance. She got to know her as a good nurse and a good person. She watched the comforting way Brianne interacted with patients and families and she tried to emulate her. "I just felt closer to her after that. She's a genuine person who makes people feel better just by speaking with them, and I want to learn how to have that quality, too," Lara said.

After the 9-year-old's death, the trauma team could have used the Relationship-Based Care committee's debriefing room—the calm space Lara had wanted to set up for staff members to catch their breath after traumas—but it still didn't exist. The committee hadn't met in months. Lara thought she knew why. Originally, management had promised the committee that they would find coverage for the members to attend meetings. But the administrators didn't do so for the last few meetings, effectively canceling them. Even the huddles had dissolved after a couple of weeks because only Lara, Rose, and Holly attempted to gather the group when they were on duty.

Without meetings, the committee couldn't get anything done. The administrators also refused to provide any resources for the debriefing room. Now that the managers had essentially squashed the idea, Lara was out $50 for the paint she had purchased.

One day, Lara was in the resuscitation room, where nurses sent the sickest patients or performed CPR. Five other nurses, all African American, walked in, including Makayla. Makayla was obsessive about bringing her own cleaning products to the ER to make sure her area was clean, although outside cleaning products were not permitted in the hospital. Nurses knew when they were in Makayla's assigned zone because they were knocked sideways by the overpowering smell of bleach. Apparently, someone had complained, because Makayla told the other four nurses, "And one of our *latte* nurses felt the need to write me up that I had wiped down the area to make sure it was clean." The other nurses clucked sympathetically.

For the moment, Lara didn't say anything because she was outnumbered. There were only three white nurses left in the ER. When the black nurses left, Lara called Makayla back. "Makayla, I have to talk to you," Lara said, speaking slowly to think through how to avoid putting Makayla on the defensive. "I respect you as a nurse and I know that you work hard. But I have to tell you, your comment about latte coworkers is racist. It wasn't cool and I was sitting right here. I'm surprised to hear a comment like that coming from you."

Makayla balked. "Oh no no, oh my gosh, no. I call people my mocha sisters and my latte sisters, but it has nothing to do with color!"

Nevertheless, for the next month, Makayla went out of her way to be nice to Lara. Normally, Makayla was the type of nurse who shopped online while other nurses ran around taking care of patients. Now she leaped up to help Lara, greeting her enthusiastically. Lara wasn't going to waste energy resenting Makayla, so she let the incident slide.

• • •

Lara was giving report on the phone when she heard one nurse say to another, "Your girl's marked off the schedule permanently."

"That bitch is not my girl," the other nurse replied.

Lara put her hand over the mouthpiece. "Hey, you guys, you shouldn't gossip without me! Hold on!"

After Lara hung up, they told her what had happened. The day before, Fatima had been in other nurses' rooms again, hovering around patients. To the other nurses, her behavior was simply annoying. To Lara, this was an obvious sign of an addict; she was hopping from room to room in search of narcs. One of the nurses Fatima tried to "help" happened to be Ursula, who notoriously preferred to work alone, which Fatima, a night shift nurse, wouldn't have known.

Fatima saw an order for Dilaudid and took the medication from the med room. She charted that she gave the patient the medication, then apparently put it in her pocket.

Two hours later, the patient was still rolling around in pain. "Did anyone give you pain medication yet?" Ursula asked. "I see it was ordered."

"No one's been in here yet," the patient said.

Ursula looked up the patient's file and saw that someone had taken out Dilaudid under the patient's name. She rounded up the charge nurse and the nursing supervisor and they pulled Fatima into an office. They told her their concerns.

"No, no, I was just helping medicate the patient," Fatima said.

"*Did* you medicate the patient?" the supervisor asked.

Fatima tried to evade the inquiry.

"You need to answer this question: Did you give that patient the pain medication that you took out under his name?"

Again, Fatima gave a nonanswer.

"We believe you are taking narcotics. This has been a concern for a while. We need a urine sample."

"No," Fatima said, changing tactics. "I have the pain medication right here! I just didn't have the chance to give it yet." Ostensibly, she went to pull the patient's vial from her pocket. Lara wondered later if Fatima had been so nervous that she didn't think about what she was doing. The average Dilaudid dose was 0.5 milligram to 1 milligram. Fatima pulled out three 2-milligram vials.

"We're going to have to ask you to leave if you won't give a urine sample."

Fatima wouldn't provide the sample. She quit on the spot.

After the nurses told Lara the story, Lara tried to refocus their slant so that the narrative wasn't about Fatima's character. The South General nurses didn't know about Lara's own addiction. "Wow, she's got a horrible disease," Lara told them. "I hope she's going to be okay. I'm going to say a prayer for her because I'd hate for her to overdose."

Her coworkers were more empathetic toward Fatima than Lara had expected. "Drug addiction is more rampant than people would like to admit, and everyone knows it," Lara theorized. "It's not like 'Oh my God, what a shock.' It happens a lot."

Lara had mixed feelings about Fatima getting caught. She felt bad that she had not gotten through to Fatima in time. But she also was relieved. "When I got caught, because I was so scared, there was a weird sense of relief," she said. "So I'm relieved for her, too. She can move forward."

The same week, Nicola, a younger nurse, approached Lara for advice. She had been cited for drunk driving over the weekend. Lara supposed that a mutual friend must have told Nicola that Lara didn't drink. "I don't know what to do," Nicola said. "I don't want to drink anymore, but I see things here and they're sad. I go home and I don't know how else to deal with the sad things or the frustration when people are mean at work. I drink to forget about the day."

"That's why I don't drink," Lara said. "I did the same thing. I didn't just have a beer. I ordered double vodka sodas to forget stuff. But it didn't really work, and then more stuff would pile on. So I just stopped. Do you want me to help find you a sponsor?"

"Nah, I'll try to stop by myself first," Nicola said.

Actually, Lara had been tempted to drink lately. Now that she was truly on her own, her worries overpowered her. It had been harder than usual to stay clean this season, because she'd paused her college classes, which had been one of her distractions. Without John at home, classes and childcare were prohibitively expensive. Trying to work out her frustrations at the gym wasn't enough. "I've been in such a funk lately that I'm thinking being dead would be better than this," Lara admitted. "I feel like I don't have enough outlets for my fears. And I'm so tired. It pops in my head, *If you drank or got high tonight it would be okay, just for tonight.* So I'm sort of on watch."

Lara still didn't feel like herself at work; her personal issues had eroded even her confidence as a nurse. Often she came to the ER hoping she wasn't assigned to seriously sick patients because she wasn't sure that she would be able to think clearly enough to help. But sick patients always came in anyway, and, despite her misgivings, Lara found that "I don't have time to be up in my head feeling sorry for myself, because people are sick and they need my attention."

The patients at South General reminded her that her situation could be worse. One day, she spent three hours entertaining a toddler while his mother was evaluated. The patient had confronted her husband about his girlfriend and he had responded by choking her, hitting her, and kicking her pregnant belly. After the evaluation, the woman returned home and did not press charges.

Lara's coworkers continued to create last-minute openings, using her as a floater to cover for nurses during lunch, or assigning her as an extra trauma nurse. Some of the other nurses confided to her that when they got divorced, they coped by working long hours, too. "We're going to see more of you here," one of the women told her. It was nice to know that her colleagues had her back. Lara regularly volunteered to work twelve-hour shifts on three consecutive days.

On the nights that she cried herself to sleep because she felt like "a horrible mom" for missing so much of her children's lives, she reminded herself repeatedly that she was doing what was best for them. "I'm going to meetings to get mentally focused. I'm going to work to pay the bills and to cover their health insurance," she told herself. "This is making me a better person so that I can be the best mom for them."

The Code of Silence

Lara was an outstanding nurse who recognized that Fatima had an addiction. Her own troubles aside, why didn't she act sooner to try to save her colleague from what has been called "one of the most devastating diseases in the nursing profession"?

Many nurses speak about a "code of silence," an implicit vow of loyalty and protection that includes a reluctance to intervene when a fellow nurse's job or reputation may be at stake. When they observe incompetence or suspicious behavior, some nurses might look the other way if a coworker is generally skilled or if they sympathize with her professional stresses or difficulties at home. This "don't talk rule," as it has been called, is akin to "What happens in the unit stays in the unit." According to materials from a nurse home-study program, nurses "bend rules or . . . may not report other nurses for fear of being perceived as snitches or labeled as whistle-blowers. These nurses may be concerned about retribution for reporting, such as having their own work scrutinized and criticized. Some nurses do not want to become involved because confronting someone who may become angry, deny the problem, or plead for another chance can be difficult." Lara hesitated for all of these reasons.

If they report a nurse for substance abuse, nurses worry that their colleague will lose her job or her license and/or be arrested. The public, as well as fellow healthcare providers, can be quick to stigmatize substance-impaired nurses, perhaps more readily than they condemn people in other fields. As the home-study material explained, "Society, in general, views nurses as angels of mercy; nurturers par excellence; or the lily-white, starched presence of yesterday's movies. Being placed on such a pedestal has its consequences when a nurse becomes a 'fallen angel.' Society and other healthcare professionals are quick to demonize this fallen angel as a 'bad person' who now steals our grandmother's pain pills."

It's easy to see why the stigma persists: Disturbing examples abound in the news. In several states, nurses (and other healthcare providers) have been caught stealing drugs from hospitals or nursing homes for personal use. In Texas, an army medical center nurse used his own syringe to steal fentanyl, a painkiller, from vials that the center then used for other patients; he infected at least sixteen patients with hepatitis C. Nurses across the world have stolen narcotics and replaced or diluted them with tap water or saline solution, leading patients to receive saline instead of pain medication during surgery. A nurse at a nursing home in England was charged with killing a patient and taking her medication. The nurse became hooked on painkillers when she was prescribed medication for her migraines.

Because of a lack of self-reporting, it is difficult to pinpoint a reliable statistic for the number of nurses who are chemically dependent. The American Nurses Association estimates that 6 to 8 percent of nurses currently are impaired at work because of drug or alcohol abuse. While nurses abuse alcohol at the same rate as the general population, studies have found that addictions to prescription drugs, specifically, are between five and 100 times greater among nurses, a wide-ranging estimate.

What's more surprising than the number of drug-addicted nurses is their quality of work. Research shows that often the nurses who become addicted are skilled, achieving, respected medical professionals—the admired super-nurses, not the inconsistent employees, suspect from the start because of checkered pasts.

A *Journal of PeriAnesthesia Nursing* study reported that 67 percent of nurse anesthesia students with substance abuse problems were in the top third of their graduating class, while less than 5 percent were in the bottom third. Another small study described chemically dependent male nurse subjects as "intelligent, calm, and controlling individuals who were considered competent leaders in the clinical setting and whose peers enjoyed working with them." The study subjects were highly ranked nursing school students, all of whom considered themselves perfectionists and received excellent evaluations from their supervisors.

Smart, driven nurses may be more likely to become addicted to prescription medications because they "believe they have the knowledge and ability to control the use of dangerous drugs when, in fact, they do not," the *Journal of PeriAnesthesia Nursing* researchers guessed. They may be less inclined to admit to themselves or others that they are addicted because they don't believe they can fall that far. It took Lara months to realize that her stomachaches were related to an addiction; she might have made the connection immediately if she were assessing a patient instead of herself.

Like Lara, nurses are much more likely than the general public to have a family member who has struggled with alcoholism. People who have cared for an afflicted relative may be inspired to enter nursing because it is a helping profession. But this background may also be a factor in the odds of becoming addicted. If the disease runs in their family, they may be more susceptible. And if they think of themselves as someone who helps others, rather than someone who should ask for help, they might not recognize their own downward spirals in time. ER, OR, PACU, and ICU nurses, who might see unexpected deaths and tragedies more frequently, experience substance abuse in larger numbers than other nurses. As in Lara's case, the drugs can both energize them and seemingly help them to cope with these traumas.

Certified registered nurse anesthetists (CRNAs) may be even more vulnerable than other nurses to chemical dependency. Experts estimate that the addiction rate among CRNAs and anesthesiologists "has reached staggering levels," at more than 15 percent. Nurse anesthetists are at a higher risk for substance use disorders because "they're playing with rocket fuel," said CRNA Art Zwerling, an American Association of Nurse Anesthetists (AANA) peer assistance advisor. "The stakes go way up because folks are working with and diverting drugs that are much more powerful." People can become hooked on fentanyl, which is eighty times more potent than morphine, from just one exposure. "It's also that we work in isolation and the production pressure in anesthesia is horrendously escalated," Zwerling said. "People have bad times on call, remember how comfortable their patient looked when they were given fentanyl, and see that as a potential stress reducer."

Jan Stewart, a CRNA for twenty-eight years, was the president of AANA and a nationally recognized lecturer. The AANA called her "a dedicated professional whose expertise knew no bounds and who was committed to the mission of providing high-quality, compassionate care to all patients. She was acclaimed by many as a leader among leaders and a friend to all." Following back pain so intense that she needed surgery, Stewart eventually became addicted to painkillers. She died at age 50 of an overdose of sufentanil, an opioid hundreds of times more powerful than morphine. That's how many nurses, like anyone, become addicted: They have a legitimate prescription whose effects become irresistible.

Perhaps the most persuasive reason that CRNAs and critical care nurses are more prone to addiction is the same reason that nurses are more vulnerable than the public. They have easier access to the drugs. It seems intuitive but it's worth mentioning: Studies show that nurses who have easier access to these substances abuse them more often. (Doctors' substance abuse is also linked to their ease of access as well as the frequency with which they prescribe the drugs.) The effect of access is twofold. The drugs are simple to get, and the nurses' familiarity with them instills a confidence and a "pharmacological optimism" that they can self-medicate without becoming addicted. They believe they are more invulnerable than the general population.

Actually, the opposite may be true. Medical professionals tend to get sicker than the average drug addict because the medications they have access to are more powerful and habit-forming than street drugs.

How are they able to steal from hospitals, nursing homes, hospice centers, and other workplaces? Lara's initial strategy of taking only drugs that were to be wasted is an inconspicuous method. Other nurses take patients' doses for themselves and chart that they gave it to the patients, or they document, for example, that they gave a patient two pills when they actually gave only one. They might sign out drugs for people who have already been transferred or discharged from the unit. They can steal prescription pads and forge prescriptions, take samples from supply closets, back-date medical records, write verbal orders that a doctor didn't give, or take advantage when coworkers forget to log off drug-dispensing machines. Or they get creative. A nursing home RN in Florida ate the gel from two narcotic patches meant to relieve pain for a burn victim and a patient with muscular dystrophy. He gave the patients placebos.

When the addicts aren't obvious, like Fatima sticking her hand into a sharps box, their behavior may go unnoticed for months to years. Because these are often highly skilled nurses, they are, for a time, able to work competently under the influence. "Often, it's our best people," Laurie Badzek, director of the ANA's Center for Ethics and Human Rights, has said. "They have such good clinical skills that they can be impaired and still be functioning at a good level. But eventually, it catches up [with] them."

Even when managers do suspect drug abuse, they don't necessarily act immediately. Hospital administrators might wait because they want to catch the employee red-handed, assemble a file's worth of evidence, or avoid reacting in a way that might draw public attention. Many employers don't provide candid references for employees (even fired employees) because they are afraid of lawsuits or desperate to shoo them out of the workplace. Addicted nurses can then job-hop, expanding their access to the narcotics they crave.

Coworkers who observe suspicious behavior might not be certain what they saw, what it means, or what to do about it. As of 2013, nurse anesthesia programs are required to include chemical dependency content in their curricula. Other nursing schools "should incorporate prevention and education," according to the American Association of Colleges of Nursing, but the AACN doesn't monitor whether schools comply. Students become nurses who may not be adequately educated about the dangers and prevalence of chemical dependency, how to recognize when colleagues might be impaired, and how to help them. This lack of awareness "enables an abusing nurse to continue and prevents colleagues from documenting and reporting the suspicion," nurse Debra Dunn wrote in an article for the Association of PeriOperative Registered Nurses. "This passive environment condones the code of silence. Embedded in nursing culture is the practice of covering up for a colleague with a perceived problem, which can actually exacerbate the original problem rather than help the individual concerned. . . . Usually, by the time a nurse is caught and confronted, most of the people in the unit knew there was a problem."

Nurse addicts may hide their secret for as long as possible, because they don't realize they can get help without losing their license or they keep believing they can quit without assistance. They often continue to steal medications until they get caught. When they are caught, the consequences can be steep: License suspension is the most common result, and civil and criminal penalties are possible. Prosecutors can demand that a nurse not only surrender her license, but also that she never again work in healthcare. If a nurse turns herself in, however, she has a chance to save her livelihood. Nursing boards are usually more interested in helping nurses to rehabilitate and return to the workplace than juries, who are more inclined to kick nurses out of the field.

Eventually, most nurse addicts will have two choices: get help or get caught. "The good news is if the nurse enters treatment, they're covered by the American Disabilities Act, so that helps to protect their license," said Al Rundio, president of the International Nurses Society on Addictions and a practicing nurse himself. "But if they get confronted by the DEA prior to getting in treatment, they're not covered by ADA so their license is more at risk. The longer you let it go on, the bigger the problem becomes."

Certainly the focus on reparative programs rather than punitive measures is not without controversy. A relapse could endanger an impaired nurse, her patients, and her workplace. And not every rehabilitative program succeeds. A *Los Angeles Times* and ProPublica investigation revealed that participants in a California nursing board program continued to work while impaired, including more than eighty nurses whom the board deemed "public safety threats." Even when the board expelled nurses from the program, the reporters found, "The board takes a median 15 months to file a public accusation—the first warning to potential employers and patients of a nurse's troubles. It takes 10 more months to impose discipline." California eventually instituted stricter rules, and ended an anonymous rehabilitative program for doctors following complaints that doctors in treatment were bungling surgeries.

While all fifty states have treatment programs that protect a doctor's license, only forty-one have nondisciplinary alternative programs for nurses. Nurses with substance abuse issues have fewer resources than doctors, report more problems following treatment, and receive more frequent and more severe professional sanctions. The *Journal of Advanced Nursing* reported, "The rate at which nurses were placed on probation was not only higher than physicians prior to treatment, but was also disproportionately higher than doctors after treatment. . . . Therefore, the group who can least afford to miss work appears to be most likely to be reprimanded and may be least likely to seek costly legal representation."

Despite high numbers of addicted nurses, fewer than 1.5 percent of nurses are enrolled in substance abuse monitoring programs. Massachusetts, for example, has approximately 140,000 nurses, about 200 of whom are enrolled in the state program at any given time. "If you go by national statistics for drug abuse, you're talking eight to ten percent," said Douglas McLellan, RN coordinator for Massachusetts' Substance Abuse Rehabilitation Program. "If you apply those numbers to nurses in the state, there should be twelve to fifteen thousand nurses in our program. God only knows what they're doing."

Nurses can nudge coworkers to self-report by compassionately mentioning the topic. "The best recommendation is to know how to identify an impaired colleague and get them safely into treatment. Once the brain is hijacked by addiction, it's deeply in denial. Usually, an individual will not seek help. It's up to others," said Julie Rice, who manages the AANA Health, Wellness, and Peer Assistance Programs. (See page 317, for additional resources for nurses with substance abuse issues.)

Loyalty is admirable, and one of the bonds that make this subculture so strong. The sisterhood is more powerful, though, when nurses can ask their peers for aid, and when colleagues, unbidden, can reach out to help. Overlooking an addicted nurse's transgressions protects neither the nurse nor her patients. The ANA has stated that "it is every nurse's responsibility to acknowledge the needs of an impaired nurse and to help him or her regain full professional capacities."

In fact, experts warn that a nurse is legally responsible to turn in an impaired coworker; if a patient suffers, some states can bring charges against the nurse who didn't report her colleague. Reporting an impaired colleague can save her life—and her patients. There should be no stigma when, as one nursing administration journal phrased it, "the nurse becomes [the] nursed."

Nurses' patient advocacy can extend toward their fellow nurses when it is clear they need treatment. Getting them help may break the "don't talk rule," but ultimately, the code of ethics outweighs the code of silence.

SAM   CITYCENTER MEDICAL, April

At 3:00 a.m., Sam was documenting at the nurses station when she received a text from William. She hadn't seen him much since her schedule had shifted. She'd been surprised how much she had missed him. She glanced at her phone. He had texted, "Didn't know you went on a date w/ McCrary."

"What?" Sam yelped, and slammed down the phone. From Citycenter, Sam had gone out only with Dr. Spiros. Certainly not McCrary, an intern.

Where do people come up with this stuff? she wondered. Rumors of promiscuity had followed her at Pines Memorial, too. How did people not see that she was too awkward to be a slut?

She texted him back. "I didn't! Where is this coming from?"

When he replied, she learned that he was at a bar with several people from work, including CeeCee and Dr. Spiros.

She did not have time to stew about it. Medics brought in a trauma patient who had been shot in the leg. With no pulse in his foot, the staff assumed that the bullet had severed an artery. When the OR called down to say that the team was ready, the ER doctor told Sam to hurry the patient upstairs for surgery. Once Sam wheeled the patient upstairs, however, the OR nurse refused to take her report. "I don't know anything about this patient," the nurse huffed. "Just go in there. They'll take report." The nurse pointed toward the operating theater, the area bordering the operating rooms.

The patient, a young man in his twenties, was whimpering in pain. His bleeding was well controlled and his family was on the way. There was little that Sam could do for him because he was in a limbo between the ER and OR. Sam found two anesthesiologists in the operating theater. "Do you know who I can give report to?" Sam asked. She had to thoroughly update a nurse from the admitting department on the patient's condition before she left.

"No," said the more senior doctor. The doctor turned to the patient. "Have you ever had surgery? Did you have any problems with it? Okay, open your mouth." Anesthesiologists checked patients' mouths before surgery because if the patient had a large tongue or the roof of the mouth hung low over the throat, then intubation would be more challenging.

Sam wasn't allowed to return to her other patients until she gave report on this one. After several minutes of waiting around, she asked the male anesthesiologist about the delay.

"We're still waiting for the on-call vascular attending to get here," he answered.

"Can I get fentanyl for him while you're figuring this out?" she asked. Her patient desperately needed pain medication.

"No," the doctor said, and resumed doing paperwork.

Sam, exponentially more confident than she had been in August, stared down the more senior anesthesiologist. "Really? You want him to sit here in pain when you guys were the ones who wanted him to come upstairs and I could have gotten him pain medicine downstairs, so he's up here in pain because of you?"

The doctor sighed. "Fine," she said, and wrote the orders.

By the time Sam retrieved the fentanyl and administered it to the patient, there was still no news on the surgery status. Sam was frustrated: She had nowhere else to take him, and she had five other patients downstairs who needed her, including a woman in bad shape and bound for the ICU.

Typically, taking a patient to the OR was a quick and easy trip. If Sam had known this visit would have been so complicated, she would have asked a less busy nurse to escort the patient. Sam circled the floor, asking the anesthesiologists and the PACU nurses for the name of the person who had given the okay for the patient to come upstairs, so she could finally give report.

"Here," the senior anesthesiologist said, handing her a piece of paper. "Call this number. It's the senior surgical resident."

Sam had a feeling the doctor was giving her a task just to shut her up. Reluctantly, she dialed. "Who gave you this number?" the surgeon barked when Sam reached him.

Sam realized that the anesthesiologist had given her the doctor's personal cell phone number rather than his hospital cell. ("That was completely inappropriate! It was a doctors' pissing match," she said later.)

The surgeon ranted to her about the anesthesiologist. "Anesthesia had no right to give you this number," he fumed. "No one is on their game tonight. The OR has had problems all week."

Sam fidgeted with her glasses. *The ultimate goal is taking care of the patient, not seeing whose stethoscope is longer,* she thought. She didn't care about interdepartmental politics; and she had heard that tension between surgeons and anesthesiologists was common. Sam just wanted to get back to her patients.

"I need to go. I'll just leave the patient in the PACU with the nurses."

"That's fine," the surgeon said.

When Sam wheeled the patient to the PACU, she found a nurse surfing the Internet. "The surgeon says to leave the patient here. I have five other patients to get back to."

The annoyed nurse took Sam's report. Later, Sam learned that after seventeen hours of surgery, the patient would make a full recovery.

When he left the bar, William called Sam. He explained that someone had blurted out that she had dated the intern and a few of the residents, making her sound like the hospital tramp.

"Funny, I didn't realize I was going on these dates," Sam retorted. "Who said this?"

William sighed. "Okay, so what happened between you and CeeCee?"

"Oh. Well. CeeCee and I don't make beautiful music together," Sam said, and recounted when CeeCee had discovered that Sam said she drove her crazy.

William told her that the group had been drinking. Out of nowhere, CeeCee had declared that Sam had been hostile to her. She launched a diatribe about what a horrible person Sam was, and then claimed that Sam had dated four guys who worked at the hospital (none of whom Sam had dated). Dr. Spiros had chimed in, "Oh yeah, she went out with me, too," as if something had happened between them. Dr. Spiros was now dating another tech.

CeeCee then burst into loud drunken tears. "Why do you even like her? She's so mean!" she wailed to William. Surrounding bar patrons turned to watch her drama.

Eventually, CeeCee's friends had dragged her out of the bar before she could make more of a scene. Later that night, CeeCee texted William: "I hope you and I are okay."

Once again, Sam was beset by unfounded rumors of promiscuity at her workplace when she tried hard to avoid drama, let alone extraneous personal interaction in general. And self-absorbed girls like CeeCee didn't even get embarrassed by their own ridiculous behavior.

People had done this to Sam since high school: Because she was quiet, they projected onto her a superficial image of the character they assumed she was. Because she was opinionated and did not mince words, that character was often negative, and because she was chesty and men found her attractive, that character was presumed to be a slut. Sam tried not to get caught up in what other people thought about her. But these types of rumors motivated her to work even harder. "I need to be really good at what I do if people are going to think ill of me without even knowing me," Sam explained.

Sam didn't claim innocence; she shouldn't have said CeeCee drove her crazy when they were interns. But at least she had respected CeeCee as a nurse. Confronting CeeCee would only exacerbate the hostilities. "I feel like I should wear a plaid skirt and carry a backpack to work," Sam told a friend. "It's like high school, except for the dying people."

MOLLY   May

CITYCENTER MEDICAL

Carl, one of Molly's Citycenter patients, weighed more than 300 pounds and was missing a leg. He complained of chest pain but wouldn't let anybody treat him. When Molly told Carl, who was homeless, that his discharge orders had come through, he crossed his arms. "I'm not going anywhere because I want to kill myself," he said, smug.

Molly was unfazed. This was a popular game among homeless people so that they could score "three hots and a cot." They would come to the ER, try to gain admission to the psych ward, refuse treatment, and get a warm bed and meals. Many hospitals automatically admitted any patients who mentioned depression or suicide, even if the staff knew they were bluffing. But here was one thing Citycenter did right: Molly called the crisis counselor, who spent three minutes with Carl, then told Molly to resume discharging him.

"But I'm going to kill myself!" Carl insisted.

"The crisis team thought there was a low likelihood of that, so here are your discharge instructions," Molly replied.

"Just set them on my chest because when I go outside and kill myself, I want everyone to see them and know you don't give a shit about me."

The man leaned back in his chair, splayed his arms dramatically, closed his eyes, and pretended to be dead.

Molly shrugged. "Okay." She set the instructions on his chest and walked away. "I'll call security to come help you," she said while leaving. Carl wheeled himself out of the building.

Later that week, the hospital's CEO sent an email to the ER staff. The Joint Commission had performed a follow-up investigation and had determined that the ER could keep its accreditation. Molly was stunned. "I can't believe they found nothing!" she said.

The department had improved slightly; Molly didn't get sick to her stomach on the way to work anymore. For her, the biggest difference at Citycenter was that the ER created a dedicated trauma nurse position. Because Molly was always assigned to the sickest patients, she was now able to concentrate on Zone 1 patients without having to abandon them immediately whenever a trauma came in.

The rooms still weren't as clean as they should have been, however. Nurses were supposed to call housekeeping as soon as they discharged each patient, a practice that had quickly fallen by the wayside. And now that TJC had come and gone, Citycenter was trying to control the budget by creeping the nurse-patient ratios back up again.

Undercover observation conducted for this book during this time revealed multiple violations of TJC standards. At one visit, floors, supply drawers, carts, tubes, and equipment were spattered with dried blood; urine samples had spilled across a counter in a lab room; and bloody gauze was strewn over a sharps container. In the utility room where nurses brought pregnancy tests, a urine-soaked absorbent pad lay on the counter beneath a hospital binder.

Elsewhere, the ER didn't use proper TJC notification systems, and a tech blatantly flirted with a visitor as he held down a patient who was being catheterized and moaning in pain. And when a pregnant woman came in with vaginal bleeding, worried that she had miscarried, the ER doctor discharged her without bothering to tell her that her fetus was fine.

Molly would continue to take shifts at Citycenter, but she knew that it wasn't the hospital she was looking for. She didn't like that Citycenter and

Academy hired new grads directly into the ER and that she was considered one of the most senior nurses, with only ten years of experience. "There's no one for me to learn from," she said. And while Academy was easy, it was too easy for her to consider working there permanently: "There aren't enough sick people there for me to help."

ACADEMY HOSPITAL

Molly took a few extra shifts at Academy so that Jan, the grateful young nurse, could spend time with her long-distance boyfriend. Molly was in triage when she heard a familiar voice in the lobby. "How long have you been waiting?" a man asked other patients. "What're *you* in for? I'm suicidal." It had been only six days since Carl had visited Citycenter, at least when Molly was working.

Molly finished assessing her patient. When she finally called Carl back, he was sweet as pie. "I'm suicidal," he repeated, giving her puppy eyes.

"Uh-huh," Molly said.

"Are you a nurse?" he asked her.

"Yes, I am. I've also been *your* nurse at Citycenter."

"Really? How'd you know it was me?"

Nurses called patients like Carl "frequent flyers" or "hospital hoppers." One man called an ambulance at least once a day to visit the Pines, Academy, Avenue, or Citycenter ERs, complaining of "uncontrollable farting." Molly was incredulous that EMS was required to transport him and that ERs gave him IV fluids, food, drinks, clean clothes from the hospital's donation closet (collected mostly from staff), and a bed. Several drug-seeking frequent flyers claimed to have sickle cell disease and asked for Dilaudid. This was a shrewd tactic; nursing schools taught students not to treat sickle cell patients as drug seekers because they had legitimate pain. Many doctors went ahead and gave these patients six Percocets, then discharged them.

"Why do y'all give in?" Molly asked one of the Academy doctors about a drug seeker. "He goes to a different hospital every day of the week. I would bet my last dime he sells the pills."

The doctor shrugged. "I sometimes find it easier to give drug seekers what they want than deal with them raising hell."

Molly knew of one drug seeker who had gone to an ER every day that Molly had worked for the past six years. "I want to know how he still has Medicaid," Molly said. "That's a minimum of $600 to $800 per visit. Conservatively, that's $1.3 million to support a drug dealer and addict. I worry about what will happen to healthcare costs if we can't get our act together." When he became her patient, she used a larger needle than necessary on purpose to draw his blood; it was the only time she had ever practiced punitive medicine. Less than an hour after he left Citycenter, he showed up at another ER to get more drugs.

The ER abusers who most infuriated Molly were the homeless people who claimed they had a problem—chest pain, abdominal pain—so that the ER, as required, started a full workup. Then they would ask for a sandwich. "Some will even admit that the only reason they came in was for a sandwich," Molly said. "Are you effing kidding me? You think taxpayers should pay six hundred dollars so y'all can get a sandwich?!"

Another abuse of the system routinely occurred on weekends at Citycenter, which wasn't far from a jail. Come morning, people incarcerated for drunk driving or drunk and disorderly conduct looked for any excuse to leave their cell. Police escorted a 22-year-old college student from jail to the ER because he had slept in his contact lenses and claimed he needed eye drops. "To avoid doing paperwork, sometimes the police ask patients if they want to go to jail for being drunk and disorderly in public or to the hospital. Of course they choose the hospital!" Molly said.

ERs were packed with nonemergencies. One patient came into the ER complaining of acne. Another man showed up because his barber told him he was going bald. And then there were the patients who visited the ER simply because it fit best with their schedules. Several patients checked in because their doctor couldn't see them until the afternoon. One of Molly's Academy patients had an outpatient prescription for an ultrasound, but said, "The line was too long, so I came here." Instead of paying $200 for the exam, the patient's insurance company would now pay the minimum of $600 for an ER visit plus approximately $500 for an "emergency" ultrasound.

Molly decided to emulate another triage nurse, who greeted patients by asking, "And what's your emergency today?" While the phrasing wouldn't embarrass patients enough to leave, perhaps it would discourage them from coming to the ER the next time they had a nonemergency complaint.

JULIETTE   PINES MEMORIAL, May

Juliette was working triage with Erin when a thin man in his late fifties came in. He had pulmonary problems and his doctor sent him to the ER because of an irregular EKG. His vitals were fine. "Do you have any chest pain?" Juliette asked him.

"No."

"Any cardiac history?"

"No."

"Shortness of breath?"

"No."

Erin took the man to the adjacent lab room while Juliette began triaging the next patient. "Are you doing okay?" Juliette heard Erin say.

"I'm okay," the patient said.

"Do you feel weak?" Erin asked as she began to place the IV.

"No," the man said. "But . . . I think I need to lay my head back."

"Juliette!" Erin shouted. "You need to come in here!"

Juliette rushed to the room. The man looked unconscious. "Do you have a pulse?" Juliette asked.

Erin already had her hand on his neck. "No, I don't have a pulse."

Juliette quickly checked the man's neck. She couldn't find a pulse, either. He was barely breathing. "Agonal respirations," Juliette said. "I'm starting CPR." Juliette pushed the Code Blue button behind the chair and began doing chest compressions. Erin began airway management with the ambu bag.

They wheeled the chair toward patient rooms while continuing CPR. "We need a bed!" Juliette announced as they dashed through the double doors.

Juliette had performed solo CPR twice (as opposed to working a code with a hospital team). Once, she and her daughter were going out to dinner when a businessman collapsed on the sidewalk. Juliette did chest compressions until, finally, he came to.

That time, Juliette had been scared because she was outside of the hospital setting, without equipment and staff that could support her. She had not been afraid recently when a 50-year-old woman came into the ER for bradycardia, a slow heart rate. Juliette had asked a new tech to put in an IV, but when she returned to the patient's room, she discovered that the tech instead had gone to triage. Juliette was hooking the woman up to the cardiac monitor when the patient took her hand and said breathily, "I just want to say good-bye."

"What are you talking about?" Juliette said. The words sounded strange.

"I'm just going to say good-bye," the woman repeated. Her eyes went vapid. The monitor showed the woman's heart rate plummeting to zero. There was no time to press a code button. There was no IV to utilize.

Juliette didn't even think. She did the precordial thump, a method of resuscitating a patient in cardiac arrest: She raised her forearm to her nose and brought it down hard on the woman's chest. The woman opened her eyes and burst into tears. She seemed to know exactly what had happened. "Thank you," she whispered, grasping Juliette's hand. "Thank you."

When Juliette yelled at the tech, he blamed the new zoning rules, another Westnorth policy. "They set up our priorities so we're supposed to help with triaging," he complained.

"If I ask you to put a line in somebody who has a heart rate below forty, you need to put the line in," Juliette said.

Shortly after the tech placed the IV, the woman's heart rate rose. Later, Juliette learned that the woman received a pacemaker.

Juliette wasn't going to lose this cardiac patient, either. Her arms ached but she continued the compressions. About a minute later, his eyes flickered. He looked around in a daze. "What happened?" he asked. Juliette savored the adrenaline rush.

Erin turned to her. "He was totally gone! His eyes were rolled back, he was shaking all over before he went still!" Agonal convulsions sometimes preceded clinical death.

Carla, a nurse in the clique, walked by. "Way to save a life!" she told Juliette, who smiled.

Once the man was in a room, the cardiologist came downstairs to evaluate him. "It turns out he also passed out at the pulmonologist's office when he got some bad news, so it might have just been a vasovagal reaction," the doctor told Juliette. A vasovagal reaction is a nervous system reflex that causes a sudden drop in heart rate, resulting in less blood pressure to the brain and leading some patients to lose consciousness. The doctor nevertheless admitted the man to the hospital's cardiac unit.

When asked later what it felt like to save a life, Juliette said, "It's amazing. That's what we're supposed to be doing but it doesn't happen every day. Most days are about cleaning up poop or addressing abdominal pain or nasty family members."

At the start of her shift the next morning, Juliette looked over the charts for Mr. Morse, a 77-year-old who had come in overnight. She noticed that the night shift had made a mistake. The man had blood in his urine and low blood pressure, but the nurses hadn't done a three-way bladder irrigation. These irrigations weren't pretty, but they usually worked. If a man had a large clot in his bladder, treatment involved inserting a catheter into his penis to flush out the clot.

Juliette caught the night nurse before she left.

"The doctor didn't order it," the nurse said.

"But if he has blood in his urine, you need to make sure there aren't any clots."

"Well, I would have needed an order and it wasn't ordered."

Juliette stared at the night nurse long enough to convey that she knew the nurse had been lazy; she should have requested the order from the doctor. Juliette called urology, then explained to Mr. Morse what she was going to do.

"Mr. Morse, I have to flush your catheter with saline to get rid of the blood clots that are in your bladder," she said. After a tech inserted a Foley catheter, Juliette rolled up her sleeves. With one hand, Juliette held the man's penis, and with the other, she pushed saline from a 60-cubic centimeter syringe through the catheter until the output was no longer cranberry-colored. Periodically, she also dialed a clamp on a tube to transfuse the patient's blood. The skinny old man resisted. "What are you doing?!" he yelled. "What are you *doing* down there?!"

Juliette looked up. Mr. Morse was feebly trying to bat her hands away from his penis. Finally, he gave up. He put his hands behind his head and, with a look of bemusement, said, "Young lady, you ought to be ashamed of yourself."

Juliette laughed and again explained what she was doing. Throughout the morning, she kept returning to the room to irrigate, but sometimes she didn't get to Mr. Morse quickly enough. When his catheter got blocked, his sheets would saturate with fluid. Mr. Morse would try to escape the wet sheets. The staff would find the man naked and halfway out of bed while undergoing both a blood transfusion and a three-way irrigation.

Her coworkers were annoyed with Mr. Morse, but Juliette liked him. He was funny, sweet, and slightly senile. "I wanted to make him better," Juliette said later. "He required so much work, but I didn't mind because he was sick and he needed help."

She was checking on another patient when out of the corner of her eye, she saw Priscilla treading cautiously down the hallway. *Uh-oh*, Juliette thought. She left the patient's room to investigate. There was Mr. Morse, naked in the hall, a bag of blood hanging from his arm, and a catheter hanging from his penis.

"That's it, Juliette, you have to put him in restraints," Priscilla said.

Juliette escorted him back to his room. She wasn't going to put the poor man in restraints. Juliette stayed past the end of her shift to take Mr. Morse upstairs to the cardiac unit. He would undergo surgery the following day to find the source of his bleeding.

The next afternoon, Juliette called the urologist from home to ask what had happened to Mr. Morse. "He made it," the doctor said. "We were able to close off the bleed."

Nursing involved deaths and inevitable disappointments, hostile visitors and slacking coworkers. But just often enough, something wonderful happened to remind a nurse why she loved the field.

During her next shift, Juliette was meticulously sanitizing her cell phone when someone from the hospital's professional development committee found her. He handed Juliette a certificate and her clinical ladder portfolio. "Congratulations! You got the promotion! You're a clinical level four!"

Juliette grinned with pride. A step up on the clinical ladder was almost comparable to an extra degree after her name, and clinical level 4 was considered a major accomplishment. She had put in time and effort to develop her expertise and prove her work ethic. A $2,000 bonus and a raise accompanied the promotion but, to Juliette, the promotion wasn't about the money. It was about recognition of a job well done.

CHAPTER 8

DON'T GET SICK IN JULY:
Nurses' Secrets—What Patients Need to Know About Their Hospitals and Their Health

"Nurses are frequently put in situations of conflict arising from competing loyalties in the workplace, including situations of conflicting expectations from patients, families, physicians, colleagues, and in many cases, healthcare organizations and health plans."
—*CODE OF ETHICS FOR NURSES*, PROVISION 2.2

"Somewhere along the line, when we lost the long white skirts, pleated blouses, and nursing caps of yesteryear, we also seemed to have lost the public's respect. I would gladly go back to the nursing days of Florence Nightingale and Clara Barton to have the respect they had from society. I wish I could start a revolution for ER nurses specifically; we are the rock stars of nursing, but are treated like the red-headed bastard stepchild."
—A NORTH CAROLINA ER NURSE

"So many things are just simply bullshit. I don't know why I was surprised. I guess I always thought that when it came down to *people's lives*, things like making money no matter what wouldn't be so important."
—A TEXAS ER NURSE

LARA   SOUTH GENERAL HOSPITAL, June

A divorced South General nurse in her late forties was trying to get pregnant through IVF. Afraid to give herself the injections, she asked Lara if she could come to her house and inject the daily shots. Lara agreed without hesitation. The nurse repeatedly tried to pay her for her time. "I'm not taking your money," Lara told her. "Just tell me, how did you talk to your first husband when you guys were separating? What did you tell him? What did you wish you didn't say? Help me with advice."

Friends called Lara all the time to ask medical questions or to have her look at their injuries. Before she had kids, Lara slept over at her friend's father's house for two weeks because the family couldn't afford a twenty-four-hour nurse and the man had painful bone cancer. "I'd never accept money for stuff like that," Lara explained. "I do that in a heartbeat."

She loved that people felt they could ask her opinion and that she could almost always help them. Being a nurse was more than a job. "It's kind of who I am," she said. "Nurses can truly make a difference in someone's life. In the ER, even if it's not a true emergency, an accident is something a person will never forget. That ER visit for stitches could be one of the worst times for people, and a nurse can make it a little better for them, putting them at ease, alleviating some of their fear. Even a pillow or blanket for someone's grandma can make a difference. It may sound silly, but that makes nursing special."

Now that the bills had started to come in and she was paying them, Lara had begun to grasp how well she could manage life as a single mom. She could support her family. She couldn't spend as much time at home with her children as she wanted to, but she was doing her best, and she knew that her kids were safe when she left them with John. She had started to emerge from her funk, though she was still disappointed that she wouldn't be able to go to PA school. She put her bachelor's degree classes on hold, unsure of when she'd be able to continue them.

At work, she was able to focus more on her patients. One morning, Lara was working trauma and precepting a nursing student when an ambulance brought in a heavyset woman in her forties. While driving, the woman had told her spouse she didn't feel well, then pulled over and went into cardiac arrest. The medics had briefly brought her back to life twice by the time she arrived at South General with no pulse. She was blue from midchest up.

Dr. Alisa Hawkins, a well-respected ER doctor, ran the code. While the team performed CPR, she reviewed several possible algorithms that could have caused the heart attack. Dr. Hawkins stuck a needle in the patient's chest in case fluid had pooled around the heart.

"It's not fluid," Dr. Hawkins said. "Did we cover our Hs and Ts?" ("Hs and Ts" was a mnemonic device to help medical professionals run through possible causes for a cardiac arrest.)

"We did," Lara said.

"Could be a blood clot in the lung," said the doctor. "Does anyone have any ideas?"

"What do you think about t-PA?" Lara asked. Tissue plasminogen activator could save a patient by dissolving a clot or it could cause a patient to bleed out and die. Typically, the procedure required the patient's or family's written permission. In this case, the patient was technically dead anyway.

"Yeah, let's do it," Dr. Hawkins agreed.

The other nurses backed away from the bedside, suddenly busying themselves with other things. Lara looked around. She hadn't given t-PA in more than a year. "Wow, really, guys?" Lara said. "Okay, I'll do it."

As the others continued CPR, Lara explained to her student what she was doing. "Usually you give a bolus [a single dose] of t-PA first intravenously, and if the patient is still alive, you do the second half over thirty minutes. But we don't have that kind of time, so we're doing a straight push over three minutes," she said. She encouraged her student to take a turn performing CPR, which she had never done before. "It can be creepy to do CPR because you often break ribs even when you're doing it right, so I want you to know what that feels like," Lara told the student. Lara stood by the intravenous drip, slowly depressing the plunger of the syringe of t-PA while instructing the student how to set up the remaining medication. Afterward, the student thanked her effusively.

The patient, as expected, didn't make it, but Lara found that she had completely regained her medical confidence. "I felt like it came back and flowed," Lara explained to a friend, relieved that she was back on her game. "I didn't feel like I was struggling to think through anything. That was nice, because my fear at work was missing something on a patient. As a team, we didn't miss anything. T-PA might have helped, so I was glad I thought of it. Even though the patient died—really, she came in already dead—I walked out of there knowing I did every single thing I could possibly do to try to save her."

• • •

A week later, Lara was having a tough morning. If getting through a divorce was a process that took two steps forward and one step back, then today was definitely a step back. She dropped the kids off at school and cried on the way to work. *This sucks*, she thought. *I'm an old single mom and now I'll have to date again.*

Now that she was single, she supposed she could do what many nurses she knew had done: They kept an eye on the firefighters and policemen who brought patients in to the ER. At her former hospital, at least half a dozen nurses had married men they had met that way.

Lara had always been drawn to men in these positions, both because their uniforms were a turn-on and because they understood what it was like to be a nurse. "They're protectors and caregivers," Lara said. "Maybe it's the whole men-in-uniform thing. Firemen stay in shape, and they have that sensitivity about saving lives. You feel safe when there's a fireman or policeman around. They know what it's like to look into the eyes of a parent whose kid just died. They understand."

Still, Lara was scared to return to the dating world. How would she find the time to get to know someone when her life revolved exclusively around her kids, job, meetings, and workouts? Puffy-eyed and sulking, Lara moped into work at 11:15 a.m. "Are you coming from the breakfast?" Holly, that day's charge nurse, asked her.

"What breakfast?" Lara asked. "I'm just coming in to work a couple hours."

"You were supposed to be at the breakfast for the finalists," Holly said. Lara didn't know what she was talking about. "You're a finalist for Nurse of the Month!" Holly said.

Lara laughed uneasily, thinking this was like an "Oh, you're mom of the year" joke.

"The ER director sent you something in the mail." Holly was serious.

"I moved," Lara said.

For the rest of the day, Lara bounced between excitement that her work had been recognized and guilt that other ER nurses' work had not. Her nomination was the talk of the department. Someone had taped a copy of the letter listing the finalists to a medicine cabinet for everyone to read. The ER nurses hadn't even known the honor existed, because in the history of the award, no ER nurse had been a finalist.

Lara sensed some resentment from her coworkers toward the ER management. "If our managers can nominate us, why haven't any of us been nominated all this time?" they said. "I work my ass off!"

The other nurses mostly teased Lara. They kidded that she missed the finalists' breakfast on purpose because they knew that socializing with "management types" made her uncomfortable. Lara joked back that administrators must have "just been feeling sorry for me because I'm such a pathetic loser in a pathetic place right now."

Another nurse snorted. "If that was the case, I would have been nominated a long time ago."

Lara poked her head into the ER director's office to say thank you.

"Girl, you work hard. It doesn't go unnoticed," the director said.

The boost came at just the right time. Until the nomination, Lara hadn't realized how badly she had needed some sort of validation that at least something was going right in her life.

Two weeks later, when Lara arrived at work, Holly said, "You're the hallway nurse from eleven to twelve, but then you're going to the luncheon." Nurses nearby snickered.

"A luncheon? I'm not going, guys," Lara said.

"You have no choice. You won the award!" Holly said. She purposely had not told Lara she won until the last minute, so Lara couldn't duck out.

Lara was stunned. Word spread quickly, as usual in the ER. Within an hour, everyone was referring to Lara as Nurse of the Month. "Hey, Nurse of the Month, can you help me in Room Nine?" "Can you roll this patient off the backboard, Nurse of the Month?" Only one nurse sneered at her, nastily sniping things like, "I'm going to take my patient up, if that's all right with *you*, Nurse of the Month."

Lara laughed it off. As great as it felt to win, she was a little mortified that she had been chosen above equally deserving coworkers.

At noon, Holly and the education coordinator found Lara in the hall. "I'm going to watch your patients for you," the education coordinator said, clapping Lara on the back.

In the elevator, Lara squirmed. She was no good at chatting up bigwigs. She envisioned sitting across from them, stumbling to make conversation.

When Lara poked her head into a fancy doctors' conference room she had never seen before, the head of the hospital stood up and came over to her, his arm extended. "Hello!" he said, shaking her hand. A handful of department heads and three nurse finalists from other departments were seated at a table laden with catered food. *Wow, I would've looked really jerky if I hadn't shown up*, Lara thought.

As the hour progressed, she relaxed. The hospital chief was laid back and friendly. Mostly the group talked about the hospital. The chief discussed upcoming events and how much he appreciated the employees. But he kept coming back to the ER, which he seemed particularly excited about. "The ER holds this hospital together," he said.

Lara listened with pride. "That made me feel grateful I was a part of it," she told a friend. "I could have lost my license for my ridiculous behavior in the past, so this was a nice reminder. It got me energized to keep doing what I'm doing."

The chief presented her with a trophy engraved with her name. Because it was too large to fit in her locker, Lara left it at the nurses station. But her coworkers moved the trophy to wherever Lara was working. If she was in a patient room, when she left, the trophy would be waiting for her at the door. If she went to the meds room, the trophy would magically appear in the hallway outside of it.

Despite the Nurse of the Month teasing, most of Lara's coworkers were gracious. "You really deserve that," one told her.

"I can see why you got it," said another.

After work, Lara reflected to her friend. "I love nursing. I think I have the coolest, best job in the world," Lara said. "I probably feel more passionate about it now than I ever have, because it got taken away from me. I am so lucky I didn't go to jail. I am so lucky to be here with my amazing kids. Most nurses who did what I did lose their licenses or don't get to return to an area that would be a trigger, like the ER. I am never going to stop being grateful that God gave me another chance to be a nurse."

When she took the trophy home and told her children about it, they were so proud of her that they carefully placed her award on the shelf that displayed their soccer trophies.

SAM   CITYCENTER MEDICAL, July

Since the charge nurses had begun to assign Sam regularly to Zone 1, the area with the sickest, most interesting patients in the ER, she was happier at Citycenter. Zone 1 procedures ran relatively smoothly on the night shift that could have been disastrous during the day. One night, the ER had two coding traumas simultaneously in the trauma bay, a CPR in progress on a patient with no pulse, and an unresponsive trauma patient. All eight nurses on duty came to work on them. Half the nurses were back-to-back, facing the gurneys; their bottoms kept bumping into each other as they worked. They were able to save one of the patients. Had this situation occurred during the day, Sam believed they would have lost both because the situation would have been even more chaotic.

Doctors on either shift made mistakes, particularly the new ones, particularly in July. One day, Sam watched with horror as a surgical intern inserted a chest tube into one of her patients and dropped the needle—a tree trunk of a surgical needle—onto the floor. "I'll pick it up later," he said, at Sam's look. After the procedure, the surgeon strode toward the door.

"The needle!" Sam reminded him.

He briefly glanced around, said he couldn't find it, then left the ER. It was a generally understood courtesy that doctors, nurses, and techs took care of their own sharps. Too often, new doctors didn't clean up after themselves, or wouldn't handle patients' urinals, "as if they were too cool for school," in Sam's words. She was tired of these doctors "acting helpless when they're really just lazy." She paged the surgeon. He called her back ten minutes later.

"You need to find that needle," Sam told him.

"I'm busy on the floor," he said.

"I don't care. The patient has HIV and hep-C. None of the nurses or cleaning staff are going to accidentally get stuck by that needle and get hep-C because your dumb ass dropped it and you won't come find it."

"I might be an hour."

"That's fine, but you better come down and find it because I am not your handmaiden."

Shortly thereafter, the surgical team's four medical students were in the patient's room on their hands and knees. Sam scoffed. Who did the surgeon think he was? It was hardly safe for people to crawl on the ER floor. They found the needle within five minutes. The surgeon did not return downstairs.

There were a few physicians Sam enjoyed working with, like Dr. Geiger, who now would come to Sam specifically for assistance. But too many young doctors were careless. Recently, while a new surgeon was working on a patient, the connector between the chest tube and the drainage chamber came apart and fell onto the floor. The surgeon picked it up and put it back into the sterile chest tube. Sam stared openmouthed.

"Do you want another one? How about we change that out?" Sam said.

"Oh, well, yeah. Of course," the doctor said, as if she had planned to all along. Sam ran to get another drainage chamber.

On her night off, Sam called William. He had ramped up the teasing lately, for no discernible reason. She wondered whether CeeCee had blabbed again, in which case Sam wanted to clear the air with him.

"I didn't pee for at least eight hours last night," Sam said by way of introduction.

"Me neither," William said.

Sam smiled. "The fact that this conversation seems perfectly normal to us is odd in itself."

"Hey, to do this job well, you need to be dedicated."

"Yeah, in between getting berated and fighting with the lab, actually getting to help people is kind of awesome."

"You have to keep it all in perspective," William said.

Sam took a breath. "So what's the deal?" she asked. "You're acting like you're twelve. Get your head out of your ass."

"I'm interested in you, Sam."

Sam almost dropped the phone. "Um, I guess I hadn't noticed that." Her heart pounded. Her dream guy was interested in her? This was the stuff of movies, not the kind of situation that happened in Sam's real life.

"Well, yeah."

"You have a girlfriend and I'm not going to be your little side fling."

William paused. "Actually, things weren't going so well. We broke up a couple of months ago."

"Oh." Gears turned. "You're single?"

"Yes, I am."

Sam processed this information. "I wish you'd told me that sooner. This whole time I thought you still had a girlfriend."

"I don't talk about my personal life at work, so there's no way you would have known. And I didn't know if you felt the same."

"Well . . . maybe we should hang out," she said.

"How about now?"

Within half an hour, he was at her door. They stood there for a moment.

"Hi," she said.

"Hi," William answered. They grinned sheepishly at each other.

Ten minutes later, they were settled on Sam's couch, watching a movie. When William slid his broad muscled arm around her shoulder and leaned toward her, Sam's mind raced. *Okay, sure, I guess that's what we'll do now.* As she kissed him back, she realized it didn't feel awkward at all.

Nurse Confessions: Behind-the-Scenes Secrets from the Front Lines of Healthcare

As a fly on the wall of a hospital, you can learn a wealth of healthcare secrets, some of which are entertaining and some of which could save your or a loved one's life. In front of an undercover reporter conducting research for this book, an exasperated attending physician at Citycenter shook her head as she corrected a colleague's error. "Just trying to get through July," she muttered. Her reason for saying so exposes a major secret about hospital life. Here is that secret, and others that nurses want you to know.

Don't get sick in July.

Every year in teaching hospitals at the start of July, medical students become interns, interns become first-year residents, and each successive class of residents moves up a level. These new doctors are immediately thrust into direct patient care. As the National Bureau of Economic Research reported, "On day one, new interns may have the same responsibilities that the now-second-year residents had at the end of June (after they had a full year of experience)."

This upheaval causes what healthcare workers call "The July Effect" in the United States and "August Killing Season" in the United Kingdom (where the shift happens in August). The changeover harms patient care, increasing medical errors, medication dosage mistakes, and length of hospital stays. Most strikingly, in July, U.S. death rates in these hospitals surge 8 to 34 percent, or between 1,500 and 2,750 deaths. University of California San Diego researchers found that fatal medication errors "spike by 10 percent in July and in no other month." In the U.K., August mortality rates rise by 6 to 8 percent as new doctors are tasked with surgeries and procedures that Britons say are "beyond their capabilities." Patients in English hospitals have a higher early death-rate when they are admitted on the first Wednesday in August than patients admitted on the previous Wednesday.

Nurses always make vital contributions, but it is during these months in these hospitals that their vigilance is particularly paramount. Experienced nurses have seen more than inexperienced doctors. They know more about the hospital's equipment and pharmacy system than someone new to the unit. "Nurses are correcting every error and preventing major mistakes every day," said a Maryland solid-organ transplant nurse.

The residents who know enough to know what they do not know, and, therefore, listen to and seek out nurses for advice, are not the problem here. But too many residents, enamored of their MD status, won't ask for help. "I've had doctors give orders for meds to be given IV that should never be given IV. And residents have asked me what a med was," said a Washington State ER nurse. "They need to be guided and given lots of hints: 'Would you like me to call the doctor who specializes in that? Would you like me to order that test?' I don't think they realize everything the nurse does for them and the patient. We cover their asses."

Some patients who must be hospitalized in July for particularly complex procedures might consider avoiding teaching hospitals. Approximately 25 percent of U.S. hospitals are teaching hospitals, which patients can identify by checking the "About Us" page on a hospital's website.

There are dead people in there.

If you see a large gray box in the hospital hallway, that's not meal services. It's probably a container holding a deceased patient, a Pennsylvania nurse said. "The morgue is never labeled that, either. They'll call it something like 'Anatomical Pathology,' so if someone passes by, they won't think there are dead bodies inside."

We know secrets about your doctors.

Nurses have much to say about the doctors with whom they work. Perhaps more than anyone else, they are certain which doctors they would trust with their lives and which ones to steer clear of. "If you want to know if a medical facility or a doctor is any good, ask a nurse [away from that facility]," said a Washington State nurse. "Unless she doesn't like you, she will tell you the truth."

Some of their observations include:

- After the procedures, when witnesses dwindle, doctors aren't necessarily on their best behavior. An Arkansas nurse watched a cardiovascular surgeon check whether his female patient was awake. The doctor pulled down the sheet and twisted the patient's nipple. "My reflex was as if he had done this to me: As soon as he touched her, I smacked him on the arm. He gave me the dirtiest look," the nurse said. "A lot of nurses would like to smack their doctors once in a while."

- "Sometimes residents practice procedures on a patient after a code [such as using a needle and catheter to remove fluid from the sac around the heart]. We put a stop to this in our hospital," said a nurse in the South. This practice does not occur as often as it used to. Before simulators were sophisticated enough for doctor training, physicians would "spend up to eight hours practicing on the deceased, which prevented family from coming in, and they did not know why," a North Dakota nurse said.

- "The highest-rated heart surgeon at my hospital, according to *U.S. News & World Report*, is the one I would least want to have operating on my family member," said a nurse in the Northeast. "It seems that more of his cases come out of the OR with bleeding complications. The consensus among the nursing staff is that this happens with him more frequently than our other surgeons."

- "Some physicians, especially psychiatrists, make rounds at night or very early in the morning so they don't have to talk to the patients," said a Texas nurse.

- "Doctors don't always tell the truth, they often blame others to protect themselves, and some doctors are lazy. They want nurse practitioners to do the work and they bill for it [in the hospital]," said a Michigan nurse. "I've seen a lot of mistakes: misplaced lines, nonsterile technique, lying to patients or withholding information, wrong medication dosage. There was an incident where equipment in the OR was not used correctly and it affected the patient. No one told the family, but staff knew."

Some doctors and nurses are placing bets about you.

Several nurses confess that they have wagered on patients. Guess the Blood Alcohol is a common game, where actual money changes hands. Other staffs try to guess the injuries of a patient arriving via ambulance. And surgeons have been observed playing "games of chance" during operations, placing bets on outcomes of risky procedures.

Hospital codes can vary, but the meanings are fairly common.
Different "codes" mean different things at the hospitals that announce them over the loudspeaker, but here is a sampling of what they can stand for (some hospitals use different colors to refer to these scenarios):
- Code Blue: patient in cardiac arrest
- Code Pink: infant abduction (all exits are secured)
- Code Red: fire
- Code Orange: hazardous material spill
- Code Silver: hostage or weapon situation
- Code White: communications equipment or computer system failure
- Code Green (or Condition Green): combative patient
- Code Gray: tornado warning/severe weather; a combative or violent patient or visitor

Depending on the hospital, a bomb threat can be a Code Gold, Code White, Code Black, or Code Yellow (among others).

Sometimes hospitals don't want patients to guess what a page means.
Some hospitals further disguise codes to announce bad news. A page for Dr. or Mr. Firestone can indicate a fire. Code Strong signals hospital security that a patient or visitor is becoming aggressive. "MSET" (Medical Surgical Emergency Team) alerts staff to an unresponsive patient. At some hospitals, Code Lavender means that a doctor or nurse is overtaxed; at Ohio's Cleveland Clinic and Hawaii's North Hawaii Community Hospital, a rapid response team including a chaplain and a holistic nurse offers the healthcare provider Reiki, light massage, healthy snacks, water, and a lavender bracelet so that he or she remembers to take it easy.

Actually, Code Lavender, which is called approximately once or twice a week, is meant to achieve what Lara had hoped for with the debriefing room. Originally, Cleveland Clinic's healing services team was created in 2008 for patients. "Then we started getting called more and more often for staff. If you care for one nurse, you've cared for twenty patients," said the

Reverend Amy Greene, director of spiritual care. Healing services is most often summoned for staff after an unexpected death. The team arranges backup coverage and finds the nurse or doctor a quiet corner in a break room or broom closet where she can listen to meditative music, talk to a chaplain, or simply find a few moments of peace.

The break lasts approximately ten minutes, which is enough to recharge someone, Greene said. "Compassion is self-perpetuating and reinvigorating, and it doesn't take that long. Symbolically, this says that what happened to you is important, you're important, and the institution has your back. Caring for the caregivers is much more important than we thought in times past."

We have our own secret codes, too.

The most universal code that nurses call among themselves is a Code Brown, an elegant designation for an inelegant situation: a defecation mess. If you hear nurses referring to "liver rounds," they are probably talking about happy hour. Non-gastrointestinal doctors who say they are doing "G.I. rounds" are likely taking a break to eat.

Some people impersonate nurses, and you have no idea.

A medical/surgical nurse who has worked in a pediatrician's office warned that when you call a doctor's office to speak to a nurse, you might not actually reach one. "Parents call to ask the nurse a medical question about their child. The medical assistants, who *are not* nurses, pick up the phone, say, 'Hello, this is the nurse,' and then give advice," she said. "This is illegal and dangerous. Parents have no idea this is going on. MAs have taken a one- or two-year certificate training program, may not have a college degree, and do not have a license. I've heard them give incorrect advice. We worked hard to get where we are and it makes me mad when people think they can easily do our job. We have a two- or four-year college degree and a Registered Nursing License. If you are calling in to a doctor's office, make sure you know who you are speaking to." Ask whether you are speaking to a licensed nurse or to a medical assistant.

Sometimes we goof around with the medical equipment.

When a department is slow (more likely on the night shift), hospital staff members have several props with which to entertain themselves. Nurses told me about wheelchair-racing down the hall, playing darts with needle syringes and rubber-glove balloons, having squirt gun fights with saline syringes, and bowling with (empty, clean) urinal jugs for pins. A Louisiana nurse and her coworkers do lunges down the hall at three in the morning to stay awake during the night shift. On slow nights in a Virginia ER, nurses used to pull clothes out of the donation box and have runway fashion shows. "The little things you do with coworkers can make your shift exponentially better," said a Minnesota travel nurse. "We listen to music all night, do the wobble wit (a group dance like the electric slide) at the nurses station, or have catwalk competitions down hospital hallways."

We gossip about our patients . . . when they deserve it.

Plenty of nurses confessed that they gossip about their patients, although they take care to respect the patients who respect them. "If there's something really different, salacious, or disgusting, we love to tell our coworkers," said a Washington State nurse. One story involved a mentally disturbed patient who went into the bathroom, cut off his penis, and threw it across the waiting room. Most patients don't have to worry, though. A Maryland cardiovascular ICU nurse said, "The funniest stories involve the crazy patient who did something with poop."

We might use a larger needle than necessary.

In a practice that is not often discussed in the medical profession, some nurses occasionally use larger needles than necessary to "punish" obnoxious patients, as Molly did with the drug seeker.

Sometimes we break the rules.

If breaking a rule will help a patient or protect a colleague, some nurses will break it. A Midwestern nurse at a hospital that refuses to give nurses overtime has clocked out before she was finished so she wouldn't get written up for working overtime, and then risked being penalized anyway by returning to the unit to care for her patients for free. "That used to never happen, to work in a place where you're afraid to make a mistake or you'll be fired," she said. "Overstaffing the next shift is a mistake, ordering too many or too little supplies is a mistake, not answering the phone within the first few rings is a mistake."

In an Indiana NICU, "personal interaction is against policy," a nurse said. Nevertheless, "When the kids are hurting or dying and the parents aren't there, we will sing, kiss, rock, and love on the babies. We pull the curtain for privacy. You can't help but smooch their tiny feet. That spot behind their neck is especially a sweet place to nuzzle. They love it."

Sometimes we lie to you.

Nurses occasionally lie to protect a patient's feelings or to make him feel more comfortable. A New York nurse told *Reader's Digest*, "When you ask me, 'Have you ever done this before?' I'll always say yes. Even if I haven't."

"We usually know the results of your tests before the doctors talk to you. We can tell when a loved one will have a bad neurological outcome but can't tell you," a Virginia pediatric nurse said. "We usually know what we would do, but can't tell you what it is. We have to give you information in a nonbiased fashion so that you can make those decisions, even if we are dying to tell you what to do." Even if patients specifically ask nurses, "What would you do in my situation?" some healthcare institutions have told nurses they cannot answer directly.

We are gross.

Nurses use toilet humor and are known for telling disgusting medical stories over meals (to the chagrin of non-nurse dining companions). And when they are out in public, "we are secretly looking at people's arms to determine where we would start an IV," an Arizona nurse said. "Sometimes if I'm out with a group of nurses, we're like, 'Wow, look at those veins. I could hit those from across the room.'"

At Pines, medics once brought in a 90-year-old man who had passed out after choking. A nurse grabbed a pair of forceps and pulled out a piece of chicken the size of half a deck of cards from his trachea. By then the man had gone too long without oxygen. Once his time of death was announced, Molly helped clean him up and tidied the room. "Then I washed my hands and immediately went and ate my lunch: leftover chicken!" she said. "Nurses are gross."

Your DNR might be ignored.

Nurses in several states confirmed Dr. Clark Preston's statement to Juliette that a family member can override a DNR, or Do Not Resuscitate order. While some nurses said that at their hospital, patients with signed, current DNRs are not resuscitated, several nurses told me that saving patients with DNRs "happens all the time." The most common scenario occurs when an elderly or chronically ill patient with a DNR requires resuscitation and a family member tells the medical team to "do everything you can" to save the patient. Particularly if the family member has power of attorney (POA), nurses said he can change the plan of care.

"Theoretically we're supposed to honor the DNR, but oftentimes the family will want the patient treated because they see the DNR as 'giving up.' We tell the families that the DNR means the patient didn't want to be worked on if they're in this situation. If the family tells us to do everything, though, then usually we have to, because the POA has the legal right to make medical decisions even if it overrides the DNR. Even if there isn't a POA present, the next of kin still have the right to make decisions," said a travel ER nurse based in Texas. "Families want us to 'do everything,' and if we let the patient die, we're accused of killing them by refusing care. Because a POA can decide for the patient, it gets tricky if we try to honor the DNR. Basically it's a lose-lose scenario."

Medical providers can override a DNR because of a family dispute "and not really risk punishment," said Arthur Caplan, Division of Medical Ethics director at NYU Langone Medical Center. If a DNR is vague or was filled out many years ago, physicians might doubt whether they can trust the document. "Think of a DNR as something that tells you a person's wishes, but it's not a binding order. Sometimes it can't be binding because it's confusing. Sometimes the family's screaming a lot and we don't want to cross swords with them," Caplan said. "Sometimes the nurses don't feel involved in these discussions with the physicians and don't know why they decided not to treat further, so the nurses line up with the family. I have seen nurses fighting with each other about a DNR."

It's unlikely that the medical team will be penalized for overriding a DNR written with a patient's consent, Caplan said, "because if you're trying to keep someone alive, no lawyer will take that case." If the medical team abides by the DNR, despite the family pushing them to override it, the family could sue, but would most likely lose. However, "Hospitals are afraid of being sued unnecessarily, so they tend to do what families want. Usually the patient with a DNR is pretty sick, probably not even talking. The family's talking a lot. The easier route is to just do what they want. Forget a lawsuit; hospitals just don't want to get into a fight. There's a lot of deference to families who make a lot of noise, particularly families who are rich. I'm not sure every family counts the same."

If there is time, hospital ethics committees can review cases in gray areas, such as when family members disagree. A New Mexico travel nurse said that physical fights break out among families over this issue. "People get desperate at the end," said a California travel nurse.

The outcome may depend on the physician's comfort with discussing the DNR process with family members, said a Canadian critical care nurse. "Patients have told me they wanted a DNR because they 'can't take it anymore,' but doctors have overridden the patients' decision because they said I was 'playing God' by advocating the patient's request to die peacefully," she said. When a Maryland hospice nurse told a physician that her patient had an advance directive for "no life-support measures in an end-stage condition," the doctor replied, "I am not a lawyer," and resuscitated the patient anyway.

The hospice nurse said that the waters would be less murky if doctors told patients' families, "Your loved one filled out a form after a conversation with her physician that said she would want only comfort measures at this time. We would like to honor those wishes."

Nurses also wish that healthcare providers did a better job of explaining resuscitation efforts to families, and that family members had more honest end-of-life discussions with each other. "I think if people better understood exactly what 'do everything' entails, they would be less likely to demand it," said the Texas travel nurse. "Performing CPR is probably going to break multiple ribs, [some patients] will almost certainly die in the ICU after a prolonged barrage of horribly toxic medicines, and we can put someone on a ventilator but their anoxic brain injury means they're never waking up again. If we could show families how much more horrible it is to prolong treatment of a dying person, perhaps they would choose differently."

There are "codes"... and there are "slow codes."

Some medical teams have a hush-hush way of dealing with discrepancies between a patient's DNR and family members' demands. In some hospitals, as a Missouri nurse told me, "there are lots of unsavory things that the polite public would make hay with," including the slow code, a little-known term to the general public. Various units have different designations; at a Canadian hospital, medical teams distinguished between a full code, which they called "code 55" and a slow code, or "code 54."

Some physicians will unofficially call a "slow code," which will never appear in a patient's chart, if a coding patient is elderly or chronically ill. The signal notifies a team that they are not expected to revive the patient but should go through some of the motions anyway. "Responders literally walk slowly, are slow to respond, give medications slowly, or hesitate to intubate so that the patient is unlikely to be revived," said a Midwestern nurse.

"It's often for the sake of a family who needs to see us doing something, anything," said the Texas travel nurse. "We do [these things] when it's painfully obvious someone is so far gone they can't be saved, and occasionally when the patient is a DNR. The CPR and meds are the same, because it's a dangerous line to cross if you withhold standards of care, but if it's a young, healthy guy, we might code for 45 minutes, whereas with the elderly terminal DNR we will only code for 10. Usually we do a round of CPR, check for cardiac motion on the ultrasound, and then call it."

A Midwestern nurse said the slow code is "not ethically appropriate" and used only by certain teams. As a Washington State PACU nurse explained, "Pounding on the chest of an extremely frail, elderly person is torture, not lifesaving. In instances when family members insist that we do all to keep them alive, it's understood among the staff that the patient is a 'slow code' and no one hurries to get a crash cart. We do, of course, make the patient as comfortable as possible."

We do not treat all patients equally.

Nurses work hard to give patients the best healthcare they can. But not every patient gets the same treatment. Respectful patients might get faster, kinder service than the pain-in-the-ass down the hall; grateful, thoughtful patients might get some additional perks: extra snacks, the newest DVD releases from the library, the best magazines from the waiting room, additional diapers in the postpartum ward. "I'm always happy to get something for the patient if it will make them more comfortable or make them smile," said an Arizona pediatric nurse. "When an able-bodied parent asks me to fill the water pitcher because they don't want to walk to the galley to fill it themselves, I get just a little pinched. The hospital is not a hotel, and I'm not your personal butler."

The secret is simple. If you're not nice, said a travel nurse in Colorado, "rest assured that every single person involved in your care will know about it. While we will never cut corners on medical care, you can be damn sure we won't be doing you any favors or even acting as if we like you. You'll get your extra cup of soda or warm blanket a lot quicker if you're not a dick. Also, we won't talk about you in the nursing station if you're nice. We reserve the trash talk for the mean ones."

And sometimes we are told to treat certain patients better.

Many hospitals treat VIPs better than the average patient, saving deluxe private rooms for celebrities and officials who know about them. While some luxury rooms are available to any patient who can pay, like those in the Johns Hopkins Hospital's Marburg Pavilion, others are kept secret.

Nurses described accommodations that look more like spacious luxury hotel suites than hospital rooms, with kitchenettes, beautifully glass-tiled bathrooms, and other amenities. In one Washington State hospital, when a VIP comes in, the staff combines two rooms to make a large one. They are instructed to bring in a large-screen TV and the "VIP furniture." After the VIP is discharged, a nurse there said, the furniture is removed and stored until the next VIP admission. "They do this for rich and influential people and we nurses are disgusted by it. Nurses are taught to treat each patient as an important person and to give our best care to each one of those patients. Personally, I find it insulting to our profession," she said.

A Washington, DC, hospital has a VIP unit devoted to patients such as visiting foreign dignitaries, senators, and professional football players. "It doesn't have typical hospital furnishings; the rooms are much bigger, with fancy bedspreads, decorative pillows, and lavish curtains," said a Maryland nurse who used to work at the hospital. "The patients are served excellent food—much better than the food on the regular floors—and the nurses cater to their every whim. It's a restricted floor, with no access from the regular elevators. Most people don't even know this floor exists."

In California, celebrities have been offered their own private nurse; one nurse said that her hospital "definitely bent over backward for anyone they considered important." In other states, some administrators give nurses special instructions when VIPs arrive and will personally check in on the patient. When the nurses give report, they are supposed to remind the incoming nurse that the patient is a VIP.

VIP care becomes problematic when those patients unnecessarily take up resources that more critical patients need. "Sometimes they will get a one-on-one nurse or we are all told to give them extra-special treatment," said a New Jersey nurse. "They can't hold back a room in the ICU, but I have seen critical patients who should be next to the nursing station moved so that a relation of a board member, a big donor, or celebrity could have the better room even if their condition didn't warrant that level of observation. At another local hospital they had an entire VIP section set aside; those rooms were not to be used for the riffraff."

Every hospital at which a Virginia nurse has worked had "a couple of rooms, if not a floor, dedicated to VIPs, which is often hidden. At one hospital, there was a room specifically maintained only for the use of a very famous person with a very crappy heart. They'll get the best food, the nicest rooms, the most accommodating physicians, and the nurses who are easiest to push over. The hospital left the VIP section completely empty unless a VIP was present. No intermingling. Politicians have such a warped sense of how the healthcare system works, because they never have to be part of the actual system."

This discrepancy in care frustrates nurses, who observe firsthand when patients with similar health concerns have extremely different experiences. "Some people abuse the system and take up more of the doctor's time, utilizing more resources and even taking up ICU beds. Sometimes they even dictate staying in the ICU extra days," said a Washington, DC, pediatric nurse. "It doesn't seem fair that one family is having a cushy experience, while the other is sleeping upright in a chair crammed in the corner just because they aren't famous."

We know you better than your doctor does.

Nurses want patients to remember that from the moment patients enter a hospital to the moment they leave, nurses—not doctors—will be more intimately involved with their care. "The doctor is at your bedside for all of three minutes unless you're getting intubated or coding. The nurse is the one rapidly assessing you at the door, immediately determining what interventions need to be made, so that when the doctor does come into the room he has something more intelligent to say than, 'Well, we're going to get some labs and an X-ray,'" a North Carolina ER nurse said. "I get you undressed, on the monitor, cleaned up if needed. I will wash the blood and vomit out of your hair, and not gag or make you feel embarrassed that you're sick. I'm the one who will go to the doctor and tell them you are having nausea, pain, or a neuro status change because suddenly you think it's 1988. That will be the reason that you get a head CT, and we find a brain bleed and contact the neurosurgeon. And then I will be at your bedside for the next three hours while we wait, reassuring your mother. You will hardly ever see the doctor. You will always see the nurse."

Sometimes we are forced to stay at work against our will.

Nurses told me about regularly being expected to stay 30 minutes, an hour, or 90 minutes past the end of their shift without pay. But inclement weather is an entirely different beast. "Our last snowstorm, they wouldn't release the nurses until enough of the next shift made it in to cover the hospital," said a Midwestern nurse. "During these times, we work, sleep, and shower at the hospital just to work another couple of shifts. If we can't make it in, they'll get us with a snowmobile if they have to. They've had army reservists drive out in their Hummers to get us. They make us stay against our will. Sucks when you have kids at home or are a single mom without a strong support system."

Nurses don't necessarily choose to work fourteen- to sixteen-hour shifts. "When nurses have attempted to refuse this overtime, we have been told this would be considered 'patient abandonment.' Nurses are not willing to abandon our patients," an Ontario nurse told the Canadian Federation of Nurses Unions.

Don't get sick on weekends, either.

Depending on the hospital, weekends and nights can be riskier for patients, some nurses said. "Half of this hospital is unavailable during those hours. A STAT echocardiogram isn't always STAT," said a Midwestern nurse. "There isn't maintenance available, so you have to wait for Monday to get things fixed, which can be frustrating when it's a procedure light that could help you out, or you have to move a patient because the monitor broke. If you run out of supplies, you have to make do until Monday."

If a hospital's technicians don't work weekends, nurses might have to send special labs to outside techs, which can delay a patient's care. Because some organizations' housekeeping services are reduced on weekends, nurses have to take time away from patients to clean patient rooms or hunt down equipment themselves. If a hospital needs to work on the computers or the water system, the outages can also cause increased wait times. "It's risky sometimes because of the staffing issues. We can't staff for the what-ifs," said a NICU nurse. "At night, our NICU nurses go to ER and Peds to draw labs and start IVs. That takes nurses off our unit and we're temporarily understaffed. If there is a code or a delivery when this happens, it can be bad."

Sometimes we put alcohol in your feeding tube.

If a patient with a history of alcohol abuse needs open heart surgery, a Maryland Cardiac Surgical ICU nurse said, he or she might get alcohol (supplied by the pharmacy) with hospital meals or through a feeding tube to prevent alcohol withdrawal symptoms such as elevated heart rate, anxiety, and shaking. A nurse in an Oklahoma cardiac unit who has administered this treatment to a patient said that, on physician's orders, the pharmacy brought 60 ml of bourbon each night to the nurse and watched her pour it down a nasogastric tube. While this method is considered "old school"—hospitals more often give patients Ativan—"it is funny to say that you gave your patient a shot of bourbon as a medication order," the nurse said.

That's going in your chart.

Ever wonder what nurses are writing in your patient chart? If you say something offensive or off-the-wall, nurses chart it. If your family member creates issues, that goes in the chart, too. "I always chart when a patient is difficult or belligerent. I keep it objective and write direct quotes; it's funny to have to type 'Fuck you, bitch' in medical documentation," Molly said. Nurses chart everything because if a patient later sues the hospital, the evidence can diminish the patient's credibility. Along those lines, Molly added, "If you claim to know someone, be someone, or say you're going to sue, it doesn't increase your chances of getting better service."

You might not need the surgery your doctor says you need.

"Sadly, doctors and doctors' offices bully people into having tests and procedures they don't really need, especially the elderly," said a Tennessee travel nurse. Similarly, "If I could talk to my patients *before* open heart surgery, I would probably advise thirty percent of them not to have surgery," said a New York nurse. "Our fee-for-service healthcare system incentivizes doctors and hospitals to advise aggressive, high-cost treatments and procedures. Doctors undersell how much rehabilitation the successful recovery from heart surgery requires. Most patients tell me they didn't know the recovery would be as difficult as it is. Every time I see patients over eighty-five opt for an aortic valve surgery because they were becoming short of breath on exertion, I scratch my head because many of these high-risk patients will not get back all the faculties they had before the surgery, and some won't even make it out of the hospital."

We cry over you.

They might not do it in front of patients, but nurses do cry about the people they treat, whether with patients' families or on their own. "Because I'm a burly man, [people think] I am not affected as much, but I am," said an Oregon murse. "Sometimes I cry on the way home from work."

Some stories are too sad for even the most composed nurses to bottle away until after the shift. Nurses in Kansas, California, and other states told me about child abuse cases that led them to sob in the break room. A young Illinois nurse was taking care of a woman in her nineties and learned that "even when a patient can't respond and their eyes are closed, they can probably still hear you." While the nurse was talking to the patient, her preceptor laughed at her. "She can't hear you and she'll never open her eyes again. Stop wasting your time. We have a lot of other patients to get to," she said and walked out the door. The nurse took the patient's hand, squeezed it, and said, "I believe that you *can* still hear me, and I promise to take good care of you." The woman lightly squeezed back. "I knew she heard me and I lost it right there. Even when patients may not be there all the way, they are still someone's mother, father, sister, or friend, and deserve to be treated with respect," the nurse said.

TV shows don't get it right.

In reality, nurses manage many of the duties that viewers see doctors performing on TV, such as inserting an IV or catheter. "I laugh when I see shows like *House* or *Grey's Anatomy*, where doctors are pining at the bedside of patients, giving them medications, or administering treatments. Doctors do nothing of the sort," says an Arizona clinical education specialist. "They come by once a day, take a short look at the patients, review their chart, make orders, and leave."

A New York hospital night-shift nurse said that sometimes his patients don't see a doctor or a PA overnight. The nurse diagnoses the patient, determines the course of treatment, then treats the patient himself, sometimes without even calling the PA to approve the orders for fluid boluses, antihypertensives, diuretics, and other medications. "We reserve calls to the PA for fairly urgent matters, and handle whatever other issues arise ourselves. This can mean doing things that are beyond our scope of practice, but most of the PAs appreciate the uninterrupted sleep and will generally cosign any orders once they make their rounds in the morning."

One major difference between TV and real-life hospitals is that many patients who survive in the shows would die in real life. A Texas clinical nurse specialist said, "In almost forty years, I can count on less than ten fingers the number of patients I've helped resuscitate who walked out of a hospital under their own steam. Even in a hospital, ninety-five percent of all codes fail to resuscitate the patient in an unwitnessed arrest" (if a person is found without a pulse and no one saw him/her collapse).

Some supervisors ask us to do things for which we're not trained.

One reason an Air Force nurse left civilian nursing was because her supervisor skimped on her unit's training. When an oncologist decided to admit patients to her unit who needed twenty-four-hour chemotherapy treatments, a nurse gave the staff a brief talk on the chemotherapy administration. "After that talk, we were expected to hang the agent [administer the medication] whether we felt comfortable with it or not," she said. "I told my supervisor I did not feel comfortable administering the agent to any patients and she told me I was trained to do it. I told her a brief talk does not validate my competence to hang the drug. To protect the patient, I refused to do it. People who treat these patients have years of experience on an oncology unit, generally. I was working on a multiservice unit with ten to twelve patients at a time and could not care for the patient receiving the chemo appropriately. I didn't want to administer the medication if I couldn't monitor it effectively. From that day on, I was criticized for not wanting to do anything out of my realm of comfort."

You make us value life.

Many nurses say that their work makes them appreciate the fragility of life. "Recently a perfectly healthy man slipped on the floor and severed his spinal cord. He will be dependent on others the rest of his life," a Minnesota travel nurse said. "Think about not being able to hug your child, feed yourself, or scratch an itch. If every human spent even an hour on a nursing unit, it would change their perspective on what's important. Before every hike I take, I dedicate it to one of my patients who will never be able to hike again. It's a gratitude I never knew before I became a nurse."

For nurses, each individual patient death is precious and, collectively, the deaths a nurse observes become a kind of *memento mori*, reminding her to cherish life. This appreciation is one of the threads that weaves nurses together. "Nursing keeps me grounded in my own mortality even when I'm helping someone die," a former Army nurse in New Jersey said. "It's a holy profession."

We will try to do everything we can to help you.

California nurse Jared Axen was holding a dying hospice patient's hand when he began to sing an old hymn. The woman, who didn't speak English, hadn't been responsive in days. But when Axen sang to her, she squeezed his hand, a response that soothed the woman's family. Six years later, Axen, a classically trained musician, sings to some of his patients every day. "It gives them their humanity back," he said. "Music is a common language that helps me connect with my patients." Many patients also claim to feel better and to need fewer pain medications, Axen said. "It's become a vital tool for my patients and their families."

. . . And to save you.

In 2012, Emory University transplant nurse Allison Batson donated a kidney to 23-year-old patient Clay Taber, a recent Auburn University graduate. The 48-year-old nurse, a mother of four, told the media that her children were around Taber's age, so his sudden rare illness, Goodpasture's Syndrome, hit her hard. Batson, a hero, saved his life, and Taber now considers her part of his family. "I wasn't even supposed to be on her floor, but the floor I was supposed to be on was full. And now we joke that we're kidney-in-laws," Taber told me. "I'd been on dialysis almost a year-and-a-half by the time I got the transplant. It was definitely something I never expected her to do. Just how selfless she is, willing to do something for a stranger, to change my life on a dime, was very heroic. I like to say she's an angel sent down to help people."

LARA   SOUTH GENERAL HOSPITAL, July

Lara was attempting a new exercise as she worked out at her gym's boot camp for the third time this week. Because she wasn't taking her college classes, she had stepped up her already frequent exercising, determined to throw her energies into something that would give her a natural high.

"Take this," her trainer said, handing her a forty-five-pound plate. Lara was skeptical; forty-five pounds was a lot of weight for a five-foot five-inch woman weighing 123 pounds. As she swung the plate from between her legs to overhead, she felt a horrible burning sensation in her stomach.

"Something doesn't feel right," she said.

"Wimp!" a boot camper called out.

"Wimp-ass!" shouted another. The trainer laughed.

"Oh my God, my stomach is killing me," Lara said. This wasn't a sore-muscle kind of feeling. It felt like someone was tightly squeezing the area near her belly button. Determined not to lose face, Lara finished the set of fifteen reps and moved on to her next exercise.

At work that afternoon, Lara noticed a bulge in her lower abdomen. She knew what it was right away. So did her coworkers. Every once in a while, she tried to push her intestine back where it belonged. "Girl, your shit is sticking out!" the nurses told her. "Quit pushing it back in!"

When Lara finally saw her primary care doctor, he diagnosed the hernia and sent her to a surgeon. "I have two things to tell you that you're not going to be happy about," the surgeon told her. "One, you need surgery. Two, you're not going to be able to exercise for six weeks afterward."

Immediately, Lara's mind began whirling. *I'm going to get painkillers! I get a free high!* she thought. For the next two weeks, she was appalled at how quickly her thoughts corkscrewed into old, familiar patterns. *This is so exciting!* a little voice exulted. *Maybe I should ask for the prescription ahead of time so I don't have to get it after surgery. Maybe I should go pick it up now!*

A few days before the surgery, Lara still hadn't told anyone about it. At work, the vials beckoned once again.

JULIETTE   PINES MEMORIAL, July

Care at Pines had continued to falter. The Westnorth Corporation had decreed that instead of having a second trauma doctor on call in case multiple traumas came in, which often happened with car crashes, the ER physician would be considered the second trauma doctor. The new policy alarmed Juliette. "The ER doctors have never, ever covered trauma," she explained. "And now, in addition to covering patients in the ER, they're also going to have to cover trauma? The hospital is doing that just to save money. They're sacrificing the patients."

One morning, Wendy, an older part-time nurse, came sauntering through the ER, flashing a large diamond ring. "I'm engaged!" she told an ER volunteer. "Guess what? I got engaged!" she announced to the secretaries. She navigated the department throughout the day, telling everyone except for Juliette. She kept walking by her, pretending Juliette wasn't there.

Wendy hadn't spoken to Juliette for about a year now, ever since a disagreement over a patient. A woman had come into the ER with a dislocated ankle. When Dr. Hughes, a resident who picked up ER shifts only occasionally, went into the patient's room, Juliette was across the ER, in the bathroom. At the sound of a bloodcurdling scream, Juliette raced to her patient's room to find that the resident had pulled her ankle into place without offering any pain medication.

Juliette gasped and rushed to the patient's side.

"It's okay," the doctor said to Juliette as he turned to leave the room.

"He just relocated the ankle," another nurse said.

"Without pain meds?" Juliette said. She turned to the patient, who was incontinent because of the agony. "I am so sorry he did that to you without any pain medication."

"What are we giving her?" Juliette called out to the doctor.

"Dilaudid."

Juliette rushed to the medication dispenser, pulled the medication from the machine, then ran back to the patient.

"Thank you," the patient whispered, and reached for Juliette's hand. Juliette sat with her for a few minutes, then changed the patient's gown.

As the patient settled in to rest, Juliette took the other nurse aside. "Why wasn't she medicated?" she asked.

"We asked for pain meds and the doctor said it was fine, she didn't need it."

"Juliette, hallway please," the doctor said from outside the room.

"We had the pain meds to give her," Juliette told him.

"I had to do it right away," Dr. Hughes said. "There wasn't time."

"No, we could have medicated her," Juliette said.

The doctor shook his head. "Next time that happens, you need to call me out of the room and tell me you have a problem with what I'm doing."

"Fine, but I believe what you did was wrong," Juliette said.

From the nurses station desk, Wendy, openmouthed, watched the conversation like a Ping-Pong match. "I can't believe you said that to the patient and were disrespectful to Dr. Hughes!"

"My first responsibility is to the patient, Wendy, not the doctor," Juliette said. "The patient deserves care."

At 65, Wendy was a nurse from a time when nurses stood up to give their seats to the doctors. "The doctor deserves respect and you shouldn't speak to him that way," Wendy scolded.

"Doctors aren't God," Juliette told her. "They need to be called out when they're wrong."

Wendy hadn't spoken to her since. Meanwhile, Dr. Hughes and Juliette, who had a good professional relationship, easily resumed working together with no problems at all.

• • •

Juliette was eating lunch with Molly on their day off when Molly mentioned that she had seen Bethany at a nursing conference. "She said something that you're not going to like," Molly added. Juliette looked at her, puzzled.

"This is going to hurt your feelings," Molly said. "This is going to upset you. But I have to tell you."

"Okay," Juliette said. She figured she had angered somebody at work. It wouldn't be the first time.

Molly paused. "Well, Bethany said that in her interview for senior charge nurse, Priscilla told her, 'I heard the only reason you were applying for the job was so Juliette wouldn't get it.'"

"But I didn't even apply!" Juliette said.

"I know. Bethany said you two were friends and she never thought that, much less said that," Molly said. "But then Priscilla said, 'Between you and me, I would never hire Juliette for senior charge nurse.'"

Juliette sat back hard in her chair. "Wow" was all she could say. Her eyes welled. She hadn't applied for the job because she had no interest in it. She liked being charge nurse on occasion, and coworkers had told her she was great at it, but she didn't want a full-time supervisory job. Her heart was bedside, with the patients, doing the job she loved.

Molly continued, "I wanted you to know what she said because Priscilla is not the same person to your face as she is behind your back. I know that you've trusted her and that you've been confiding in her. I thought you should know what she is saying to your colleagues about you because I'm worried she'll tell people about your private stuff, too."

Juliette was dumbfounded. She had believed that Priscilla liked and respected her. Priscilla had never written Juliette up, never called her into her office, never told her she was performing poorly at any aspect of her job; rather, she had frequently encouraged Juliette to be charge nurse. How was Juliette supposed to become a better nurse if her supervisor wouldn't tell her what she was doing right or wrong? "Why would she do that to me? If Priscilla really felt that way, why wouldn't she have told me during my evaluation? Why would she tell someone else?" Juliette wondered. "Priscilla was totally unprofessional, and it makes me angry and upset. The number of times I have been in Priscilla's office and shared various confidences, felt that she was on my side, believed in me, thought I was a good nurse. To find out she said this to another employee is hurtful and a betrayal. And I didn't even want the job! All I wanted was clin 4. She's gossiping and trying to create fights. It's staff-splitting. It's wrong, it's damaging, and I can't possibly respect her after this."

Priscilla's slight was not only a personal betrayal from the one person left at Pines who Juliette had considered a confidante, but also a reflection of a toxic environment where cliques, gossip, and vendettas affected both staff morale and patient care. Good nurses were underappreciated and Juliette was a good nurse. "Priscilla is an ineffectual manager on so many levels. Her duplicity is too glaring to ignore, and Charlene's poor managerial skills combine to make a miserable work environment. The emotional drain isn't worth it anymore," Juliette said.

During her next shift at Pines, Juliette found Bethany in the med room looking for supplies. "Bethany," Juliette said, "I heard from Molly that Priscilla told you she would never give me the senior charge nurse job."

"She did!" said Bethany, looking relieved. "I told Molly because I knew she'd tell you and I didn't feel comfortable telling you that directly. Priscilla said she wanted to make sure I knew she'd never give you the job. But you didn't even apply!"

"I'm just astonished she would say something like that," Juliette said, disappointed that the gossip was true.

"It's so completely unprofessional," Bethany said, shaking her head. "What are you going to do?"

"I don't know. I've been done with this place for so long anyway." Juliette thanked Bethany and went on with her workday.

That evening, Juliette called Erica, the senior charge nurse who had resigned in November. She explained what had happened. "Can you believe she said that?" Juliette asked.

"I can absolutely believe she said that," Erica replied. "I heard things that she said about me in that office. There's an endless cesspool of information flowing from that back office to the ER. She fosters a sorority girl atmosphere with the gossip and the backstabbing, which is why I couldn't wait to leave."

"If I go agency, would you write me a letter so that I can update my recommendations?" Juliette asked.

"Of course I will."

The next day, Juliette came to a decision. Molly had been trying to persuade her for months that she would be happier if she went back to the agency they had worked for previously. It was finally time to give up on Pines. Like many talented nurses continually defeated by poor working conditions, Juliette quit.

Juliette found Priscilla in her office. "I'm resigning and this is my two weeks' notice. I'm going agency so I can look for work closer to home," Juliette lied. She saw no reason to tell Priscilla the truth. As Molly would say, how would you get that horse back in the barn? Juliette was proud of her work, doctors and nurses complimented her on it, and it had been good enough to make her one of the few Pines ER nurses to achieve clinical level 4. If the nursing director couldn't respect that but wouldn't tell her to her face, then it was simply time to move on.

"Okay," Priscilla replied. She said nothing further. She resumed her paperwork and Juliette never saw her again.

The doctors had a different reaction. "I'm sorry to see you go," Dr. Kazumi told her.

"That's really bad news," another doctor said.

On her way out of the building, she told Dr. Preston that she was leaving Pines. "Well, you've finally done it, Clark. You've driven me off."

"I knew it wouldn't take long," he joked back.

Juliette smiled. There were some people she would miss at Pines. Her eyes watered.

"They're jackasses if they don't treat you right," he said, squeezing Juliette's shoulder.

"I love you; that was really nice," she said.

"I'm not such an asshole."

Juliette hugged him. Then she unfriended the clique on Facebook.

MOLLY   July

THE FERTILITY CLINIC

On a warm summer morning, Molly wearily listened to Jennifer, her fertility clinic nurse, list the names and prices of the medications she needed for IVF.

"Man, it's expensive to buy a baby," Molly half-joked. "We need all of those?"

"Yes. But I can give you some," Jennifer said. "We have some leftover medications from people who had more than they needed, and I can also put together some samples from the drug companies for you. That should save you about four thousand dollars."

"Are you serious?" Molly exclaimed. "Thank you, thank you, oh my God, thank you." She hugged Jennifer.

Jennifer smiled. "We nurses need to stick together!" she said.

Exactly thirty-six hours before the egg retrieval operation, Molly had to give herself an ovulation trigger shot. While her previous injections had been subcutaneous shots with small needles, this was a large needle that she was supposed to inject into her thigh muscle. She had only one chance to get it right. Because Trey had to work that night, Juliette had offered to do the injection, but Molly didn't want her to have to get up at 2:30 a.m. Molly sat on the toilet seat, her hand shaking. *Schoolchildren can do their own insulin injections but the almost 40-year-old broad who gave countless shots to other people today is a huge wuss.* Needles didn't bother her; she worried she would hesitate, flub the injection, and lose that expensive dose. As a nurse, she knew what to expect, but as a patient she felt vulnerable.

Molly counted to three, exhaled forcibly, and jabbed the needle into her thigh. Success. She was so amped with relief that she couldn't get back to sleep. She toyed with the idea of calling Trey, who was at the station, but he was trying not to emotionally invest too much in the process in case it didn't work. His self-preservation was probably wise. Nonetheless, for a few minutes, she let tendrils of daydreams hazily curl into the image of a baby.

The next week, Molly and Trey were in a surgical room with an ultrasound and video monitor. The screen displayed a picture of two embryos, one with eight cells and one with four. *Those could be our babies!* Molly thought, mesmerized. She turned to look at Trey, who was silent as usual, but noticeably wide-eyed, staring at the picture, too.

The embryologist presented her with a photo of the embryos in a small paper frame. Molly didn't want to get her hopes up, not with her low chance of success. But she couldn't stop staring at the picture.

CITYCENTER MEDICAL

At Citycenter, a woman came into the ER with a severe allergic reaction to nuts. Molly was in the medication room when another nurse, who was new to the ER, came in to get the epinephrine that a resident ordered. The nurse stared at the vial. "Can I ask you something?" she said to Molly. "The new resident ordered point-three milligrams of one to ten thousand epi. That doesn't seem right."

"It's not. It's one to one thousand given subcutaneously," Molly said. She showed the nurse the dosage in the hospital's drug guide and pulled out the proper vial. Molly was swamped with her own patients but accompanied the nurse to the allergic patient's room. This was a high-risk situation with a high-risk drug and she didn't want to put the new nurse on the spot in front of the resident.

"I'm giving one to one thousand," the nurse told the resident, who was in the patient's room.

"No, you've pulled the wrong vial," the resident insisted.

Molly spoke up. "If I were giving one to ten thousand, I would have to give three milliliters instead of point-three and you don't give that volume subcutaneously."

Molly glanced at the patient, whose lips had swollen practically to the size of Twinkies. Epinepherine was risky because too high a concentration could put the patient in cardiac arrest; too low wouldn't reverse the allergic reaction. This patient didn't have time for the doctor to make the wrong call. Molly drew up the dose from the correct vial and injected the medication while the resident argued with the other nurse.

Once the resident saw what Molly was doing, she stalked out of the room.

"Go get the attending physician," Molly told the other nurse.

The attending confirmed that Molly had been correct and the resident's order had been wrong. Nobody thanked the nurses.

This was typical. If a nurse made the wrong call, she could get fired. If a resident made the wrong call, the nurse could get fired simply for carrying out her orders. And when the nurse made the right call, residents often took the credit. One afternoon, a Citycenter patient came in with an obviously broken leg. Because Molly couldn't feel a pulse, she used a Dopplar machine to check for blood flow. When the brand-new resident came in, she told him what she had done.

A moment later, the attending physician entered the room. "What's going on?" he asked.

The resident's chest puffed. "Obvious fracture. I got the Doppler and found a pulse," he said.

"Good job!" the attending said.

"How can they take credit for my work right in front of me?" Molly wondered later. "They want so desperately to look smart in front of the attendings. How hard would it be to use the word 'we' rather than 'I'?"

Residents weren't the only doctors who made medical errors, of course. At Avenue Hospital one day, an ER doctor had prescribed a clot-busting medication used for heart attack or stroke patients. Molly had never given this medication before, but the dose seemed high. When she asked the doctor to double-check, he pulled out his calculator, re-entered the patient's weight, and said, "It's right."

Molly sent the order to the pharmacy. When the medication was ready, she started the medication pump, which began working extremely quickly. *That doesn't seem right*, Molly thought, and stopped the pump. She opened the drug book the hospital kept in every room, but the medication wasn't listed. Molly returned to the doctor and told him she didn't think the dose was correct.

"It's right," he said again. Molly verified the dose with the doctor a total of six times.

By the time Molly brought the patient to the ICU, the entire dose had been administered.

"When did you start this?" the ICU nurse asked.

"Twenty minutes ago," Molly said.

The nurse's eyes widened in alarm.

The next day, the ER nurse manager called Molly into her office. The ICU nurse had written an incident report about the dose, which had been wrong. The patient could have died. "I have to write you up because it was a medication error," the nurse manager said.

"Y'all can ask the doctor, the pharmacy, all of the people I asked for information on this medication that I tried to confirm the dose," Molly said.

"Yes, but you were the one who gave the medicine," the nurse manager said.

Molly didn't confront the doctor because she learned that the doctor told the patient what had happened and had accepted responsibility (which didn't change the fact that the incident was documented in Molly's file).

At another hospital, Molly remembered when a doctor ordered the wrong medication for a patient. As per protocol at that hospital, the patient's nurse acknowledged the order on the computer and clicked a button when she had given the medicine. Later, when the nurse returned to the computer to update the patient's chart, she saw that the medication order, which she had already administered, was gone.

In the fallout, the doctor claimed he had never ordered the medication. The hospital fired the nurse. The nurse responded by filing a lawsuit, forcing the hospital to research the records. After four months, the hospital admitted that the doctor had lied, and agreed to rehire the nurse. "But the doctor is still there! He wasn't fired!" Molly said. "They blindly trusted the doctor over the nurse. That kind of thing happens all the time."

CHAPTER 9

WHAT MAKES A HERO:
Why Nurses Do What They Do

"Nursing is a calling, a lifestyle, a way of living."
— THE NIGHTINGALE TRIBUTE, DEVELOPED BY THE KANSAS STATE NURSES
ASSOCIATION TO HONOR DECEASED NURSES

"Nurses are the glue that holds healthcare together. They live to assess, treat, coordinate care, and advocate for patients, and they do it all under the most direct of pressures with the littlest of concern for their own health or well-being. There is no one less self-concerned than a nurse. They are the implementation masters of coordinated care."
— A VIRGINIA WOMEN'S HEALTH NURSE

"It's incredibly fulfilling. As a nurse, you have the opportunity to provide hope and comfort to people on what is often one of the worst days of their lives. I feel whole when I am caring for others, teaching them to care for themselves, and helping them heal."
— A WASHINGTON, DC, CARDIOTHORACIC SURGERY NURSE

"I'm Right There Wearing a Dress": Why Murses Are Nurses

At six feet two inches, with 230 pounds of muscle and a 32-inch waist, WWE wrestler Dean Visk was enjoying a successful second career when he decided to leave professional wrestling because he missed nursing so dearly. "I thought to myself, 'I'm a healthcare professional.' The WWE is wonderful, but I felt like nursing was my calling," he said.

Visk originally got into nursing because, as an amateur bodybuilder, he was interested in the prerequisite anatomy, chemistry, and biology classes. He was a full-time behavioral health nurse for five years before moving to Cincinnati to work part-time as a nurse while training for the WWE. He trained for four more years before the WWE offered him a contract. The other wrestlers didn't mock him for working in a predominantly female field; instead, he said, they were impressed that he had such a stable career to fall back on.

Now Visk is an outpatient facility nursing director who continues to wrestle on the side for charity functions (and tells patients who recognize him, "I don't fight anymore; I heal"). "I've had nothing but positive experiences in nursing," he said. "If it's a sisterhood, then I'm right there wearing a dress with all the other nurses. I've always been taken into the sisterhood without any issues."

Out of 3.5 million nurses in the United States, approximately 330,000 are male. The highest percentage is concentrated in anesthesia: 41 percent of CRNAs are male, while 9.6 percent of registered nurses are male.

Because murses are so dramatically in the minority, some of them have had to deal with lingering public stereotypes that they are gay or effeminate, which both devalues gay nurses and contradicts an *American Journal of Men's Health* study finding that male nurses "hold a high degree of masculinity."

"You know what's not fun in your early twenties? Being well-dressed, walking up to a girl at a bar, sparking a conversation, and then telling her you're a nurse," said a Virginia murse who has contended with these stereotypes. "I had to work backward to prove my heterosexuality. Now that

I'm older, in a long-term relationship with a woman, and generally more confident, I don't really care what people think. But those first few post-graduation years were rough."

An Oregon critical care nurse said that his favorite jibe about his job is "So, you're a male nurse, huh?" He likes to reply, "Yep, I tried to be a female nurse, but couldn't afford the operation." (He added, "I am not effeminate. I am a dude.")

Comments about being gay, feminine, or "not man enough" helped push one nurse to join the U.S. Army, which deployed him to Afghanistan with an active combat unit, at his request. The guys in his unit good-naturedly referred to his medical supply bag as "the murse's murse," for the male nurse's man-purse. "I got to apply and test my skill-set and medical knowledge, at times in the most adverse of conditions, producing some of the most powerful memories I will ever experience," he said. "On a few occasions, I was the first person on the scene for people who were critically wounded in battle. The opportunity to create my own valuable experiences is something that nursing offers that most other career fields don't. Nursing puts you in the driver's seat."

Most murses said that these stereotypes don't bother them, and that their sexuality, gay or straight, is nobody's business but theirs. What bothers them is when (typically older) patients assume that because they are men, they must be aspiring doctors. A Canadian ICU murse said that while he had originally planned to be a surgeon, he changed his mind during the month he spent at his father's hospital bedside before he passed away. "I realized, after seeing the effect that the nurses had on me and my family, that I could have a much bigger impact on patients by being at the bedside all the time, instead of simply writing out orders and operating on someone, but never really being there for them," the murse said. "I get offended when patients don't understand why I wouldn't want to be a doctor, or they keep asking about my 'real aspirations' in life. When that happens, I have to explain that my goal is to be a nurse, I love what I do, and I get to do more as a nurse."

A Maryland medical floor murse had been on the job only a few months when, even after he had clearly introduced himself as a nurse, the patient and patient's family continued to refer to him as "doctor" and the female physician as "the nurse." A Delaware murse explained why this is insulting not only to the doctor but also to the nurse. "It insults my profession when people think that if I say something smart, I must be a physician," the nurse said. "When I worked in the ER, patients would say, 'You're so good! Don't you wish you were a doctor?' No. I'm a nurse. It's like telling a chef he's so good, why doesn't he become an IT programmer. It is absolutely infuriating. And female nurses never have to deal with it." Dean Visk, who is finishing his master of science in nursing degree and plans to get a PhD, said that even when he becomes a Doctor of Nursing Practice, "I'll still identify myself as a nurse. I'm very, very proud to be a nurse."

On a personal level, murses' experiences as the minority gender can vary, depending on the unit: While many, like Visk, feel welcomed, others deal with occasional teasing from coworkers. Professional challenges can include "always having to take the infected patient because you're the only one who can't get pregnant," a New York NP said. The Oregon nurse echoed a common murse observation that they are disproportionately assigned to the most difficult patients and often get called in to do the heavy lifting.

But they get paid more to do it. According to the U.S. Census Bureau, male nurses ride the "glass escalator"; although they are in the minority, they receive higher wages and faster promotions than women in the same jobs. The wage gap is smaller in nursing than in other professions, however. Compared with men, women earn ninety-one cents to the dollar in nursing occupations, versus seventy-seven cents to the dollar on average across other fields.

Some men become defensive about being in a field with mostly women, but the majority of the murses interviewed for this book didn't consider the disparity to be a problem. "Yes, I'm in a job where I am surrounded by women. But guys, come on, I'm in a job where I'm surrounded by women!" said the Army nurse, who is now stationed at a base in Europe and engaged to a female physician. The murse's female coworkers and the "sixty-five sisters" in his nursing school class provided him with "access to some pretty big answer keys," he said. "I dress better than most of my male friends, I understand what I did or said to make a woman upset or happy, and I have an endless supply of opinions on gifts and date ideas."

290 | THE NURSES

The murse, however, cautioned other potential male nurses, "As a general rule, you aren't in the nursing field to get laid." Instead, "If you're the caregiving type of guy, you should join us because of the wide range of nursing opportunities. You could work in a hospital or nursing home, dabble in management and administration, you can travel, or you can stay put," he said. "Don't let the female-dominated work area intimidate you. Want to know what brings a smile to everyone in the ER? Seeing that big burly wall of muscle and testosterone who's good with kids. There's nothing like a nurse's feeling of satisfaction at the end of the day."

SAM   CITYCENTER MEDICAL, August

One night, the charge nurse found Sam in Zone 1 to give her a five-minute heads-up that a trauma was on the way: a pedestrian who was struck by a car and thrown several feet. Five minutes was a decent amount of time for nurses to prepare for a patient; typically medics didn't call Citycenter until they were practically on the back ramp. Sam arrived at the trauma bay at the same time as CeeCee. Before Sam could open her mouth, CeeCee announced, "I'll be bedside and you can document." CeeCee thought bedside nurses got all of the glory, but Sam didn't believe that one nurse was less important than another.

Sam shrugged, uncomfortable about working with CeeCee. At least CeeCee had just returned from a three-week vacation and seemed relaxed and ready to work. Sam crossed her fingers for a drama-free night.

When the already intubated patient came in, a physician conducted an assessment while various doctors hooked the patient up to the vent and inserted a chest tube. Sam recorded all of these procedures while CeeCee took the patient's blood pressure.

The moment the patient began to wake up and fight the ventilator, Sam pulled drugs from the Pyxis and handed them to CeeCee. CeeCee continued to monitor blood pressure and assist the doctors as Sam recorded. When the patient stabilized enough to move him to the CT room, Sam helped CeeCee hang units of blood before, during, and after the scan. ("The scaredy-cat doctors were all behind the glass watching us get irradiated," Sam said.) Sam was surprised to notice that she and CeeCee worked well together, managing the flow of various doctors' orders and dispensing medications.

Once CeeCee took the patient to the ICU, Sam began her hour-long stint at the computer to document the series of procedures coherently. When CeeCee returned from the ICU, she sat down for a few minutes to help. Sam hated to admit it, but CeeCee was a good nurse under pressure. She finished documenting with a newfound respect for CeeCee.

Sam had come a long way in only a year. She had realized that "everyone is going to come to the table with different opinions and personalities, but the goal is to take care of patients, so everyone getting along is important. As I learned, it's hard to be on your best behavior for twelve hours when your coworkers are pissing you off. But you work extremely closely with them. I've worked with people who've touched my butt more than guys I've dated (it's totally normal for people to take my trauma shears out of the butt pocket of my scrub pants). Patients come and go, but your colleagues can make or break your shift. So I can at least give everyone a chance."

Sam's next patient was an intubated man with carbon monoxide poisoning. She monitored his propofol, a powerful sedative that required just the right balance: enough to keep the patient sedated, but not so much as to lower his blood pressure excessively. Within a few minutes, the man started bucking the vent, agitated. His chest raised, his head strained against the stretcher, and his heart rate increased. Before the man could wake up, Sam increased the propofol. Three minutes later, the man's blood pressure dropped. She lowered the propofol. Ten minutes later, the man became agitated again. Sam called in a tech to help her hold the man's arms down so she could increase the propofol once more.

Sam paged the attending doctor. "The propofol isn't really working," she said. "I think we need something else to sedate him."

The attending nodded. "Good call. How about a Versed drip?"

Sam nodded and prepared the drip. *He actually listened to what I said! He took me seriously!* she thought.

After a few hours of standing by the patient's bedside and watching his monitor, Sam noticed that he was having longer and longer runs of bigeminy, a heart rhythm that, while not immediately threatening, could lead to more dangerous rhythms. She checked his labs, saw that his magnesium levels were slightly low, and found the attending. This doctor was a reasonable man who had worked at the hospital for decades.

"His mag is one point two," Sam said. "I think we should give him magnesium." Low levels of magnesium could cause irregular heart rhythms.

"Good call," the attending said. "Why don't we give him two grams of mag."

Sam hung the bag of magnesium on the IV pump. She was pleased. For so many months at Citycenter, the charge nurses had assigned her to zones that didn't see seriously sick patients, making Sam feel as if the staff didn't think she knew what she was doing. "Now I have a sick patient and the doctors are listening to me," she realized. "Maybe I kind of do know what I'm doing after all."

Everything seemed to be falling into place. Sam and William were happy together as a couple, but they kept their relationship under wraps at work. She didn't want to fuel any more rumors, especially when she was finally gaining respect as a nurse. Her professional reputation was becoming, in her words, "I'm a no-nonsense hard-ass. We're going to do things the right way and efficiently and don't give me any crap." She liked that reputation because it minimized drama. "If everyone is clear that's the way it's going to go from the start, then staff are less likely to sit around and have social hour."

Even she and Dr. Spiros had gradually thawed. The gossip about Sam had tapered off, probably because of CeeCee's vacation. Sure, nurses made comments here and there about Sam's supposed love life, but Sam could let those remarks slide.

A woman in her early thirties came in one night with stress-induced supraventricular tachycardia, a dangerous arrhythmia in which the heart raced at more than 180 beats per minute. To treat SVT, staff first tried getting the patient to bear down as if having a bowel movement. This was a technique aimed at activating the vagus nerve—called a vagal maneuver—to slow down the heart. If that didn't work to bring down the arrhythmia, the next step was to administer adenosine, a drug that stopped the heart for a few seconds so that it would hopefully resume at a slower rate. In the ambulance on the way to Citycenter, the medics fortunately had been able to use adenosine to convert the patient's heart rhythm back to normal.

The ER doctor told the woman to follow up with her cardiologist, and ordered some Ativan to calm her down. Sam could hear through the curtain from the next patient area as the woman explained her fears to her husband. The patient was upset because she was under stress at work, which was leading to a cycle of increasing SVT episodes. She did not want to take Ativan. Sam guessed that the doctor had not adequately described the patient's condition and treatment.

So she popped in to talk to the patient. "I thought you could use some more information," Sam said. "Stress can activate a vicious cycle: You get stressed out, you get SVT, and that makes you even more stressed. So I can only imagine how stressed you are."

The woman nodded.

"If I were given the option, I would take a really small dose of Ativan just to bring the stress down a notch. It could break the cycle," Sam continued. She explained that Ativan wouldn't affect the woman's heart rate, but was intended to calm her so that her heart wouldn't start racing again. She answered the couple's questions and talked to them for ten minutes.

Sam was not a warm, fuzzy nurse. She probably never would be. In her opinion, giving a patient "all the information is more calming to someone than patting them on the head like, 'There, there dear.'" By giving the couple thorough information about SVT and Ativan, she was hoping to provide them with "every tool they needed to make a good decision."

The woman agreed to try the Ativan. As Sam walked away to retrieve it, she overheard the woman say to her husband, "She's awesome. She gets it!"

Sam paused in the hallway for a moment to collect herself while her eyes filled with tears. She explained, "I think it meant so much to me because it wasn't intended for me to hear. This is why I got into nursing. I was able to talk to her like a human being and help her understand what we were trying to do. There's a different sense of satisfaction than when you work on an interesting trauma patient. With most traumas, you're using your brain on a clinical and tasky level but you don't really interact with the patient. Anyway, it was the nicest compliment."

Sam had assumed she needed to become a nurse practitioner in order to gain universal respect within the medical industry. As she said, "It's been my mission to make doctors and laypeople realize this isn't our grandmothers' nursing. I don't wear white and I sure as hell don't stand up when a doctor enters the room."

Now, after a year as a nurse, she could see that she didn't need the doctors' validation. Rather than view ER nursing as a stepping-stone toward a more prestigious degree, she knew that her job was about healing. She also didn't need patients' respect. Sam was a nurse to save patients' lives, not to convince them to appreciate her. But oh, what a difference it made when they did.

JULIETTE   EASTGREEN HOSPITAL, December

Juliette hesitated in front of the broad automatic doors of the Eastgreen ER, where she had landed permanently following eight weeks of agency work. After working full-time for a few months at Eastgreen, a hospital with a good reputation and a varied patient load, she had arranged a two-week unpaid vacation to spend quality time with her husband and daughter. Now, as she prepared to resume working, she remembered when she had returned to Pines after a three-week vacation and no nurses other than Molly had welcomed her back.

Eastgreen, which was not far from Juliette's home, had a much larger ER, with twice the number of Pines' staff. Juliette couldn't help but wonder if some of her new coworkers had already forgotten her name. Thus far, the experience at Eastgreen already outclassed Pines. Most of the nurses Juliette had worked with were courteous. Unlike at Pines, Eastgreen nurses were diverse; they ranged in age, race, looks, weight, sexuality, and numbers of tattoos and piercings. The charge nurses made a point of thanking nurses who worked hard, like Juliette.

Socially, Juliette and several coworkers had started a book club. She was friendly with one of the ER doctors, and she had traded dog-sitting days with another colleague. A group of nurses had even invited Juliette to go on a whale-watching trip.

Despite all of this, Juliette worried about how they would react when she returned. After all, she had trusted Priscilla, but her judgment had been wrong. She took a breath and entered the ER. The first tech who saw her gave her a hug. "Juliette, we missed you!" she said.

At the nurses station, the nurse manager stopped her. "I'm so glad you're here! How was your vacation?"

"Juliette's back?" asked the ER doctor, looking up from his computer. "Hey, I got a new puppy! Come here and see the video."

The nurse manager read Juliette a compliment from a patient evaluation that had come in while she was gone. The patient had written that she knew how busy ERs were. "Juliette took great care of us," the patient said. "It made such a difference with our stay and we just want to acknowledge the care we received."

Juliette beamed. Eastgreen wasn't perfect. There were social groups that she wasn't a part of, and staff members who were unhelpful. But already, she felt more comfortable at work than she ever was at Pines.

LARA   SOUTH GENERAL HOSPITAL, August

The day before the surgery, Lara couldn't stop thinking about the drugs. *Remember how shitty you felt when you were trying to get clean?* she pleaded with herself. *You don't ever want to feel that way again. Don't do this to your kids.*

Frightened that she would succumb to temptation, Lara went to an NA meeting and shared: "I'm going to have surgery and I'm kind of excited about getting my stomach muscle cut open because then I'll need Percocet." She was embarrassed, but the response was immediate. "It's cool you're making yourself accountable by telling us," a man told her.

"Who do you have to hold your medicine?" a woman asked.

"I guess my ex-husband," Lara said. He was the only adult whom she saw every day. She would be most accountable to him because he was watching their kids.

"Do you want me to drive you to a meeting?" asked someone else.

Lara had mixed feelings. She had been eager for the meds, and now a little voice scolded her, *You just ruined your chance.* But her relief that her NA network would not allow her to relapse offset her disappointment. Quickly, she told several people about the surgery so that they would watch out for her. But even up until the moment of the operation, Lara was scared by how thrilled she was to get cut open because she would get high.

• • •

When she woke up, Lara was giddy on her post-op pain medication. After John drove her home, Lara called in her Percocet prescription. Still high from the surgery, she decided to drive the three miles to the pharmacy herself although driving so soon after surgery was inadvisable.

Lara picked up the prescription and three bags of chicken from the restaurant next door. She balanced everything on top of the car while she gently opened the door, careful not to strain her surgery site, then loaded the chicken into the trunk. As she backed out of her parking spot, she heard a crunch. She glanced in her rearview mirror, saw nothing unusual, shrugged, and drove back to John's. After dinner, she went to her car to get the Percocet. Her plan was to keep two pills at home and give the rest to John to hold for safekeeping. The prescription wasn't in the car.

He took them from me! Lara thought. She tore into the house, where she found John in the den. "Are you messing with me? Where's the Percocet?" she asked.

"What do you mean?" John asked.

"The pain pills aren't there! Did you take them?" she asked, panicking.

"Are you hiding them?" John asked.

Lara immediately felt guilty. Had she hidden them? She didn't remember handling them, but she was still slightly loopy. *This doesn't look very good*, she thought. *They're magically not there after I said I got them?*

"Maybe your brother took them," John said. "Maybe they fell out of the car."

As she argued with her ex-husband, Lara remembered the strange crunching sound outside of the pharmacy. *Oh no*, she thought. *No way.*

She drove back to the parking lot and found the crushed bag. "No! No, no, no!" she shouted. Lara's surgery site was now hurting so badly that she legitimately needed the Percocet. She scooped up the bag. The pills were pulverized, crushed into the shattered plastic they'd come in. *I can't believe I ran over my pain medicine.*

Back in her car, Lara leaned her head on the steering wheel. It figured. The one time that she truly needed legally prescribed Percocet, she had accidentally destroyed the pills. She took a picture of the pills for evidence. Then she reconsidered. *There is no way in hell I'm going to call the doctor's office and tell them a) I was driving and b) I ran over my medicine and I need more*, she thought. Later, she explained, "People come up with the most ridiculous stories to get pills. So I had to deal with having no pain medicine because I was too embarrassed to call the doctor and have them thinking I was drug-seeking."

At home, Lara struggled through the agony and fought the urge to hunt down narcotics. Without her two major outlets—work and exercise, both of which were forbidden—she was lost. It rained every day. When the kids were home, she focused intently on taking care of them. When they were in school, she rested or watched TV, trying to ignore the pain in her stomach and the battle in her mind.

A few days into one of the hardest weeks of her life, Lara was sitting alone, tears streaming down her face because of the sharp pains. She couldn't take the hurt any longer. *I can send the doctor the picture to show that I'm not making this up*, she thought. She picked up the phone to call his office. "Oh my God, you're going to look like you're crazy because you took the picture in the first place," she told herself. "Forget it." *But the pills will take you out of this funk*, a little voice nagged. She started to dial. "The pills aren't going to take you out of the funk. You'll get a little buzz, you'll enjoy it, and then you'll be going at it again." She hung up the phone. *How am I going to get through this?*

For the next week, Lara refused to allow herself to think beyond the present moment. Forget day by day. Lara asked herself only, "What am I going to do right now?" Embarrassed and determined "not to be a drama queen," she didn't tell most of her friends about her predicament. But the people she did tell rushed to her aid. Angie, her former coworker and roommate, checked in with her regularly. Molly and Juliette brought her meals. Another nurse friend helped get the children through their nightly homework and bath routine. Friends from NA drove her to meetings every night; one even found a meeting site with no stairs so that Lara would strain her abdomen as little as possible. The South General ER nurses, who knew nothing about Lara's addiction, sent a get-well basket with flowers and candy. Rose, Holly, and Brianne had tucked in personal notes.

Four weeks later, Lara was back in the gym. She was profoundly proud that she had recovered without being seduced by narcotics. She believed she could get through anything now: overwhelmingly busy days, single motherhood, maybe even dating. She would not be presumptuous enough to assume she had beaten her demons; NA meetings were a reminder that the disease was waiting for her, that just one slip-up would send her back into its arms. So she accepted what she called "a healthy fear," which she would live with, always, because of the mistakes she'd made in the past.

Why did Lara return to ER nursing, the worst possible job for her addiction—tempting her with narcotics to administer, to throw out, to watch other nurses steal? "Because being a nurse is my passion," she said. "When all my struggles were going on, my biggest fear was that nursing would be taken away from me. It truly makes me happy."

For Lara, being a good nurse also made her feel like a good mother. "As a nurse, I feel strong, like I can protect my children. Because of my medical knowledge, I know when something's not right with them," she said. "Every parent wants to feel like they're keeping their kids as safe as possible. As a nurse I can make sure my kids are safe. And nursing pays pretty well, so my kids and I will be okay. It's not easy supporting the family by myself, but I will make this happen."

Lara wanted other nurses to know there is hope, help, and life after addiction. "You can get help and you don't have to feel like this ever again, like you're never going to laugh again, never going to feel good," she said. "It does get better and you can do this clean. You can do anything clean."

She had proven that to herself repeatedly over the past year. But now she finally believed it.

MOLLY   August

Two weeks after Molly's IVF, she decided to take a home pregnancy test, even though she had read that because of the hormones in the ovulation trigger shot, urine pregnancy tests could result in a false positive. She tried to wait for Trey, who was finishing a night shift, but the test instructions said to use her first morning urine, and Molly couldn't hold it any longer.

She stared at the stick as she waited for the three minutes to pass. The test line slowly began to develop, like an old Polaroid picture sharpening into focus. And—was she imagining it or was a second line forming, too? She tried not to get her hopes up, but she allowed a tiny string of excitement to loop around her heart.

The next day, after Molly's official blood draw at the clinic, her nurse, Jennifer, called her at home. "Molly! Molly, Molly, Molly!"

"Jennifer! Jennifer, Jennifer, Jennifer!"

"Sorry! I was so excited I couldn't get it out. It's just so great to say this nurse to nurse. I have great news for you! You're pregnant!"

"Hooray!" Molly whooped. She wanted to shout from the rooftop. She was ecstatic that something she had wanted so strongly for so many years would finally come to pass. Her mother had been such a fabulous mom. Molly's best memories of her had nothing to do with "fancy activities," she said, but centered on simply being together, much like her mother's nurse coworkers had written to Molly about how dearly they cherished simply being with her. Molly got choked up thinking about how she would now be able to build on those memories with her own son or daughter.

She was going to be a mom. This changed everything.

WORLDVIEW HOSPITAL

The agency sent Molly to a new hospital that bordered the city and the suburbs. Worldview was known for what healthcare workers colloquially called "concierge medicine": The hospital took care of people with money and high expectations for customer service. Molly arrived early to take five written tests on medication administration, safe transfer/lifting, EKG interpretation, fire safety, and patient privacy. She scored 100 percent on all of them. Afterward, the staffing office representative walked Molly to the ER and introduced her to the charge nurse. Molly was impressed; at other hospitals, busy staff had pointed her in the general direction of the ER and left her to navigate her way alone. The charge nurse gave Molly a tour of the department and assigned her to a zone.

The Worldview staff was amicable, the ER manager was ever-present and interactive, and all of the doctors introduced themselves by first name. Molly couldn't believe the contrast between Worldview and her other hospitals. The staff was happy because they were not overworked. She had only three patients at a time because two float nurses and several techs picked up some of the workload. Because the ER was relatively slow, Molly had enough time to spend with each of her patients, which made her feel like a good nurse.

Not long into Molly's shift, the charge nurse, who had been watching her, said, "You have your act together. What are your scheduling preferences? When we have needs, I'll call you first."

In the middle of Molly's shift, the computer system went down for several hours. Doctors could input orders, but other departments couldn't view them. The radiology department didn't know when the ER wanted to send in patients for exams, the lab wasn't notified when nurses ordered tests, and the Pyxis didn't have access to patients' names for nurses to pull out drugs.

At every other hospital where Molly had worked, this shutdown would have been catastrophic. But no one at Worldview batted an eye. The nurses pulled out paperwork and charted manually.

At the end of Molly's shift, the charge nurse wrote her a spectacular review for the agency's required first-shift evaluation. She marked "exceeded expectations" for each of the dozens of skills listed, and added a note about Molly's quick learning curve and willingness to take on anything. She also wrote that the nursing staffing office should make sure that Molly returned.

Was Worldview the hospital Molly had been looking for? Over the next few weeks, she took several shifts there. She learned that Worldview doctors and nurses were kind to each other and there was no nurse bullying. Patient flow was quick, with low wait times and not much volume.

Techs did their jobs without being asked, and other departments pitched in; radiology picked up their own patients, for example, rather than waiting for nurses to bring them. The charge nurse told Molly that she was her favorite agency nurse because she was independent and didn't complain.

But there were downsides to Worldview. The hospital didn't see trauma or cardiac patients, so the ER transferred the sickest patients elsewhere. And, as at Academy, the work was so slow that the job, for Molly, was boring.

Molly had come to realize that there was no Holy Grail of ERs. "I liked some of the patients at South General because they actually listened and saw the nurse as a person to learn from. I like Academy because some of the staff is really nice. I actually do like Citycenter because of the ridiculousness that happens there. I like Worldview because it's a welcome break from super-hard work," she said. She decided to continue as an agency nurse so that she could work at the variety of hospitals on her own terms.

It had been a full year since she quit Pines Memorial. She was not wrong to leave. In an arena that mattered greatly to Molly—"being held accountable and doing your job well because it's the right thing to do"— Pines was the worst of the bunch. At the same time, because of the high numbers of septic nursing home patients and highway-speed car accident victims, Pines treated some of the sickest patients in the area, which Molly valued because of the intellectual challenge. And Molly appreciated Pines' experienced nursing staff because she learned something new every week. "That hasn't existed at any other hospital," she said. "If they could stick Academy management into the Pines ER, that might be the ideal place to work."

But maybe the trappings didn't matter so much. Molly hadn't become a nurse because she wanted an ideal place to work. Ultimately, the tensions among nurses, disrespect from doctors, and bureaucratic inconsistencies weren't what mattered. Ultimately, what mattered was helping people. That was what her mom had loved about nursing. That was the priority Molly wanted to pass on to her own child. Maybe it was time to let everything else go.

One night, Molly took a shift at Avenue Hospital. At 11:00 p.m., an elderly couple came in. The man, who was on hospice care because he was dying of cancer, was having trouble breathing. Typically, hospice patients didn't come to the hospital, but sometimes families panicked and brought them in. Because Avenue had no beds available on the medical floor, the man boarded in the ER.

All night, the man drifted in and out of consciousness. His wife of sixty-eight years never left his side. At dawn, when Molly's shift ended, the patient received a medical floor bed assignment. "I'll come get him and take him up," the oncoming nurse said over the phone.

"No, I'll bring him," Molly said. "I've been with them all night."

As the elevator doors opened on the seventh floor, Molly saw the sun just beginning to glow through a tall window at the end of the hallway. She knew it would be the patient's last sunrise. She turned to him. "Would you like me to take your bed to the end of the hall so that you can watch the sunrise together?" she asked.

The man nodded feebly. His wife whispered, "Yes."

Molly wheeled the bed past the man's assigned room and parked it at the end of the hall. On the bed, the couple held each other for the last time. As the sunrise unraveled warm pastels across the sky, Molly stood silently behind the head of the stretcher.

"Oh, John, isn't it gorgeous?" the woman said to her husband.

He smiled weakly. "It sure is," he whispered. He closed his eyes and passed away peacefully in his wife's embrace, his needs met, his end loving.

That was why Molly had become a nurse.

CHAPTER 10

WHAT YOU CAN DO:
Advice and Inspiration for the Public, Patients, Families, Nurses, Aspiring Nurses, Managers, and Others

"Nurses can work individually as citizens or collectively through political action to bring about social change."

—CODE OF ETHICS FOR NURSES, PROVISION 9.4

"Our clinical skills are essential in carrying out high-level nursing care, yet the complete package that defines nursing is one human being reaching out to support another."

—A FAMILY NURSE PRACTITIONER IN MICHIGAN

A solution to many of the issues in this book, and one that would go a long way toward fixing American healthcare, is relatively clear: Treasure nurses. Hire more. Nurses are perennially the number-one most trusted profession in America, according to an annual Gallup poll rating honesty and ethical standards. They are called to an exhausting commitment in which mortals must sustain an unwavering grace at the edge of life and death, almost divinely slowing heartbeats, hurrying them along, or pounding them back into existence. Nurses are exceptional. So why aren't they treated accordingly?

As new healthcare laws funnel more patients into the system and 6 million baby boomers are reaching the age of greatest healthcare need, nurses are absolutely vital to the health of the country. Every year through the end of this century, 2 to 3 million people will age into Medicare, which increases demand for services.

While hospital finances are tight, the margins are still positive in most institutions, said ANA senior policy fellow Peter McMenamin, a healthcare economist. "Hospital finance people are skittish particularly when it comes to uncertainty, and the monster under the bed is what's happening with Medicare," he said. Hospital administrators fear further Affordable Care Act cuts in payments to hospitals, which could explain why hospital industry employment numbers that were increasing in 2012 and 2013 were virtually flat in 2014. But over the next several years, hundreds of thousands of RNs and APRNs are expected to retire. "A hospital that now may be seeing two to three longtime staff members retiring [per] year, eventually could be holding retirement parties once a month," McMenamin said. "Hospitals should be looking at the longer run. If they wait five years to get back into the job market, they're going to be competing with all the other hospitals that waited five years and they'll be competing for the same cohort of experienced nurses. If they start hiring new nurses today, they could be developing their own experienced workforce. It's a sound long-term strategy."

It's also a way to quickly improve patient care. Researchers have proven that patient-to-nurse ratios directly affect patient mortality; medical errors and adverse events; patients' length of stay; risk of heart attack, hospital acquired pneumonia, or infections; failure-to-rescue rates; patient falls;

readmissions; nurse retention; and patient satisfaction. Lightening patient loads reduces nurse stress, burnout, bullying, and exhaustion.

The bottom line is that hospitals could save money, patients, and nurses by investing in staffing. Policymakers could help by providing grants, fellowships, and other subsidies for additional nurse hires.

Before hospitals implemented the checklist mentioned in Chapter 5, medical professionals couldn't imagine reminding physicians to wash their hands. When infection rates dropped to zero, the checklist ably demonstrated that small changes can have big payoffs. Here are additional tips to help people receive—and staff provide—better healthcare.

For hospitals and managers
Involve nurses in decision making.

Directly involving nurses in decision-making processes is a good strategy for developing efficient policies, making nurses feel like valued workplace contributors, decreasing occupational burnout, and increasing morale. As frontline healthcare providers, nurses have important insights and day-to-day perspectives that can inform everything from patient-care procedures to workplace policies. Currently, many workplaces do not include nurses in these strategic meetings.

Appoint a contact person to objectively handle nurses' concerns.

Inter-office politics affects patient care, as evidenced by Dr. Bitch's and other doctor bullies' power plays over nurses. One strategy to curb bullying is to establish a contact person or inter-staff committee to whom nurses can report disruptive behavior without risking retaliation, according to the *Online Journal of Issues in Nursing.* This point-person could also handle reports of assaults by patients and visitors as well as concerns about physician mistakes. Nurses will be far more effective at checking doctors and caring for patients if they are expected to speak up. They must feel empowered to protect their patients. Hospitals can develop protocols for nurses to report urgent concerns to an administrator who can and will intervene. As the Institute for Safe Medication Practices suggests, workplaces should have a no-retribution policy for employees who report worrisome or disrespectful behavior.

Provide debriefing/counseling resources.

It's unrealistic to expect even seasoned nurses to recover immediately from handling trauma victims or unexpected patient deaths or complications. A range of resources could help nurses cope with tragedies and/or manage burnout, second-victim syndrome, and other longer-term work-related emotional issues. Accessible on-site counseling would be ideal. Debriefing sessions can help to find lessons, meaning, or closure after certain patient cases.

Some hospitals have trained colleagues across departments to provide support, comfort, resources, and counseling referrals to any staff member dealing with a difficult situation; a liaison is on call at all times. At the least, hospitals could provide a quiet room in which nurses can relax and compose themselves. Ohio nurse practitioner Barbara Lombardo has suggested soothingly colored walls, comfortable chairs, and relaxing music to relieve stress. Advocate Lutheran General Hospital in Illinois gave nurses a small budget to furnish a retreat in a break room; the nurses purchased a massage chair and some puzzles, if only to refocus coworkers' thoughts with a brief distraction.

Compassion fatigue, stress, burnout, and other mental health issues not only wear nurses down but also drive them out of the field. Administrators' efforts to prevent these issues could demonstrate care for their employees and save money in absenteeism and job attrition.

Use first names.

In many workplaces, nurses are called by their first names, while doctors are not. Requiring doctors, nurses, administrators, and other staff members to call each other by their first names is a no-cost strategy to reduce the appearance of hierarchies among the professions. One of the reasons Pines Memorial nurses liked working with Dr. Preston was because they could call him Clark, which blurred the doctor–nurse tiers. "Using a colleague's first name can help break down artificial barriers that may impede effective communication," the ISMP recommends. This simple way to help equalize the playing field could help to decrease disrespectful and disruptive behaviors and lessen the "us versus them" attitude.

Prioritize security.

Getting assaulted by patients and visitors should not be tolerated as "part of the job." Hospitals have had success by assigning uniformed security personnel to make frequent rounds in patient care areas. The Joint Commission recommends wand-screening visitors for weapons or conducting bag checks. Some hospitals also might consider installing metal detectors. Within six months after Detroit's Henry Ford Hospital began using metal detectors, staff had confiscated thirty-three handguns, ninety-seven chemical sprays, and more than 1,300 knives.

By requiring staff to report all violent acts and threats, administrators can track the events, deduce patterns, identify frequent aggressors, and better prevent future incidents. As mentioned in Chapter 3, the computer database identifying violent patients at the VA Medical Center in Portland, Oregon, reduced attacks by 91.6 percent. If other hospitals implemented this successful program, countless nurses could be spared injury and suffering.

OSHA states that "at a minimum, workplaces should ensure that no employee who reports violence faces reprisals . . . [and] place as much importance on employee safety and health as on serving the client." Separately, all states should make it a felony to assault any healthcare professional on the job.

Talk about substance abuse.

The most important step employers can take to reduce narcotics addiction among their staff is to make sure that addicts can easily get the help they need. "A lot of nurses get caught and no complaint is filed. Whatever was driving them to use comes back at their next job and they steal drugs again," said Douglas McLellan, RN Coordinator for Massachusetts' Nursing Substance Abuse Rehabilitation Program. "The best thing is for nurse managers to file the complaint, get the nurse into a program, and let her be monitored."

Prevention strategies could include more vigilant monitoring of medication disposal and placing posters in staff areas that list signs of possibly impaired colleagues and ways to help them. All nursing schools should teach a unit on chemical dependency and intervention strategies. This type of instruction would help to prevent addiction and lessen the stigma associated with chemical dependency. Addiction is an illness, not willful misconduct. If healthcare providers view nurses with chemical dependency issues as patients with a treatable problem, they may be more likely to assist them rather than stigmatize them.

Don't automatically or exclusively fault nurses for medical errors.
Nurses are blamed for medical errors too often when doctors or hospital policies are at the root. If a medical error occurs because of a nurse whose unit was short-staffed at the time, the hospital should accept some responsibility. Even when nurses do make a mistake, as in the case of Kimberly Hiatt, the nurse who committed suicide after her hospital blamed her for an infant's death, rather than scapegoating and/or firing them, administrators could tap them to help devise a system that would prevent similar errors. As an American Association of Critical Care Nurses study points out, "A mistake does not mean a bad practitioner . . . not correcting a mistake does." When Montreal's Jewish General Hospital launched a "no shame, no blame" campaign to track errors, staff was able to reduce bed sores (which can develop quickly when a patient can't change positions on his own) from 25 to 6 percent.

For the public
There are many things that loved ones can do to improve a patient's healthcare. Here are some tips that nurses mentioned most frequently in our interviews.

Appoint one family spokesperson.
Several nurses, as well as the networking website allnurses.com, offered an excellent suggestion to streamline hospital visits: Families or patients can designate one family member to communicate with nurses. This tactic saves nurses from having to take time away from patients to repeat themselves to various loved ones and ensures that one visitor is completely informed. Family members can write down all of their questions and

the spokesperson can ask them, then relay the information to rest of the visitors.

Ask questions.

Patients and family spokespersons shouldn't hesitate to ask doctors and nurses questions about their care and about the specifics of and reasons for procedures. "Even if you're worried about annoying a doctor or nurse, if you have questions, you should ask them," said a psychiatric nurse in Hawaii. "The patient and patient's family need to know enough about what's going on to advocate for the patient's well-being. It could save your or your family member's life."

When asking questions, avoid asking "Why," which can put healthcare providers on the defensive. Instead of inquiring, "Why did you give him that medication?" try "Help us to understand why he's getting this medication," a Texas family nurse practitioner suggested. Also, double-check the identification information on your armband or make sure your family/visitors know to check it for you. "Patients get better care when their family is involved, actively," said a Virginia nurse practitioner.

Try to keep a list of questions so that you can ask them at one time; you can even write them on the whiteboard in the room. And don't be intimidated to ask the doctor. "Countless times, the doctor has asked if there are questions, the patient and family timidly say no, and as soon as he leaves, they turn to the nurse and say, 'What does that mean?'" said a Washington State nurse.

The best time to ask a nurse questions might be during the nurse's second visit of her shift. At the start of her shift, she might be particularly busy visiting each patient; by the second pass-through, she should have more time to focus on your questions.

Be prepared.

To speed up wait times, maintain a written medical history complete with current prescriptions and dosages, vitamins, over-the-counter medications, allergies, diagnoses, and contact numbers so that you can hand a copy to your healthcare provider. Or take cell phone photos of medication labels and lab and diagnostic results so that they are handy at all times. In triage, be specific about the type and location of your pain or complaint.

Your hospital is not as clean as it could be.
Bring hand sanitizer and antibacterial wipes. Use them.

Stay with the patient.
"It is really important to have someone stay in the hospital with you. Nurses may not always be able to keep a close eye on each of their patients," said a Pacific Northwest PACU nurse. "Sometimes, the aggressive patients needing more nursing care take time from the quieter patients. It's like the squeaky wheel gets the grease." A Washington State nurse instructor suggests that relatives take turns so that someone is with the patient at least sixteen hours per day.

It's helpful for the patient if you can be in the room for the doctor's daily rounds. Ask the staff what time these rounds occur and let them know that you plan to be present for them.

Watch carefully when staff members enter your (or your loved one's) room.
Not all doctors and nurses remember to wash their hands when entering a patient room. Nurses encourage patients and visitors to speak up if someone forgets. "I would just be direct about it: 'Could you please wash your hands?'" said a physician for the U.S. Navy. "You might append it with something like, 'I'm just nervous about catching something in the hospital while we are here.' We all still slip up, so the reminder is actually appreciated, not awkward."

Do as much as you can for yourself and for the patient.
Bring or find your own food and drink if you are staying with a patient rather than asking the nurse. If you want to help the nurse, ask what you can do for the patient. "It's hard to lose control when someone is sick, and many times, visitors want to do something. Let us know that and we will gladly give you a task," said an Oklahoma nursing supervisor. For example, visitors can keep a record of the patient's fluid intake and output on the whiteboard.

Family members can give patients baths, brush their teeth, take them on walks, participate in therapies, and handle feeding, for example. "I've given a bath to a child while the parents sat there and watched," said an Arizona pediatric nurse. "Nurses do not give magical baths. We give fast ones when we are busy. Any type of care that can be done by the family is not just a help to nurses; it aids in the healing process. Who better to care for someone than the people who love them most?"

Understand that a nurse's schedule is complicated.
Even if your hospital medications are due at 6:00, you might not receive them at exactly that time because your nurse could have several other patients with medications due simultaneously. "When we're passing meds on schedule, we usually have to get all of our patients medicated right then. 9:00 a.m., 12:00 p.m., 3:00 p.m., and 9:00 p.m. are very common massive medication times," said a North Carolina ER nurse. "We usually have six to eight patients and some need ten medications. Some patients can take only one pill at a time, or all of their medications may have to be crushed and put into applesauce and painstakingly fed to them."

Also, your nurse may be late answering your call light because "she was just holding the hand of a patient breathing his last breath; someone who just lost their mother, father, or spouse was crying on her shoulder; she was elbow deep in stool; or she was being verbally and physically abused by a drunk," said an Illinois ICU nurse.

Most of all, be respectful, grateful, and kind.
Hopefully, this book will help the public to understand what nurses go through to provide the best possible healthcare. "Most nurses bust their asses taking care of their patients," said a Maryland medical/surgical nurse. "Hospital administrators are cutting aides, receptionists, and other ancillary help, forcing nurses to do more work without more pay. Nurses are skipping lunches, getting UTIs from being too busy to go to the bathroom, and staying long past their twelve-hour shifts to finish documentation. Be nice to your nurses. They work so hard with little thanks. It means a lot when patients say thank you." And if you want to go the extra mile, bring them treats.

If that's not convincing enough, patients and visitors who are unkind can delay processes like repeat pain medication, a Washington, DC, nurse said, "because the nurses don't want to deal with them."

Write to the administration about your care.
If you have a wonderful nurse, write him or her a note; even better, write her supervisors about how much you appreciated the nursing care.

For aspiring nurses

Nursing is the fastest-growing occupation in the country, according to the Bureau of Labor Statistics. Between 2014 and 2022, the United States will create 574,000 new jobs for nurses, many of them in the growing sectors of home health services and outpatient centers. The field needs more smart, dedicated workers. "The profession is exciting and fulfilling. This is a tremendously fabulous time for nurses because of the vast opportunities that exist," said Terri Weaver, dean of the University of Illinois College of Nursing.

This book describes some negative issues in nursing in the hopes that readers will lobby hospitals and lawmakers to fix these problems. But it is crucial to know that despite these issues, nurses love their jobs and will enthusiastically persuade potential recruits to join the field. Please read the nurses' testimonials at the end of this chapter to learn more about the rewards of the job.

One resource for aspiring nurses is Johnson & Johnson's Campaign for Nursing's Future. The campaign, which focuses on recruitment and retention of nurses and nurse educators, aims to "make nurses feel really good about what they do," said a spokesperson, and raises funds for scholarships, fellowships, and grants. The campaign's website, Discovernursing. com, offers steps to take to become a nurse, day-in-the-life videos, career development help, and other interactive tools for nursing students and managers.

For additional advice for aspiring nurses, I asked several nursing school deans what they tell their students and new graduates. Here are some of their tips.

Know your options.

Nursing is a practically limitless field. "Choosing nursing as a profession means that you will have career choices for a lifetime without changing professions," said Joan Shaver, dean of the University of Arizona College of Nursing. "We practice everywhere—hospitals; retail clinics; community centers; home care; urgent care; hospice; in the military, corporations, and government; in the air, on the water, on the road, on the Web; and more."

Nurses can also work as scientists, engineers, policy makers, lawyers, researchers, professors, administrators, and businesspeople. "As you learn the basics of nursing practice, observe and learn about where nurses work, their opportunities and impact, and what patients need in each. Your preferred forte will emerge," Shaver said.

In a hospital, shadowing on various floors "gives you a chance to see how the nurses interact with each other and physicians," said the Oklahoma nurse supervisor. "We have senior nursing students who will work as nurse techs and float to different floors to check them out. There are so many different job opportunities for nurses that it helps to take some time at the beginning and check out different options."

Kathleen Potempa, dean of the University of Michigan School of Nursing, recommended that all aspiring nurses "consider no less than a baccalaureate program, which is now required for work at many top hospitals and clinics," she said. "Studies show that baccalaureate-prepared nurses are first in line for jobs, are best prepared for the challenges of the field, and are exposed to a wide range of options for learning and research."

Nursing involves more than you might have thought.

Students commonly arrive at nursing school expecting to learn about performing certain tasks. "They have the same perception as the public, that nurses 'do things' to people. That's actually only a very small part of what nurses do," said Bobbie Berkowitz, dean of the Columbia University School of Nursing. "Most of nursing involves thinking critically, understanding the human condition and how people respond to illness and health, being a mediator, helping people understand what's happening, and minding the environment and the technology. These are skills that are often hidden from the public. We try to help students understand that nursing is more than giving an injection. It's a lot more complex than that."

Never stop learning.

For nurses, learning is a lifelong goal, said Mary Kerr, dean of the Frances Payne Bolton School of Nursing at Case Western Reserve University. Linda Norman, dean of the Vanderbilt University School of Nursing, agreed. "Be avid readers of the latest evidence out there related to health-care delivery in your practice. You don't stop that reading and learning when you graduate. To be a great nurse, you've got to be able to know what is the best evidence for the care that you're providing," Norman said.

Be a team player.

"We've got to get away from the doctor–nurse game. Today's world of healthcare is all about teams; nurses work with a lot of other decision makers," Norman said. "Nurses need to be comfortable in their own professional skin, and we've got to be able to appreciate everybody. We have to be able to appreciate the physicians' position, but they've got to be able to appreciate nursing and that the nurse's role has changed drastically over even the last five years."

On giving advice . . .

"Never give advice unless it's asked for and always give it when it is," said Judith Karshmer, dean of the University of San Francisco School of Nursing and Health Professions. While some nurse faculty members tell students never to give advice to families or patients, Karshmer had a different take. "People take advice from a lot of different sources. When patients or family say, 'What do you think I should do?' if they are asking for expertise from a nurse, it is your responsibility to provide that."

For nurses

Find your A-team.

"The best coping resource is my fellow nurses. We are dragged through the mud together during these tragic events; who better to debrief with? And my boyfriend, who listens to me go on and on, particularly after a really hard shift," said a New York pediatric ICU nurse. "I think that's one of the most important things for a nurse. You need to figure out who your A-team is outside of work and allow yourself to rely on them, because you can't hold this stuff inside your chest forever."

One popular resource for nurses is the social-networking site allnurses.com, which offers several discussion forums. "It's a platform for nurses from around the world to come together with like-minded people, share experiences, get support, and ask questions," said founder and CEO Brian Short. "A lot of nurses come home from working a tough shift (a patient dies, something bad happens). They don't really have support systems at home that understand what they just went through. On allnurses.com they can jump on and find thousands of people who understand."

Volunteer.

"The point of the profession is to improve the overall health of society. One way to do that, which I have found particularly satisfying, is volunteering with a health organization," such as on an interprofessional board, Terri Weaver said. "It's an indirect but effective way to impact a population of patients. Being involved in such organizations also showcases what nurses can do. Volunteering is a way to influence the perception of lawyers, businessmen, and other leaders, so that they witness the critical thinking and font of knowledge associated with nursing and realize that nursing is more than the stereotype."

To be a good nurse . . .

"To be a good nurse you have to have 'tits,' the female version of *cojones*," a Texas advanced practice nurse advised. "It's not about you, it's about the patients. What do you need to do to get their needs met? That requires self-confidence and lack of fear of humiliation by MDs (and PAs, who can also be horses' patoots). You have to be able to tell a physician that their orders aren't safe, or the patient's allergic to X, or that they need to come assess the patient."

Find a comfortable way to share.

"Many times patients wanted to connect more closely to me, but I held back after the first few times I invested emotionally" in patients who died, said a Washington State nursing professor. "It's hard to be caring and not give up part of yourself. My solution was sharing one or two things (over and over again) that seemed to meet the need of personal investment for the patient without surrendering my whole self. I learned how to use my 'polite face' with patients getting bad news, so I don't show emotion. I teach it now to my students: eye contact, relax face, and breathe. It works when they are angry at you, their illness, pain, or death, and helps the caregiver be the bridge to comfort for the patient."

Consider becoming a mentor.

Nurses nationwide told me how valuable their mentors and mentees have been to their development as a nurse. A Virginia nurse practitioner said she thinks of her mentors as "second moms."

Seasoned nurses offered several tips for being a good mentor. "I think the key components of good mentors are (1) patience: allowing a nurse to struggle and not to expect an answer immediately; (2) challenge: teaching a nurse to think out a process, task, or situation by reviewing the pros and cons; and (3) interest: helping a nurse both professionally and personally as she deals with new stresses and responsibilities," said a clinical nursing instructor in the upper Midwest. "Learning to be a nurse is like learning to be a mom. It's holistic, complicated and requires desire, knowledge, and a willingness to accept criticism. These are hard for some people, but so very important."

A Missouri clinical instructor said that mentors should be open to the idea that a mentee might have different needs than a mentor expects, and that those needs might change. "So be adaptable. Have a sense of humor, listen attentively, give the learner a chance to problem-solve or identify the possible options," she said.

Take "you time."

Flight attendants remind passengers to secure their own oxygen masks first before helping others. Similarly, nurses should remember to take care of themselves, even if only to take better care of their patients. This can help them to find joy or comfort in even the toughest weeks. "After a bad day, I go home and take twenty minutes all to myself. Sometimes I sit and cry and sometimes I just reflect on the day. After those twenty minutes, I let it go," an Oklahoma LPN said.

Help coworkers with substance abuse issues.

If you or a coworker have a substance abuse issue, check with your state nursing association for peer assistance, alternative-to-discipline rehabilitation, or diversion programs. For signs of an impaired colleague, and treatment recommendations, see www.aana.com/GettingHelp. For resources searchable by state, visit Webapps.aana.com/Peer/directory .asp. While the AANA's comprehensive directory is intended for nurse anesthetists—and the Peer Advisors volunteer only for CRNAs and student nurse anesthetists—many of the resources and state assistance programs can help all nurses. The AANA's pages provide one of the best one-stop shops for nurses seeking help.

The ANA's Impaired Nurse Resource Center also includes some links to organizations specializing in addiction: Nursingworld.org /MainMenuCategories/WorkplaceSafety/Healthy-Work-Environment /Work-Environment/ImpairedNurse/Impaired-Nurse-Resources.html.

The Massachusetts Nurses Association's guidebook on interventions advised colleagues to begin this delicate conversation with: "I am not asking you to confirm, deny, or explain the reasons for the observed behaviors. I am here to share concerns and offer possible resources for your consideration." The guidebook added: "It is important that the nurse understands that his/her options will become limited and their license will be in jeopardy if substance use continues." Coworkers can then inform the nurse about the availability of family medical leave and direct her/him to a peer assistance program.

Create moments of connection.

Canadian nursing professor Beth Perry studied exemplary oncology nurses to determine how they avoided compassion fatigue. She found that the nurses who created and appreciated "moments of connection" were energized by these occasions: "Those meaningful connections occur in moments often created by shared humor, therapeutic silence, touch, keeping the promise to never abandon—small gestures lovingly given that change the patient's sense of well-being and have a positive effect on the nurse as well."

Lobby for staff education on lateral aggression.

When Martha Griffin, director of nursing education and research at Boston Medical Center, taught a group of new nurses how to recognize lateral aggression and what to do about it, every nurse who was bullied confronted her aggressor, and in every case, the bullying stopped. Educating staff about what constitutes lateral aggression both empowers the victims and alerts the bullies to the ways their colleagues might be interpreting their behavior. This awareness and preparation can improve nurse retention rates.

Reach out to colleagues.

In some cases, alleviating hostilities among nurses could be as simple as making an effort to bridge generation or seniority gaps. "Experienced nurses can feel threatened by new nurses and resistant to changes recommended by new nurses. At the same time, new nurses don't recognize the significance of experience," said a Midwestern nursing professor. "As a Clinical Nurse Specialist, I was the one to orient new employees, and found that having sharing sessions off-the-clock, whether at coffee, lunch, or after work, decreased this. Unless nurses are allowed to share their understanding of how and why things are being done, the not-understanding becomes anger and disgruntlement. Both sides need to learn how to bring up something new and be willing to work together on change."

Remember why you love your job.

At Barnes-Jewish Hospital in St. Louis, part of the program to mitigate compassion fatigue includes an exercise in which participants share verbally with each other the reasons they chose their career. Similarly, it might be helpful for other nurses to remind themselves why their field is rewarding. Here are some perspectives on why nursing is wonderful.

"I absolutely love what I do. When patients and families come into the hospital, they are at the very least concerned, and at the most extremely frightened. There is nothing more satisfying than sitting down with a patient and discussing their diagnosis and what they can expect from their hospital stay. You can see them relax; they are so thankful that you simply took the time to sit and listen to them. I also love helping patients recover from surgery because you can directly see how your care helps them make a full recovery."

—A MINNESOTA TRAVEL NURSE

"Helping someone fills up that part of me that makes me able to give some more. I love figuring out what the matter is, that collaborative effort to make a nursing diagnosis and plan. I like that I have never been unemployed. I will always have the dignity of work that is fulfilling."

—A WASHINGTON STATE NURSING INSTRUCTOR

"There is not a day at work where a life is not changed by something I do, whether it's a decision on how to staff the floor, answering another nurse's question so she can understand what to do, or helping to settle a family issue."

—AN OKLAHOMA CLINICAL SUPERVISOR

"Nursing is that challenge which can make you a better person than you could have imagined being. It is a continuous education requiring curiosity, flexibility, ingenuity, resourcefulness, faith, compassion, and humor."

—A MISSOURI CLINICAL NURSING INSTRUCTOR

"I think nursing is the only occupation that is ridiculously crazy, challenging, and sometimes out of control, while at the same time the most rewarding, fulfilling, and inspirational occupation. It amazes me how many people's lives I have been able to touch in a meaningful way."

—A MARYLAND ONCOLOGY NURSE

"I love working in an environment where I can see the effects of my work in real time—instant gratification! I never leave feeling like I wasted my time at work. I like the mental puzzle of trying to figure out what's going on, but I also really appreciate the physical aspect of working with my hands. I learn something new every day; no day is 'just another day at the office.'"

—A CALIFORNIA NURSE PRACTITIONER

"I strive never to let my patients die alone. If family can't come, I do my best to stay and be their final companion in life. We are aware of the enormity of this journey. Our job is to help them not be afraid, feel alone, in pain, or anxious. I think nurses do this job well. There is joy in nursing, too: to see a patient's pain or infection disappear; a patient and their family's joy as they walk several feet for the first time. How can you not love nursing?"

—A WASHINGTON STATE CARDIAC NURSE

"There are very few jobs that each day some or most of the things you do for your clients make their day better. You always make a difference."

—A MISSOURI PUBLIC HEALTH NURSE

"My favorite times in nursing are when I've been able to help the spirit of the patient, from letting a kid cover me in Silly String to rocking a baby who was taken from her birth parents for maltreatment. It's the moments where I feel a connection between souls that I love the most. I also love to share my knowledge. When I teach a family something and I see the lightbulb of realization click on, that's a very rewarding feeling."

—AN ARIZONA PEDIATRIC ONCOLOGY NURSE

"As a nurse, you wake up every morning and say to yourself, 'Today I'm going to do the work of my life.' Behind every great doctor is an even greater nurse."

—AN OHIO OUTPATIENT NURSE

"I have never had a boring day as a nurse. Mostly I feel privileged to be involved in the lives of others and to work with them toward a better future. I have practiced for thirty-nine years, and I still have so much joy and energy every time I go to work. That's truly the sign of being in the right profession! We're like a secret club because we're privileged to share intimate life stories with our patients, and this level of awareness makes us a bit wiser about the true nature of people. There isn't much that surprises us about the human body, and we feel free with each other to discuss topics that are clearly off limits in other social groups. Our shared tragedies and losses help us deal with our own grief and sadness. I would say we are a hardy group."

—A MICHIGAN NURSE PRACTITIONER

"I love some of the stories I get to take home with me. It's also pretty cool to see some of the amazing things that medicine can now do. I've seen people brought back from the dead (Code Blue that ends well). Once, I got to have my hands inside a man's face, literally, like opening a real-life anatomy textbook. Where else do you get to do things like that?"

—AN ICU NURSE IN CANADA

"We are strong and opinionated. [Our unit has] worked together for so many years that we are like sisters. We finish each other's sentences, watch each other's children, and vacation together. We have a strong bond and love for each other. We spend more time with each other than most of our family members. We have nearly zero turnover. We are very close and comfort each other often."

—AN INDIANA NICU NURSE

"I love my job, and I hope people find comfort in knowing there are still people out there who love what they do."

—A NEW YORK ACUTE CARE NURSE

Wall of Heroes

This book is also dedicated to the selfless, hardworking nurses, past and present, whose stories would be enough to fill many more books. The inspirational nurses listed here were nominated by fellow nurses, who pay the highest compliments to their coworkers, mentors, relatives, or instructors. All of them deserve our heartfelt thanks.

Marion Acker, LPN, Mississippi • Deborah Ackerman, RN, BSN, Arizona • Suzanne Adams, RN, ASN, Utah • Kristen Albert, RN, Kansas • Cindy Alexander, RN, Kansas • Jodean Allen, LPN, Arkansas • Rebecca Almeida, BSN, Massachusetts • Christine Amidon, BSN, RN, NCSN, Indiana • Daynabelle Anderson, BSN, California • Jada Anderson, LPN, Indiana • Myrtle M. Anderson, RN, Washington • Judy Andrews, RN, CCRN, Maine • Laura Ardizonne, CRNA, DNP, DCC, New York • Howard Armour, CRNA, MS, Pennsylvania • Patricia Armstrong, ADN, Connecticut • Sylvia Arroyo, RN, MSN, Florida • Patricia Prentce Austin, retired USAF Major, BSN, MSN, North Carolina • Joyce Backus, RN, Kansas • Shayla Badgett, ASN, Florida • Becki Brown Baker, RN, BSN, MSN, Tennessee • Shayla Bakke-Caravia, RN, BSN, California • Amy Bales, RN, Indiana • Lee G. Balos, CRNA, Georgia • Virginia Rose Bamford-Perkins, RN, MSN, Maine • Alysia V. Barber, RN, BSN, Maryland • Jamacia Barker, LPN, Mississippi • Jenifer Barney, RN, Kansas • Brian J. Bauhs, CRNA, MSN, New York • Theodora Belz, RN, New Jersey • Wendy Beaudoin, BSN, MSN, NP, Canada • Sharon Beautz, RN, BSN, Maryland • Nancy Beckman, CRNA, RNC, MS, Michigan • Donald Bell, CRNA, MS, MSNA, Tennessee • Kim Bell, RN, New Jersey • Sheryl Bellinger, RN, BSN, MEd, Colorado • Patricia Benner, RN, PhD, California • Connie C. Bennett, LPN, Florida • Estella Bennett, LPN, Ohio • Robert J. Berger, CRNA, ARNP-A, MSNA, LTC, USAR, Iowa • Beth Bergeron, RN, New Hampshire • Anita Bertrand, CRNA, MS, Texas • Joy Biard, RN, Kansas • Antoinette "Peg" Black, RN, Wisconsin • Lisa Blackwelder, BSN, MSN, FNP, Texas • Jamie Blalock, APRN, FNP-C, Georgia • Diane Blanchfield, RN, MS, North Carolina • Gloria Jean Blenkhorn, LPN, Maine • Jo Ann Blevins, RN, Kansas • Eileen Bole, RN, Kansas • Tammy Fitch Borger, RN, BSN, Virginia • Pam Bormann, RN, New Hampshire • Loretta (Ann) Bostic, DNP, CRNA, West Virginia • Blair Bowers, BSN, Georgia • Catherine Boyts, RN, Kansas • Dr. Beverly Bradley, RN, PhD, California • Olympia Branch, LPN, Mississippi • Shirley A. Braun, RN, BSN, Florida • Cathy Bray, RN, Indiana • Jeanne Brennan, RN, Pennsylvania • Maria Brilhante MSN, FNP, MSRN, New Jersey • Hazel Brown-Johnson, Brigadier General, RN, BSN, MSN, PhD, Washington, DC • Marie Brophy, RN, BSN, MSN, Arizona • Laura L. Brown,

RN, BSN, Ohio • Sharon Brown, RN, Washington State • Katina Brownridge, RN, Mississippi • Jack Brueggemann, CRNA, Kentucky • Jo Buddrius, RN, MSN, New Mexico • Paula Bunde, RN, Kansas • Kelly Bunker-Taylor, RN, Maine • Charmon Burch, LPN, Alabama • Dana Burch, RN, New Jersey • Tashikkea Burns, RN, Alabama • Elizabeth Burridge, RN, Massachusetts • Kelly Bushnell, RN, BSN, Florida • Elizabeth Butler, RN, ACLS, NRP, Texas • Melody Anne Butler, RN, BSN, New York • Delores Byington, LPN, Oregon • Sally Caltrider, MSN, RN, Vermont • Lauren Calzonetti, RN, New Jersey • Pat Campanella, RN, BSN, California • Angela Sanders Campbell, RN, BSN, Mississippi • Tia Campbell, MSN, RN, NCSN, FNASN, Virginia • Annathea Canning, RN, Canada • Guy Caraffa, CRNA, Arizona • Agnes Carr, RN, Washington, DC • April Carter, RN, Mississippi • Frances Charles, RN, West Virginia • Julie Chase, RN, New York • Carl A. Cheramie, CRNA, MHS, Louisiana • Tony Chipas, CRNA, PhD, South Carolina • Diane Christoffer, ADN, Arizona • Tricia Christoffer, ASN, Virginia • Angela P. Clark, PhD, RN, CNS, FAAN, Texas • Gary Clark, CRNA, EdD, Missouri • Kristy Clendenin, RN, Texas • Keeshia Clouds, CRNP, Alabama • Peter Cockram, CRNA, Michigan • Ferne M. Cohen, CRNA, New Jersey • Marie Coker, CRNA, MS, Michigan • Hermine Endelkofer Colasanti, RN, Colorado • Robert J. Colcord, CRNA, MHS, Indiana • Margaret M. Cole, APRN, Connecticut • Ann Coller, RN, BSN, Indiana • Stacy Colson, RN, Indiana • Cindy Connellan, RN, Kansas • Noreen Conway, RN, Ohio • Angela Cook, RN, England • Renee Cooper, RN, Mississippi • Leigh Copsey, RN, New Hampshire • Robert N. Corbeille, CRNA, New Hampshire • Betsy Corrigan, MSN, RN, Maine • Judith Coward, RN, BSN, Utah • Lynda Lee Huse Crayon, RN, BSN, Florida • James Cuddeford, CRNA, Nebraska • Cynthia Cunningham, RN, BSN, Arizona • Lynn Curran, CRNA, Rhode Island • Deborah Currie, RN, Canada • Olive Cyrus, DNSc, MS, North Carolina • Leslie Dalaly, RN, BA, BSN, California • Karen A. Daley RN, PhD, MPH, FAAN, Massachusetts • Jessica Damon, RN, New Hampshire • Judi Dansizen, MSN, APRN, CNS, Illinois • Dr. Patricia D'Antonio, PhD, RN, FAAN, Pennsylvania • Kim Dare, RN, Kansas • Kristine Dascoulias, RN, New Hampshire • Julie Davidson, RN, Kansas • Susan Davis, RN, Tennessee • Leonardo De La Garza, BSN, Texas • Darla Denny, RN, Kansas • Mary Devlin, CRNA, BA, Pennsylvania • Janet Dewan, CRNA, PhD, Massachusetts • Monika Dewar, MSN, RN, Texas • Cindy DeWaters, RN, BSN, MSN, CCRN, Arizona • Judy Diaz, RN, Washington, DC • Saundra C. Dicicco, RN, BSN, Florida • Sheila Dickens, RN, West Virginia • Kathy Dietrich, RN, Illinois • Gail Dixon, RN, Florida • Brenda Dixon-Smith, RN, BSN, MSN, PhD, retired Army major, Oregon • Kristine Djuric, BSN, RN, Massachusetts • Saundra Dockins, CRNA, BA, Kentucky • Evelyn Dogbey, BSN, MSN, PhD, Pennsylvania • Andrea Dossey, RN, NNP, Texas • Anna Michelle Dozier, BSN, Florida • Jamie Dozier, RN, BSN, Florida • Joan Dozier, RN, Florida • Suzanne Dozier, MSN, Kentucky • Terri Dresch, RN, Colorado • Marissa Drummond, RN, BSN, California • Faith Dugger, RN, Mississippi • Nan Duncan, RN, Oregon • Belinda Dundon, BSN, MSN, NP, Canada • Dawnah Durkee, RN, Kansas • Patricia Edgecomb, LPN, Maine • John (Jack) Edmondson, CRNA, MS, Tennessee • Scott

Elder, CRNA, Idaho • Karen Eldridge, BS, RN, Maine • Tina Elwood, RN, Kansas •
Alice Peterson Erspamer, RN, Illinois • Cindy Evans, RN, ADN, Michigan • Sandra
Fails, ASN, Oklahoma • Rebecca P. Fairly, CRNA, Mississippi • Theresa Faivre, MSN,
RN, Illinois • Lucille M. Fennell, RN, US Army Captain, Montana • Mary Ferenz,
RN, New Jersey • Phyllis Mary Sinclair Ferguson, RN, Louisiana • Lauren Fink, BSN,
RN, California • Jane Firth, RN, BSN, MSN, North Carolina • Jennifer Fitzgerald,
RN, Vermont • Jeni Fitzpatrick, RN, BSN, Oregon • April Fitzsimmons, RN, New
Hampshire • Dave Fletcher, CRNA, MA, California • Kelly Fletcher, RN, New
Mexico • Jen Flippin, RN, BSN, North Carolina • Karen Florey, RNC-LRN, Texas •
Linda S. Foley, CRNA, Florida • Dr. Loretta Ford, EdD, PNP, FAAN, Professor
Emeritus, Florida • Barbara "Foof" Forfar, RN, New Jersey • Gail Foster, BSN,
California • Janine Fowler, RN, Kansas • Carol Fox, RN, BSN, New York • Bucky
(Buck) M. Frost, CRNA, Alaska • Kim Funk, RN, Indiana • Lisa Ann Gallup, MS,
BSN, RN, New York • Cheryl K. Gamble, CRNA, MSN, Delaware • John F. Garde,
MS, CRNA, FAAN, Illinois • Melissa Gaunce, RN, Ohio • Malgosia Glanda, RN,
ADN, Massachusetts • Timothy P. Glidden, CRNA, MS, Nebraska • Stacey Goddard,
MSN, Maryland • Brittney Golden, RN, Alabama • Lois Gombar, RN, Illinois •
Ronna Gore, RN, Mississippi • Ellen Graham, RN, Massachusetts • Dr. Carol Green,
RN, BSN, MN, PhD, Kansas • Susan Gregory, RN, ADN, Massachusetts • Aline
Grischkan, BScN, Canada • Linda K. Groah, RN, MSN, FAAN • Liz Guiterrez, RN,
Texas • Heather Gulish, RN, MSN, NP, Michigan • Shirna Gullo, DNP, RN, MSN,
BSN, Alabama • Jewel Gummer, RN, BSN, Oregon • Allison Hagen, RN, New Jersey
• Cherith Hager, RN, ADN, Colorado • Joel Hague, BSN, Pennsylvania • Gary Hahn,
CRNA, BSN, Virginia • Jehannah Hakim, RN, BSN, California • Dr. Bethany Hall-
Long, PhD, RN, MSN, BSN, Delaware • Donna Hallas, PhD, PNP-BC, CPNP,
PMHS, FAANP, New York • Heather Hamza, CRNA, MS, California • John Hanlon
Jr., CRNA, DNP, ARNP, New Hampshire • Tiki Hansen, BSN, RN, Maine • Kelly
Harmon, RN, Indiana • Ivan Hart, DNP, FNP-C, Kansas • Adrienne Hartgerink,
CRNA, DNP, Virginia • Felicia J. Haskins, BSN, MSN, Delaware • Ellen Haynes,
RN, Florida • Katherine "Licia" Hedian, RN, NP, CNM, DO, West Virginia • Kay
Heley, RN, Kansas • Kim Miller Hendrix, RN, Indiana • Karen Henken, RN, BSN,
MSN, Pennsylvania • DeShaunda Henly, RN, BSN, MSN, Florida • Ursula Shriver
Henry, RN, South Carolina • Jan Herren, RN, Arkansas • Amy Hicks, MSN, CNS,
North Carolina • Sharon Hindman, RN, Florida • Carla Kaye Hobbs, CRNA, APRN,
Kentucky • Mallory Hoffman, RN, BSN, Michigan • Denise Honn, RN, Kansas •
Mary Hopkins, RN, New Jersey • Diane Horner, RN, BSN, Indiana • Anne Hoskins,
RN, Kansas • Debbie Houser, LPN, Mississippi • Anne Howland, RN, New Hampshire
• Vickie Huff, RN, Mississippi • Cathy Hughes, RN, Wisconsin • Mel Hungerford,
RN, BSN, Georgia • Debra Hunsucker, RN, BSN, Virginia • Denise Indermuehle,
RN, California • Renee Irving, RN, California • US Air Force Captain Dayla Jackson,
RN, BSN, USAF, North Carolina • Falane S. Jackson, RN, BSN, Florida • Gena
Jackson, RN, Mississippi • Josie Jackson, RN, Arkansas • Kristi Jackson, RN,

Mississippi • Nicole Jackson, RN, New Hampshire • Richard G. Jaco, CRNA, California • Candice Janek, RN, Texas • Shirley Jensen, RN, Massachusetts • Brynn Jerles, RN, BS, MS, Indiana • Frances Jimenez, RN, MA, Colorado • Dr. Lucille Joel, RN, PhD, FAAN, New Jersey • Julie Johnson, RN, Kansas • Kathleen H. Johnson, DNP, MN, NCSN, Washington • Margie Johnson, RN, Mississippi • Marie Audrey Johnson, RN, Illinois • Julie Johnston, RN, Kansas • Nancy Johnston, RN, BSN, Florida • Bernice Jones, MN, Professor Emeritus, Oregon • Iberis Jones, RN, Virginia • June Jones, RN, Michigan • Roxanne Jones, RN, Kansas • Rubynelle Jordan, RN, BSN, Maryland • Lindsey Kabrud, LPN, Minnesota • Lauren Kaiser, RN, New Jersey • Kaci Karas, RN, Texas • Sarah Wilcox Katz, RN, BSN, Nevada • Sally Keating, RN, Kansas • Cindy Keilman, RN, New Jersey • Sharon Kendall, CRNA, South Carolina • Maia Kern, RN, New York • Kimberly Kerr, RN, BSN, MSN, Ohio • Maryann Kerr, BSN, RN, MSN, Indiana • Marsha King, BSN, RN, MSN, DNP, Indiana • Tim Kinnetz, RN, PS, Iowa • Melissa Phipps Kirby, RN, ADN, Virginia • Bonnie Kirtley, RN, Tennessee • MaryAlice Klaus, RN, New Jersey • Jamie Knight, RN, Kansas • Jennifer Kobylski, RN, BSN, Virginia • Robin M. Koeppel, MSN, RNC, CPNP, California • Mary-Beth Koslap-Petraco, DNP, PNP-BC, CPNP, New York • Martha Kral, CRNA, BSN, Georgia • Jaclyn Krostek, BSN, RN, Pennsylvania • Virginia Krostek, BSN, RN, New Jersey • Nikia Krouse, RN, New Jersey • Charity Kumpf, LPN, Indiana • Teresa Labrador, RN, Kansas • Kathy Lamb, RN, BSN, Pennsylvania • Dawn Landers, RN, New Hampshire • Elizabeth Lane, BSN, RN, Maine • Sharon Lane, ADN, Arizona • Patricia Lang, LPN, Minnesota • Rebecca Lang, BSN, RN, Indiana • Missy Lathem, RN, Mississippi • Sue Leach, RN, BSN, MSN, North Carolina • Heidi Leonard, RN, MHS, CDE, Canada • Joanne Lesiewicz, RN, New York • Fran Lewis, RN, PhD, Washington • Carol Goldenstein Lillie, RN, BSN, California • Ambur Lindstrom-Mette, DNP, FNP, RN, Arizona • Delores Linnenkamp, RN, Maryland • Rita Marie Linnenkamp, RN, Maryland • Rosemarie Linnenkamp, RN, Maryland • Nelda Welch Lively, RN, BSN, MHA, Texas • Glenda Lochridge, RN, Arkansas • Marilyn Logan, RN, Kansas • Ruth E. Long, CRNA, North Carolina • Daniel Longo, CRNA, BS, Michigan • Katie Loper, RN, Mississippi • Lianne Lopez, RN, BSN, MSN, California • Carry Lovelace, RN, MSN, BSN, Oklahoma • Danilo Lovinaria, CRNA, DNP, MS, MBA, Minnesota • Barbara Ballo Lowinger, RN, BSN, North Carolina • Joni Mee Lowsley, RN, Kansas • Chrystal A. Lucas, RN, BSN, MSN, Pennsylvania • Victoria Luther, RN, BSN, Indiana • Cissy Lux, BSN, NP, Texas • Daisy Moore Lydy, RN, BSN, MSN, Oregon • Claire MacDonald, RN, New Hampshire • Kathleen M. Madej, CRNA, Alaska • Uriah Magill, CRNA, MSN, North Carolina • Tak Yue Mai, RN, BSN, Florida • Marti Major, BSN, Illinois • MaryJane Maloney, RN, New Jersey • Carolina Marles, RN, New Hampshire • Kim Martin, RN, Kansas • Kimberly Martin, LPN, Georgia • Luis Martínez, RN, MSN, Puerto Rico • Wilhelmina Maslanek, BSN, MSN, Pennsylvania • Sandy Mason, RN, New Hampshire • Tommie Mathieu, CRNA, MS, Connecticut • Joy Mattsson-Boze, RN, BSN, MBA, Texas • Susan Matwiejczyk, RN,

BSN, Michigan • Suzanne Maynard, CRNA, MSN, Alaska • Frank Maziarski, CRNA, MS, Washington • Elizabeth McDaniel, ADN, Ohio • Ryan W. McDonald, CRNA, MSN, Washington • John P. McDonough, CRNA, EdD, Florida • Michelle Royal McDowell, DNP, RN, CPNP, Arizona • Charlene McKean, LPN, Indiana • Kristy McKindley, RN, California • Judy McMullen, RN, BSN, Kansas • Amy McNaught, RN, BSN, Maine • Chris McPherson, RN, Kansas • Florence McQuillen, CRNA, Minnesota • Michelle Meader, RN, New Hampshire • Ozella Meaders, RN, BSN, Oregon • Jane Meadows, RN, ADN, Tennessee • Melissa Mellace, RN, New Jersey • Bozena Michalzcuk, RN, New Hampshire • Judith Michoma, RN, BSN, Minnesota • Eileen Milano, RN, New Jersey • Lindsey Minchella, MSN, RN, NCSN, FNASN, Indiana • Sharon Mingo, BSN, Pennsylvania • Dr. Rosalie Mirenda, RN, BSN, MSN, PhD, Pennsylvania • Peggy Moellers, RN, Kansas • Joyce A. Moore, RN, MSN, Ohio • Donna Morris, RN, Kansas • Jamesia Morris, LPN, Mississippi • Marilyn Mortimer, RN, Kansas • Tom Muller, CRNA, Arizona • Idalia Munoz, RN, BSN, MHA, MSN, California • Helen Shea Murphy, RN, MSN, Massachusetts • Charlene Myers-Reid, RN, ADN, Pennsylvania • Angie Nachman, RN, BSN, Texas • Anne H. Napier, EdD, RN, MSN, CNS, Maine • Patricia Nerad, RN, BA, BSN, MHA, California • Nancy Nicolay, RN, Kansas • Phillip Noel, CRNA, BSN, Virginia • Jennifer Noll, RN, Kansas • Mary Norgren, RN, NCSN, Colorado • Paula Nuchols, LPN, Indiana • Lyna Nyamwaya, RN, BSN, Minnesota • Mary Ann Ogonowski, RN, MSN, LDAC, Maine • Karen O'Hara, BSN, RN, Pennsylvania • Nancy O'Hara, LPN, Pennsylvania • Maggie Olsen, CRNA, Georgia • Carrie Olson, RN, BSN, California • Victoria Ombuna, RN, BSN, Minnesota • Grace Oppong, RN, Canada • Victor J. Oskvarek, CRNA, Illinois • Mary Koster Pabst, RN, PhD, retired US Army Nurse Corps Lieutenant, Illinois • Nancy Pankratz, RN, BSN, Canada • Gina Pardo, RN, New York • Dolores B. Pasierb, CRNA, Oklahoma • Stephanie Patschull, RN, California • Janet Peluso, RN, Georgia • Warren L. Penrod, retired USAF Master Sergeant, BSN, MSN, FNP, Indiana • Sherry Perkins, RN, Maryland • Bridget Petrillo, CRNA, APRN, California • Maria (Hutchinson) Petty, BSN, MSN, CRNP, Massachusetts • Mary Broady Petty, RN, BSN, Indiana • Bethanne Pezzuti, RN, New Jersey • Nina Pham, RN, Texas • Gayle Phillips, RN, BSN, Oregon • Pat Polise, RN, Kansas • Graciela Phlatts, RN, New York • Helene Pietrangelo, RN, New Jersey • Pamela Pol, RN, BSN, New Jersey • Jeff Pope, CRNA, Colorado • Patricia Powell, LPN, Mississippi • Leisa Prasser, RN, Indiana • Patrick Price, CRNA, PhD, Minnesota • Venza Mae Price, RN, New York • Stacey Propper, MSN, RN, Maryland • Patricia Pruden, RN, Egypt • Janet Puglisi, RN, BSN, Colorado • Kathie Purcell, RN, New Mexico • Ernest A. Quier, CRNA, California • Diana Quinlan, CRNA, MA, Florida • Kimberly Radig, BSN, RN, Arizona • Cristina Ramirez, RN, Texas • Greg Ramplemann, CRNA, Ohio • Amber Ramsdell, MSN, RN, Texas • Christa Ramsey, RN, New Hampshire • Cyndy Rape, MSN, RN, ACNS-BC, North Carolina • Carlos "Rusty" Ratliff, CRNA, BSNA, Minnesota • Charles Raynor, retired US Army captain, RN, MSN, Texas • Myra Reddish-Randall, RN, MSN, Connecticut • Stephanie Requilman,

RN, BSN, California • Siri Richter, MSN, APRN, NP, Arkansas • Amy Riggen, BSN, RN, Indiana • Marilyn Ritenour, RN, BSN, Oregon • Brenda Rivera, RN, Florida • Sophy Rivera, RN, Florida • Keene Roadman, RN, MSN, Illinois • Teresa Robinson, RN, Pennsylvania • Deborah Harrison Robertson, MSN, FNP, Missouri • Bernadette Higgins Roche, CRNA, EdD, Illinois • Sarah Roder, RN, BSN, Texas • Don Roesler, CRNA, MS, South Dakota • Teggie Rogers, RN, Indiana • Patrick D. Roseland, CRNA, South Dakota • Heather Ross, RN, Mississippi • Sarah Rowekamp, LPN, Ohio • Tiffany Rowland, RN, Florida • Rita Rupp, RN, MA, Kansas • Heidi Sabado, RN, BSN, Washington, DC • Raheemah Saleh, BSN, RN, California • Anna Frances Sanders, LPN, Mississippi • Bridget Sanders, RN, Arkansas • Mutiat Sanni, RN, MSN, New Jersey • Natasha Sauceda, LVN, Texas • Aaronique Savage, RN, New Jersey • Akbar Sayed, RN, BSN, Maryland • Andrea Schlembach, RN, MSN, APN, New Jersey • Laura Schneider-Look, CRNA, Maine • Paul Schneider, RN, MSN, CRNA, Maine • Mary Schmitt, BSN, MSN, APRN, New Hampshire • Georgia Schnitkey, RN, ADN, Ohio • Amanda Kaye Schoenrock, Minnesota • Rose Schrempp, RN, Kansas • Heidi Schutte, RN, Kansas • Julie Scott, RN, Kansas • Melissa Sealey, RN, New Mexico • Heidi Seizys, RN, New Mexico • Anne M. Shannon, LPN, Florida • Karen Sharp, RN, BSN, Illinois • Farhan Shaukat, RN, BSN, Virginia • Jay Shelton, RN, Kansas • Marjorie Shelton, RN, Tennessee • Lisa Sheppard, RN, MSN, IBCLC, Ohio • Jan Sherman, RN, NNP-BC, PhD, Missouri • Shirley Sherman, LPN, Minnesota • Laura Shirey, RN, Arkansas • Danielle Shockley, RN, Kansas • Brian Short, ADN, RN, Minnesota • Jessie Shumpert Jr., LPN, New Mexico • Paul Silbernagel, CRNA, North Dakota • Latricia L. Simmons, RN, BSN, Florida • Leah Singletary, RN, BSN, Georgia • Evangeline Smith, LPN, Alabama • Gwen Smith, RN, MSN, Virginia • Melinda Smith, RN, BSN, Georgia • Patrick Smith, RN, BSN, MSN, Washington • Valerie Joy Smith, RN, MSN, BSN, California • Betsy Snook, RN, MEd, BSN, Pennsylvania • Tracy Snow, RN, Indiana • Alice Sollenberger, FNP, Colorado • Brent Sommer, CRNA, BS, California • Tammi Sontag, LPN, Florida • Grace Sotomayor, DNP, CNO, North Carolina • Brenda Splawn, RN, MSN, NP, Georgia • Danny Stanton, CRNA, BSN, Maryland • Rebecca Stanton, RN, BSN, Maryland • Ann Steffney, RN, MSN, New Jersey • John (Jack) T. Stem, CRNA, Ohio • Roxie Stempel, LPN, Arizona • Janet R. Stewart, CRNA, ARNP, Washington • Judy Stilwell, MSN, EdDc, Arizona • Jennifer Stinson, RN, Texas • Gregory S. Stocks, RN, EJD, Maryland • Alison Stone, RN, Arkansas • Linda Stone, CRNA, MSN, North Carolina • Arlene Stonelake, RN, Pennsylvania • Jeffrey R. Story, CRNA, MSN, Mississippi • Kellye Stroman, RN, South Dakota • Shelbe Sundeen, RN, Oregon • Jessica Switzman, CRNA, MS, Maryland • Thomas Szczygiel, CRNA, MSN, Pennsylvania • Melissa Tanner, RN, Mississippi • Betty Tate, RN, BSN, Maryland • Doris Taylor, RN, Texas • Robert Teasdale, RN, retired US Navy Lieutenant, New Jersey • Lorraine Thayer, RN, MSN, APN, New Jersey • Stacey Thein, RN, Kansas • Sharon Thomas, ADN, Texas • Michele Thompson, RN, Indiana • Vilma Thompson, RN, New York • Megan Tinling, RN, BSN, Oregon • Patty Toland, RN, Texas •

Carol Torpey, RN, MSN, Washington • Jan Tracy, RN, PhD, New Jersey • Carla Trout, RN, Nebraska • Cheryl Truzzi, RN, BSN, Washington • Sandra K. Tunajek, CRNA, DNP, North Carolina • Lemonia Tzimou-Vlisnaki, RN, BSN, Greece • Chad A. Utterson, CRNA, Colorado • Lawrence C. Van Atta, CRNA, Utah • Chris Vanderwal, RN, BSN, Iowa • Christine Varner, RN, New Jersey • Susan Varner, RN, Kansas • Amy Velez, RN, New York • Cassandra Villa-Lugo, RN, ADN, Texas • Rebecca Villanueva, RN, ADN, Texas • Amber Vinson, RN, Texas • Elizabeth Visintine, CRNA, Texas • Kristine Vosters, RN, BSN, Wisconsin • Barbara Waldron, BSN, CRNA, Georgia • Elizabeth A. Walls, RN, MSN, MBA, CNA, Pennsylvania • Cherri Ward, RN, BSN, Texas • Maureen B. Kelly Ward, CRNA, Pennsylvania • Angela Warner, RN, New Jersey • Bobbi Watson, RN, ADN, Illinois • Estelle Watts, MSN, RN, NCSN, Mississippi • Mary Watts, BSN, RN, Tennessee • Laura Way, RN, Kansas • Pam Webb, RN, BSN, Indiana • Ron Wegner, CRNA, ARNP, Florida • Amber Welch, RN, Florida • Barbee Whisnant-Burgess, RN, MSN, North Carolina • Marina Whitcomb, LPN, Vermont • Kelly White, RN, Indiana • Sheri White, RN, ADN, Washington • Robert R. Whitmore, CRNA, MS, Kansas • Anita Whittington, RN, Mississippi • Terry Wicks, CRNA, MHS, North Carolina • Lynne Widlund, RN, BSN, Oregon • Nikki Wiggins, RN, BSN, Oregon • Alicia Wilburn, RN, Mississippi • Bradley Wilburn, RN, Mississippi • Jennifer Wildung, RN, Kansas • Ernie Wildman, RN, Kansas • Diana J. Wilkie, PhD, RN, FAAN, Illinois • Luanne Williams, MSN, RN, Florida • Eleanor Sigurdson Wilson, RN, Maryland • Patty Wilson, RN, Kansas • Karen Witt, RN, MSN, Wisconsin • Christopher C. Woods, RN, BSN, Louisiana • Josephine Wong, RN, PhD, Canada • E. Laura Wright, CRNA, PhD, Alabama • Eliot Wright, RN, New Jersey • Sandi Wright, ADN, Virginia • Dixie Wyckoff-Raney, RN, BSN, CPAN, CAPA, Washington • Tracey Yazvac, RN, ADN, South Carolina • Barbara Yow, RN, MEd, NCSN, Virginia • Nancy Zeliff, RN, New Jersey • Sandra Sue Zenz, RN, Illinois • Barbara Zimmerman, RN, Pennsylvania • Gloria Zak, RN, North Dakota • Arthur J. Zwerling, CRNA, DNP, DAAPM, MSN, MS, Pennsylvania

---

The author would like to thank the American Association of Nurse Anesthetists; the National Association of School Nurses; the Association of Women's Health, Obstetric, and Neonatal Nurses; and allnurses.com for some of these dedications.

The following nurses were nominated by grateful patients and doctors or proud friends and family members. Each of these wonderful men and women is somebody's nurse in shining armor.

Kristen Novack Abreu, Connecticut • Crystalyn Acosta, New York • Kerry Hancock Abdo, Ohio • Eileen Adair, Texas • Shari Adams, New York • Tina Adeldye, Washington, DC • Julie Adoranti, Texas • Fereshta Al Awadhi, United Arab Emirates

• Candy Alfano, Arkansas • Ashley Allen, Virginia • Rhonda Allen, Indiana • Peggy Amaral, California • Angie Ames, Texas • Gail Andrews, Oklahoma • Zara Astarita, Virginia • Erica Avidano, New York • Ajarat Bada, California • Kate Baddoo-Osei, Washington, DC • Rose Bagford, Ohio • Courtney Baker, New York • Cindy Balderas, Oregon • Stephanie Baldwin, Nebraska • Carol Balentine, Kentucky • Jessica Marie Balraj, New York • Yana Banerjee, Pennsylvania • Celia Bardoff, Maryland • Bobbi Coburn Barnes, Pennsylvania • Faith Donhauser Barnhart, Pennsylvania • Heather Elizabeth Baron, New Jersey • Emily Barron, Pennsylvania • Ellen Fletcher Bass, Georgia • Karen Beal, California • Susan Becker, Michigan • Courtenay Begert, Washington, DC • Katherine Belt, California • Joanne Benedict, New York • Emylee Bennett, Virginia • Gail Bennett, Canada • Rebekah Bennett, New York • Valencia Bennett, Mississippi • Lorraine Bieser, Kansas • Linda Billings, Tennessee • Alice Bird, Maryland • Lisa Bishop, Tennessee • LTJG Holly Black, Massachusetts • Kim Black, Florida • Stan Boling, Tennessee • Marie Bolivar, Nevada • Melissa Boyd, Massachusetts • Lisa Boyle, Pennsylvania • Sue Brann, Ohio • Jan Brant, Maryland • Janice Breen, New York • Linda McCleary Brennstuhl, California • Leah Brines, Colorado • Alexandra Brown, Texas • Danielle C. Bruno, Tennessee • Jane Bucoy, New Hampshire • Lynn Burchell, Tennessee • Bill Burg, Texas • Kathy Measel Burgess, Minnesota • A. JoAnn Burket, Pennsylvania • Cam Burns, Colorado • Caroline M. Burns, Pennsylvania • Meagan Burns, Colorado • Briana Bush, Utah • Shannon Butler, Illinois • Sissel Byington, California • Janet Cadogan, New York • Rosallie Torres Cajulis, Virginia • Meghan Canning, New Jersey • Jaime Cannon, Alabama • Marilyn Cappillino, New York • Max M. Careiro, Florida • Robyn Cash, Texas • Becky Castruita, Texas • Samantha Ceponis, New Jersey • Julie Cernosek, Washington, DC • Rachel Chen, California • Kristi A. Cherry, Washington, DC • Lani Ching, California • Deanna Christensen, Texas • Kristen Chun, New York • Genie Chung, Virginia • Olivia Cimino, Washington, DC • Barbara Clarke, Michigan • Eugene Clay, Mississippi • Maggie Coakley, Maryland • Nan Campbell Coleman, Virginia • Dawn Collazo, Texas • Lauren J. Connors, Washington, DC • Trish Cooper, Kentucky • Stacy Cornelius, Pennsylvania • Connie Corrigan, Pennsylvania • Ilia Cosentino, New Jersey • Diana Costine, New York • Lindsay Coursen, Washington, DC • Megan Raley Crandel, Washington, DC • Ann Suttle Crim, Tennessee • Amy J. Crocker, Massachusetts • Kate Crooks, Connecticut • Shelby Taylor Cross, Virginia • Nicole Croyle, Connecticut • Nancy Cusmano, North Carolina • Karen Daniels, Washington • Allison Danks, New York • Jocelyn Datud, Maryland • Jonabell Datud, Maryland • Joselito Datud, Philippines • Yasmin Davidson, New York • Meagan Chase Davis, Oklahoma • Shana DeBoe, Pennsylvania • Melanie Witherspoon Decap, Illinois • Tomika Dedeaux, Mississippi • Marina Dedivanovic, New York • Ciji Boone Dellinger, North Carolina • James DeMaria, New York • Kricket Detterline, Pennsylvania • Kierstin Colby Devine, Washington • Lourdes Diaz, New York • Maria E. Diaz, California • Oswaldo Diaz, California • Dorothy Dickey, Georgia • Remy Dirige, California • Nena Ditrani, New Jersey • Colleen P. Ditro, Delaware • Katharine Dixon,

Washington, DC • Patricia Dixon, Washington, DC • Aubrey D'Onofrio, Pennsylvania • Nita Murry Dotson, Texas • Jane Driscoll, California • John Drislane, New York • Roger Dulude Jr., Connecticut • Dahalia A. Dunbar, New York • Melissa Tolley Dunleavy, Pennsylvania • Katie Dunn, Maryland • Dawn K. Dust, Georgia • Diane Edman, Maryland • John Ekelund, Maryland • Jillene Eliassen, Colorado • Christy Ann Elwood, Georgia • Johanna Emory, Virginia • Leni Engels, Florida • Karen Erdmann, Washington • Maria Erspamer, Arizona • Melecia Escobar, Pennsylvania • Mary Jean Essenmacher, Michigan • Anita Ewing, New York • Lori Fadden, Pennsylvania • Megan Faircloth, Florida • Jeannette Pugh Falconer, North Carolina • Lane Gotten Faughnan, Tennessee • Deirdre Fennely, Vermont • Rose Ferrari, Massachusetts • Anne Hemingway Feuer, Florida • Jacqueline Ficht, California • Sonya Fiebig, Washington, DC • Maggie Hass Finke, Washington, DC • Carrie Flanagan, Ireland • Neome Flores, Texas • Allison Folker, New Jersey • Philomena Fonollosa, New Jersey • Susana Font-Fontenot, Texas • Mary Ford, Washington, DC • Sharda Fornnarino, Colorado • Courtney Foster, Mississippi • Diana Fox, Washington, DC • Colleen Frampton, Louisiana • Hazel Shirley Francis, New York • Loretta Francis, Washington, DC • Lisa M. Freeman, South Carolina • Jennifer Freiwald, Florida • Andrea Froehlich, New York • Denise Furey, Pennsylvania • Cindy Garrison, Arizona • Amanda Gaston, Tennessee • Binnur Genc, Washington, DC • Monica Gerhardt, Maryland • Judith Gielissen, Wisconsin • Bernadette Gleichenhaus, Maine • Marci Glenney, Georgia • Ashley Goar, Texas • Leslie A. Gonce, Pennsylvania • Angela Goodman, North Carolina • Amanda Gordon, Massachusetts • Danielle Greco, New York • Jesse Greenberg, New York • Tricia Greene, Nebraska • Sabrena Greenewald, California • Debbie Greengrass, New Jersey • Julie Shapiro Gray, Florida • Denise Gruccio, Pennsylvania • Kathy Guilfoyle, Michigan • Megan Gulotta, New York • Bob Gwozdz, Massachusetts • Rob Gwozdz, California • Carrie Hahndorf, Virginia • Bronwyn Haines, Washington, DC • Beth Hall, Pennsylvania • Julia Halper, Colorado • Amy Haltom, Louisiana • Jennifer Hamilton, Mississippi • Julie Harab, Pennsylvania • Kimberly Hansard-Bailey, New York • Julie Harrington, Illinois • Jennifer Harris, Canada • Emily Harvey, Texas • Patricia Hauser, New Jersey • Mary Sue Hawkins, Virginia • Stephanie L. Hawthorne, Pennsylvania • Jennifer Nealon Heibel, Maryland • Melissa Helmkamp, Indiana • Tara Helmkamp, Arizona • Chermir Henderson, Pennsylvania • Yolanda Herlich, California • Louise Hesse, Nevada • Beverly Hicks, Ohio • Marissa Hicks, Washington, DC • Emyline Hiraki, Hawaii • Sarah Doss Holby, Washington, DC • Susan Hollerbach, New Jersey • Katie Holmes, Texas • Beth Houck, New Jersey • Susan Howard, Virginia • Anne Howe, New Hampshire • Retona Howell, Washington, DC • Rachel Hudson, Maryland • Debbie Hulvey, Ohio • Susan Immesoete, New York • Shamaila Iqbal, Virginia • LaTonya Ivy, Arkansas • Mary Lou Jackson, Connecticut • Jaime Jacobs, Maryland • Becca Jacoby, California • 2LT Lyndsay Thomasson Jeanes, Michigan • Rodney Jersak, Canada • Philomina John, Pennsylvania • Jennifer Johnson, New York • Veronica Johnson, Georgia • Christine Carlisle Jones, Montana • Paige Jones, Pennsylvania • Shirley Ann

Jones, Arizona • Soo-Ae Jones, Massachusetts • Peachy Judloman, Washington, DC •
Geraldine Kaminsky, New Jersey • Angela Karman, New York • Ali Karpa, Maryland
• David Katz, Pennsylvania • Michelle Keays, Nebraska • Macey Keifrider, Washington,
DC • Christine Keller, Missouri • Jackie Kelley, Arkansas • Barbara Joyce Kemper,
Indiana • Cerone Kent, Washington, DC • Cheryl Kester, Kansas • Joanna Kim,
Washington, DC • Millie King, Canada • Betty Johns Kirkpatrick, US Army 1st Lt.,
Pennsylvania • Mary Zellner Kish, Pennsylvania • Kathleen Klaus, Pennsylvania •
Jessica Koduru, California • Emily Kohnke, California • Genevieve Komisarz, Florida
• Elizabeth Konieczny, Pennsylvania • Jenna Korchinski, Ohio • Cheryl Kosits,
California • Pauline Kovich, Illinois • Lorraine Krautwurst, Maryland • Challis
Krulewitz, Massachusetts • Mike Kurz, Montana • Laura Kuss, Georgia • Jason
LaForest, Massachusetts • Stephanie Langan, New Jersey • Doreen LaPlante, California
• Gilmer Latorre, California • Rosalia Latorre, California • Silvia Latorre, California •
Whitman Latorre, California • Jane Lau, Ohio • Chelsea Laufer, Pennsylvania •
Pauline Zepel Leavitt, New York • Anne Schneider Leber, Maryland • Karen Leef,
New Jersey • Christianne Supan Legasto, New York • Kristin Leonardi-Warren,
Colorado • Angie Levesque, Idaho • Cecilia Lewis, California • Cathy Licitra, New
York • Sandra Tosti Linebarger, California • Jean Linstrom, California • Terri H.
Lipman, Pennsylvania • Joan M. Loch, Pennsylvania • Deb Long, Virginia • Marlena
Lopez, Arizona • Emily Lorber, California • Jalpa Lotia, New Jersey • Gretchen Luke,
Virginia • Cailee Luttinger, Washington, DC • Megan Lynch, Florida • Patricia Lynch,
New York • Holly MacNamara, New York • Kathleen P. Madson, Washington •
Lindsey Schaefer Magnuson, South Dakota • Meg Mallari, Washington, DC • Linda
A. March, New Hampshire • Chanel Marraccini, New Mexico • Karon Martel,
Michigan • Katie Martel, Michigan • Michael Martel, Michigan • Lucile Martin,
Georgia • Mary Lou Martin, New York • Cathleen Masterson, New Jersey • Sharon
Mattern, Texas • Margaret Matthews, Pennsylvania • Cathy May, Tennessee • Dana
McCommon, Mississippi • LaVeta Darline Holmes McGary, Texas • Mary McGraw,
Texas • Sherry McGrew, Ohio • Joyce McIntyre, Connecticut • Lyndsy McIntyre,
Vermont • Angel McKinness, Tennessee • Marie McLaughlin Boyle, New York •
Amanda McNally, Idaho • Stefanie McReynolds, Michigan • Emily McWilliams,
Maryland • Cindy Melniszyn, Pennsylvania • Jan Menefee, Washington, DC • Bonnie
Miles, Maryland • Stacy Miller, New York • Valerie Millerick, New York • Jana Mock,
Texas • Paula Mocrief, Washington, DC • Jayne Moggio, Pennsylvania • Pamela
Monteiro, Minnesota • Alex Montes, Alabama • Elissa Moorer, Delaware • Marla
Mora, New York • Michelle Kolb Morgan, New York • Sherry Morgan, California •
Janna Morris, Minnesota • Amy L. Motz, Washington, DC • Jay Mounteer, New York
• Heidi Mt. Pleasant, New York • Marilyn Mt. Pleasant, New York • Sandi Mt.
Pleasant, New York • Debbie Mull, South Carolina • Tye Mullikin, Maryland •
Kathryn M. Murphy, Pennsylvania • Lynda Murphy, New York • Sheila Murphy, New
York • Rachel Murray, Virginia • Dorothy Naidu, California • Amy Nation, Florida •
Kimberly Navarro, Texas • Leigh-Ann Hill Neal, North Carolina • Katelyn Nelson,

New York • Conni Nevills, Washington, DC • Angelita Nixon, West Virginia • Mahmoud Nur, Washington, DC • Eva Oakes, Maryland • Debra K. Oberer, Ohio • Karen Obermiller, Florida • Kathleen O'Brien, Georgia • Jerek V. Obry, Wisconsin • Ashley O'Connor, Pennsylvania • Oluwatoyin Odukoya, Nigeria • Susie O'Hara, Massachusetts • Helen O'Keeffe, New York • Melanie Olson, Vermont • Victoria Ombuna, Minnesota • Alyson Timlin O'Neil, Maryland • Dianne Mitchell O'Neill, Maryland • Julie Overbey, Tennessee • Betty Overby, Washington, DC • Linda Overstreet-Peel, Missouri • Gloria Pacelli, California • Dana Musser Parker, Washington, DC • Maire Patterson, Washington, DC • Bethany Payne, Washington, DC • Barbara Peace, Texas • Raynell Pearson, North Carolina • Marian Pelligrini, Washington, DC • Katherine Penniall, California • Kate Emerson Pennington, Tennessee • Kristy Pereira, Massachusetts • Amy Peterson, Washington, DC • Phyllis Peterson, Kansas • Jaime Pfeiffer, Illinois • Dorothy Phelps, Washington • Paula Phillips, Illinois • Brenda Pierce, Louisiana • Donna Pietropaolo, Massachusetts • Michelle Pisapia, Massachusetts • Linda Plante, Colorado • Hillary Poe, Kentucky • Suzanne Leber Poll, Maryland • Marla Pollard, Canada • Pat Pollock, New York • Mary Ponesse, New York • Eileen Ponto, New York • Katie Poppert, Colorado • Hanna Rae Pordy, Florida • Lori Powers, Maryland • Joyce Pratt, Maryland • Joyce Pratt, Washington, DC • Michelle Prim, Washington • Nell Berens Prosise, California • Allyson Protil, Virginia • Emylee Protil, Virginia • Katie Quick, Virginia • Anna Quinn, Maryland • Elana Quiroga, New Jersey • Nancy Carter Raggio, Arkansas • Cindi Raglin, Virginia • Ernestine Ralls, Tennessee • Magdalene Raven, Wisconsin • Thomas P. Raven, Wisconsin • Jennifer Rea, Washington, DC • Connie Reed, Pennsylvania • Susan Sutley Reed, Arkansas • Tony Reed, Mississippi • Vera Reed, Maryland • Susie Reed-McCullough, Maryland • Deirdre (DeDe) Regner, North Carolina • Erin Reilly, Washington, DC • Chelsea Reimer, Florida • Susan Renz, Pennsylvania • Mary Reus, Maryland • Johnna Ritchey, Pennsylvania • Jeff Ritter, Washington, DC • Caroline Leber Rivers, Washington, DC • Siama Rizvi-Sayed, Maryland • Debra Robbins, New York • Venessa Robles, Texas • Carla Rockliff, New Jersey • Ruth M. Roesler, Wisconsin • Beverly Rogers, Kansas • Karen Ronan, New York • Daniel Rooney, Texas • Laurie Rosa, New Hampshire • Natalie Rosenberg, Delaware • Becky Ross, Mississippi • Lawanda Ross-Patterson, Mississippi • Nancy Roth, Utah • David Rupert, Texas • Guadalupe Rupert, Texas • Kristen Sada, California • Rebecca Sander, Kansas • Catherine Sanders, Virginia • Helen Sandoval, Maryland • Jenny Sandoval, North Carolina • Roberto Santiago, Texas • Ginny Sasser, Virginia • Hina Sayed, Maryland • Nadia Sayed, Maryland • Melanie Sayre, Virginia • Jaclyn Schaller, Wisconsin • Robin Shecter, Massachusetts • Lisa M. Schmidt, New York • Melissa Schmidt, Minnesota • Stephanie Schneider, Washington, DC • Molly Schmitt, Pennsylvania • Susan Schottland, Maryland • Larry Schramm, Pennsylvania • Bonnie Scianna, New York • Kathleen Schroeder, Illinois • Anna Basich Scott, Washington • Jennifer Scribner, Tennessee • Pam Segerson, Washington, DC • Tricia Martoncik Seithel, Arizona • Kisha Semenuk, Washington, DC • Ashley Servi, Wisconsin • Marilyn Shapiro, Florida • Miller Sherling, Washington • Carie Ayers

Siegfried, Florida • Gail Silverman, California • Jennifer Silvey, California • Taryn Singer, New York • Tracy Sivec, Pennsylvania • Allison Skornik, Oregon • Jane Slacter, Maryland • Irma Smith, Colorado • Judy Smith, Connecticut • Loretta Smith, Arkansas • Sarah Payne Smith, Maryland • Tami Smith, Tennessee • Rose Snyder, Michigan • Catherine Soriano, Washington, DC • Soo Jung Sparks, Washington, DC • Pat Spaulding, Virginia • Guadalupe Perez Stabler, New York • Catherine Steinhauser, New Jersey • Catherine Stevenson, Pennsylvania • Kelly Ann Stock, Idaho • Liz Stocksdale, Washington, DC • Peggy Touey Stohler, Pennsylvania • Margaret Stuart, New York • Sheri Stuart, California • Jen Sturges, Oregon • Janet Stutzman, New Jersey • Michelle Suddath, Texas • Peggy Surratt, Washington, DC • Mikkii Cassem Swanson, Tennessee • Lindsey Sweeney, Maryland • Cindy Talerico, New Jersey • Jean Tatten, Nebraska • Gloria Teunisse, California • Leslie Thomas, North Carolina • Lisa Thomas, Virginia • Pup Thomas, Washington, DC • Mercy Thompson, Washington, DC • Andrea R. Thornton, Virginia • Michelle Timmer, Maryland • Laura Toews, Washington, DC • Virginia "Jean" Panelo Tomaneng, California • Maria H. Torpey, Pennsylvania • Susan Tramazzo, Florida • Jenny Trawick, Washington, DC • Miriam S. Trimble, Connecticut • Lana Troung, Washington, DC • Sheila Tucker, Utah • Diane Turner, Mississippi • Susana Valles Umel, California • Suzanne Underhill, New Jersey • Carissa Urbat, Washington • Karl V. Uriarte, New Jersey • Patty Utter-Garansuay, Texas • Kristen Van Cleave, Africa • Audrey Willems Van Dijk, Missouri • Julie Willems Van Dijk, Wisconsin • Vanessa Williamson, Texas • Katie Wooten-Bielski, Pennsylvania • Barbara Van Horn, New Jersey • Linda Vann, Maryland • Elenita Velasco, California • Karen Vincent, Maryland • Leah Viogolo, New York • Gretchen Virkler, New York • Maria DeCleene Vlach, Wisconsin • Julia Volcjak, Washington, DC • Taylor Vozza, New Jersey • Maria Wagner, New Jersey • Ashlyn Wallace, Washington, DC • Katy Russell Walpole, Connecticut • Beth Metzger Walsh, California • Kara Warner, Massachusetts • Ashley Nicole Warren, New Jersey • Elizabeth Weber, Texas • Sarah Weber, Canada • Jean S. Welch, Kentucky • Kathy Wertz, Washington, DC • Laurel M. West, Virginia • Geri Westad, California • Mara Casarez Weston, Michigan • Amber Whaley, Pennsylvania • Gwen Wheeler, Tennessee • Natacha Yanick Wheeler, Maryland • Erica Emig White, Minnesota • Lucie White, Washington, DC • Maggie White, Washington, DC • Therese White, Maryland • Dale Whiting, Kentucky • Maryann Duffy Whittaker, Florida • Elizabeth Bartz Wiener, Hawaii • Carisa Wilburn, Mississippi • Sharon Wild, Colorado • Cheryl Wille, New York • Linda Williams-Patterson, Mississippi • Nadia Wilson, Mississippi • Anne Wiltshire, Maryland • Leticia Williams, Mississippi • Meghan Williams, West Virginia • Katelyn Willis, New York • Cristina Withmory, California • Natalie Yao, Georgia • Shannon Roberts Yeardley, Colorado • Kristina Thompson Yocum, New Jersey • Diane Yorke, North Carolina • DeAlice Young, Mississippi • Josh Young, Washington, DC • Elizabeth Zagar, Washington, DC • Meri Zaumseil, California • Eve S. Zeff, California • Ann Zelenak, Virginia • Vicki Zimmerman, New York • Inarose Ries Zuelke, Oregon • Susie Zuelke, Washington • Rebecca Zylber, New York

ACKNOWLEDGMENTS

Reuniting with Mary Ellen O'Neill—wise, funny, and irresistible—felt like coming home. I could rhapsodize for pages about this remarkable woman, but she told me to keep the word count no longer than the last book we did together. I also was lured to Workman by the prospect of pairing again with amazingly talented marketing guru Jessica Wiener. I wish Peter Workman, who gamely agreed to open his magical publishing doors to narrative nonfiction, were alive to see this through. On some level, he must have intuited that, for me, a publishing house adorned with Star Wars paraphernalia, Cookie Monster bookmarks, in-progress robot prototypes, and a giant stuffed chicken is the publishing house of my dreams. I thank dynamo Carolan Workman, who plays a mean kazoo, for the warm welcome.

I have been fortunate to be on the same team as the smart, wonderful Suzie Bolotin, and the fun, creative publicity duo of Selina Meere and Noreen Herits. I'm also thankful to Page Edmunds, Michael Rockliff, Claire McKean, Beth Levy, Vaughn Andrews, Becky Terhune, and Heather Schwedel. I'm indebted to the hardworking booksellers and sales reps, many of whom told me personal stories about nurses, and to Michael Prevett, Gail Ross, Howard Yoon, and Anna Sproul-Latimer for their tireless efforts.

I am so grateful to my manuscript readers, who generously spent countless hours poring over unedited text: my Mom, my husband, my sister, and my friend Laura (all errors are mine). My Dad and brother are unwavering in their support and humor, which both are crucial to my writing and well-being.

Researcher Ali Eaves, who spent a summer assisting with research and reporting, was the best right-hand woman an author could ask for; her work was vital to this book. Semester interns Shaina Cavazos and Steffi Lee cheerfully tracked down stats and sources. Dave Holbrook and Krissy Hudgins offered sharp, helpful critiques of the essay on patient satisfaction.

I am lucky to know Denise Wills, for her friendship and for teaching me to be a better reporter and writer each time we collaborate, and the G.N.O. girls: Chrissy, Charlotte, Eliza, Jesse, Laura, Yvonne, Gwen, Danielle, and always Amy L. from afar. And I send an appreciative salute to Eva, my own nurse in shining armor.

Molly, Juliette, Lara, and Sam were generous with their time, stories, and patience, particularly when we reached the fact-checking stage. I hope they are as proud of this finished work as I am to know these incredible nurses.

My Facebook readers are awesome. They are supportive, thoughtful, interactive, and interesting. I particularly want to call out Andrew P.D.G. Everett for locating an elusive article and for helping to fact-check statistical analyses, Melinda Lundquist Denton (statistical analysis), Alexandra Markus (sourcing assistance), Andrew Eppstein, and Chip Decker (medical fact-checking). You, too, can join our fun at www.facebook.com /AuthorAlexandraRobbins or follow me on Twitter @AlexndraRobbins.

Thank you to my family with all of my heart. You know how I feel. And my eternal gratitude and devotion go to my husband: my rock, my best friend, and the love of my life.

NOTES

PREFACE

Robbins, Alexandra, "We Need More Nurses," *The New York Times*, May 28, 2015.

Robbins, Alexandra, "Is nursing a talent? You can bet your life on it," *The Washington Post*, September 17, 2015.

In a 2015 survey of Massachusetts nurses The Massachusetts Nurses Association, a labor union, sponsored the study; it was conducted by an independent research firm and the majority of respondents were not members of the association.

CHAPTER 1

"Emergency nurses practice . . . " Emergency Nurses Association, Award Recognition Program. www.ena.org/about/annualawards/Pages/ENAAward.aspx.

"ER nurses have the raunchiest jokes . . ." Interview with author (henceforth designated as "Interview").

"It's like high school, except for the dying people." Interview.

Dilaudid, a narcotic five to ten times See, for example, L. Felden et al., "Comparative Clinical Effects of Hydromorphone and Morphine," *British Journal of Anaesthesia* 107, no. 3 (2011).

injecting up to 8 milligrams of Dilaudid at a time, an enormous dose, but, for Lara, just enough to keep her alert. Lara's recollection, interview.

Medical Drug Intervention program MDI is a pseudonym. To find a rehabilitation program in your state, visit http://webapps.aana.com/Peer/directory.asp. While Peer Advisors are for CRNAs and student nurse anesthetists only, many of the programs are for all nurses.

At 3.5 million strong in the United States See U.S. Census Bureau, "Men in Nursing Occupations," February 2013.

and more than 20 million worldwide Correspondence from World Health Organization spokesperson to author.

nurses comprise the largest group of healthcare providers See, for example, "Nursing Fact Sheet," American Association of Colleges of Nursing, http://www.aacn.nche.edu/media-relations/fact-sheets/nursing-fact-sheet.

women who comprise 90 percent of the workforce Interview, Office of Occupational Statistics and Employment Projections, U.S. Census Bureau. See also "Men in Nursing Occupations."

"like a secret club . . . " Interview.

"We are not just the bed-making . . . " Interview.

They are, for example, frontline reporters. Thank you to nurse Meghan Yowell for inspiring the structure and content of this paragraph.

"Nursing is not a job." Interview.

"Doctors breeze in and out . . ." Email from this nurse to author.

an "I'm-going-to-eat-my-hair-in-a-corner person." Sam's words, interview.

CHAPTER 2

"I will not be ashamed to say 'I know not' . . ." From the Modern Version of the Hippocratic Oath. See Peter Tyson, "The Hippocratic Oath Today." *NOVA*. March 27, 2001. Accessed at pbs.org.

"The intimate nature of nursing care . . ." The American Nurses Association's *Code of Ethics For Nurses* page at http://nursingworld.org.

"Lots of hot residents . . ." Interview.

I-STAT A portable device that can perform diagnostic tests at a patient's bedside.

". . . shadowy, dark corners of our profession."   Barry Silbaugh, "ACPE Foreword." In Owen MacDonald, "Disruptive Physician Behavior," *American College of Physician Executives*, May 15, 2011.

bloody handprint on her scrubs.   Abigail Zuger, "Nurses Speak Out, About Doctors," *The New York Times*, October 28, 2008.

shoving matches in the operating room   Interviews. Also see, for example, Richard Knox, "Doctors Behaving Badly? They Say It Happens All the Time," NPR, May 25, 2011.

physicians throwing stethoscopes, pens, or surgical instruments   Interviews. See also, for example, Harold Levy, "Heal Behaviour, MDs Urged," *Toronto Star*, September 15, 2004.

scissors   See, for example, Liz Kowalczyk, "Hospitals Try to Calm Doctors' Outbursts; Medical Road Rage Affecting Patient Safety, Group Says," *The Boston Globe*, August 10, 2008.

Physical abuse by physicians is on the rise.   "Unresolved Disrespectful Behavior in Healthcare," *ISMP Medication Safety Alert*, October 3, 2013.

"Are you stupid or something?"   Interview.

A Texas doctor threw a metal clipboard . . .   Interview.

A surgeon threw a scalpel at a Virginia nurse . . .   Interview.

". . . He-Who-Must-Not-Be-Named"   Interview.

The Institute for Safe Medication Practices (ISMP) . . . has reported rampant bullying in healthcare   ISMP's Survey on Workplace Intimidation, 2013; ISMP's Survey on Workplace Intimidation, 2003.

87 percent of nurses encountered   Ibid.

"Every single nurse I know . . ."   Interview.

in countries such as Australia . . .   "Workplace bullying is a serious health and safety hazard affecting nurses and midwives." See "Bullying in the Workplace," policy paper, The Australian Nursing Federation. Reviewed and re-endorsed November 2011. See also Amanda Place, "Dealing with the Bullies in our Midst," *The Age*, Melbourne, Australia, June 22, 2002.

prevalent in South Africa   Simone Honikman and Ingrid Meintjes, "Nurses are Stressed, Ill-Treated, Burdened," *Cape Times*, September 9, 2011.

Hong Kong   R.P.W. Kwok, "Prevalence of Workplace Violence Against Nurses in Hong Kong," *Hong Kong Medical Journal*, February 2006.

Canada   Lucie Lemelin, Jean-Pierre Bonin and Andre Duquette, "Workplace Violence Reported by Canadian Nurses," *Canadian Journal of Nursing Research*, September 2009.

In 2010, a nurse in India committed suicide   "Mamata Suicide Case: Nurses Set Deadline to Nab Doc," *The Times of India*, February 16, 2010.

In Korea, a 2013 survey . . .   "Half the Nurses Suffer from Sexual Harassment." *Korea Times*, February 26, 2013.

the more abuse that nurses experience . . .   Laurie Scudder, "Physician Abuse as Reported by Early Career Nurses," Viewpoints, *Medscape Nurses*, September 20, 2013.

a link between doctors' intimidation and poor nurse satisfaction   See The Joint Commission. "Behaviors that Undermine a Culture of Safety," *Sentinel Event Alert* 40, July 9, 2008.

most nurses don't speak out   See, for example, David Maxfield et al. "The Silent Treatment: Why Safety Tools and Checklists Aren't Enough to Save Lives." VitalSmarts, AORN, and AACN.

Nurses are afraid to report doctors . . .   "Workplace Violence: Assessing Occupational Hazards and Identifying Strategies for Prevention, Part 1," a CE Home Study Course by *National Nurse*, January–February 2012.

a male travel nurse . . . saw cardiologist Abdul Shadani . . .   Reed Abelson and Julie Creswell, "Hospital Chain Inquiry Cited Unnecessary Cardiac Work," *The New York Times*, August 6, 2012.

"Sir, what are we going to fix?" . . . inserted the stent.   Ibid.

Soon after Tomlinson reported . . . including several other unnecessary procedures.   Ibid.

Shadani still works at Lawnwood.   Author's 2014 phone call to Lawnwood Regional Medical Center and Heart Institute.

In 2009, two Texas nurses filed . . . that risked patient health   See, for example, "New State Law Bans Anonymous Complaints Against Physicians," *FierceHealthcare*, September 20, 2011.

taking hospital supplies to perform at-home procedures   See, for example, Betsy Blaney, "APNewsBreak: Ex-County Lawyer's License Suspended," February 2, 2012.

pushing patients to purchase herbal supplements that he conveniently sold on the side.   See, for example, "Editorial," *The New York Times*, February 10, 2010.

sewing a rubber scissor tip to a patient's thumb   See "Justice Doesn't Always Have Happy Ending," *Austin American-Statesman*, October 7, 2011.

using an unapproved olive oil solution on a patient . . . failing to diagnose a case of appendicitis   See, for example, Kevin Sack, "Doctor Arrested in Whistle-Blowing Case," *The New York Times*, December 23, 2010.

performing a skin graft without surgical privileges   Ibid.

When the board informed Arafiles . . . his supplement business.   "Medical Justice, West Texas–Style," *The New York Times*, February 10, 2010.

Arafiles tracked down contact information for the patients listed in the complaint   See, for example, "Former Winkler County Memorial Hospital Physician Sentenced for Scheme to Fire Nurses in 2009." States News Service, November 7, 2011.

and gave it to the sheriff, who got hold of them   Kevin Sack, "Sheriff Charged in Texas Whistle-Blowing Case," *The New York Times*, January 15, 2011.

to determine the nurses' identities . . . found the letter.   Ibid.

A hospital administrator fired both nurses   Ibid.

who had not signed their letter because they feared . . . retaliation.   Rick Casey, "Justice, Injustice are Served," *Houston Chronicle*, August 13, 2010.

after months of unsuccessful attempts . . .   Betsy Blaney, "Nurse Testifies Talks on Doc's Cases Delayed Often," the Associated Press State and Local Wire, June 8, 2011.

charging them with "misuse of official information" . . .   Editorial, *The New York Times*, February 10, 2010.

Charges against one of the nurses   See, for example, Betsy Blaney, "Ex-County Lawyer's License Suspended," *APNewsBreak*, February 2, 2012.

filed a federal lawsuit . . . won a $750,000 settlement   Ibid.

the sheriff, who lost his license . . . one-hundred days in jail   Ibid.

county attorney, who was sentenced to ten years' probation   "Retaliation case merits stiff sanction," *San Antonio Express-News*, February 10, 2012.

Arafiles pleaded guilty . . . five years' probation   See, for example, Betsy Blaney, "Texas Doctor Pleads Guilty in Retaliation Case," The Associated Press, November 7, 2011.

As part of his plea agreement, he surrendered his medical license   Texas Medical Board. Public Verification/Physician Profile; Ibid.

charging him with several additional violations of improperly treating patients and intimidating the nurses . . . monitored by another doctor   Mary Ann Roser, "New Texas Law Bans Anonymous Complaints about Docs." The Associated Press State and Local Wire, September 20, 2011.

Texas Legislature passed a bill . . .   "Justice Doesn't Always Have Happy Ending."

and protecting those nurses from criminal liability.   Betsy Blaney, February 2, 2012.

In 2011, another Texas law . . .   "New State Law Bans Anonymous Complaints Against Physicians," *FierceHealthcare*, September 20, 2011.

An examination of policies and calls   Calls to every state nursing board. Arizona would be a forty-second state, but its policy is hazy. A spokesperson said, "The Arizona Board of Nursing does accept anonymous complaints, but the contact info of the complainant needs to be given to the assigned investigator. The complaint remains anonymous to the nurse."

a nonpartisan Texas citizen advocacy organization   http://www.texaswatch.org/about.

"It is shameful that nurses . . ."   Interview with Alex Winslow by Eaves.

"intimidating and disruptive behaviors"   The Joint Commission, "Behaviors That Undermine a Culture of Safety."

afraid the doctor will yell at them   See, for example, Alan H. Rosenstein and Michelle O'Daniel, "A Survey of the Impact of Disruptive Behaviors and Communication Defects on Patient Safety," *The Joint Commission Journal on Quality and Patient Safety* 34, no. 8, August 2008; Interviews.

Nurses have reported . . . confrontation with a physician   Alan Rosenstein and Michelle O'Daniel, "Impact and Implications of Disruptive Behavior in the Perioperative Arena."

Approximately half of surveyed respondents . . . "intimidation clearly played a role."   "Unresolved disrespectful behavior in healthcare." *ISMP Medication Safety Alert.* October 3, 2013; *ISMP Medication Safety Alert:* Intimidation: Practitioners Speak Up About this Unresolved Problem (Part I)." March 11, 2004.

many OR nurses are too intimidated   See David Maxfield et al.

Despite mandatory safety protocols like checklists . . .   See, for example, Julia Edwards, "Nurses Afraid to Speak Up When Doctors Slip Up," *The National Journal*, March 23, 2011.

more than 80 percent of nurses . . . "and disrespect" at their hospitals.   "New research shows communication breakdowns in hospitals undercut the effectiveness of safety tools and negatively impact patient outcomes," AORN/Vital Smarts press release, March 22, 2011.

Of the nurses who admitted . . . 83 percent did not report the violation   See David Maxfield et al.

Rhode Island Hospital in 2007 . . . which side was correct   Michelle R. Smith, "Brain Surgery Errors Rack Up at Prestigious R.I. Hospital." *The Virginian-Pilot*, December 15, 2007.

most likely to jeopardize patient safety   Carla Johnson, "Group Calls for Zero Tolerance of Doctor Bullies." Associated Press Online, July 9, 2008. For more information on these issues, see Shellie Simons, Roland B. Stark, and Rosanna F. DeMarco, "A New, Four-Item Instrument to Measure Workplace Bullying." *Research in Nursing and Health* 34 (2011). See also Arminee Kazanjian, Carolyn Green, Jennifer Wong, and Robert Reid, "Effect of the Hospital Nursing Environment on Patient Mortality: A Systematic Review," *Journal of Health Services Research and Policy* 10, no. 2 (April 2005).

Botched communications   See, for example, Alan H. Rosenstein and Michelle O'Daniel, "Impact and Implications . . ."

More than two-thirds . . . or patient deaths   See, for example, Alan H. Rosenstein and Michelle O'Daniel, "A Survey of the Impact . . ."

63 percent of cases . . . communications failure   The Joint Commission, "Sentinel Event Data Root Causes by Event Type 2004–2013," April 15, 2014.

"the most significant factor . . . communication"   Arminee Kazanjian et al.

patients die unnecessarily   Ibid.

the mother of a toddler . . . to follow up with him.   Lisa Rosetta, "Abuse Protection Sought for Healthcare Workers," *Salt Lake Tribune*, October 21, 2009.

"We tried to stop the doctor . . . an advocate for the patient."   David Maxfield et al.

"Failure of MD to listen . . . outcome in newborn."   Alan Rosenstein and Michelle O'Daniel, "Impact and Implications . . ."

"When a nurse reported . . . safety and well-being."   L. L. Veltman, "Disruptive Behavior in Obstetrics: A Hidden Threat to Patient Safety," *American Journal of Obstetrics and Gynecology* 196 (2007).

attending surgeons are . . . disruptive behavior.   Alan Rosenstein and Michelle O'Daniel, "Impact and Implications . . ."

Doctors and nurses . . . neurologists.   Ibid.

The hospital departments most likely   Ibid.

three-quarters of doctors . . . affects patient care.   Owen MacDonald, "Disruptive Physician Behavior," *American College of Physician Executives.*

"despite the best efforts of many . . ."   Barry Silbaugh.

"I could teach a monkey . . ."   Interview.

Up until the mid-twentieth century . . . wait on him."   Leonard Stein, "The Doctor-Nurse Game," *Archives of General Psychiatry* 16 (June 1967).

In 1967 . . . penis envy.   Ibid.

"Nurses have spent . . . hate each other?"   Rahul Parikh, "Do Doctors and Nurses Hate Each Other?" *Salon*, May 30, 2011.

"A couple of the nurses . . . got the point."   Interview.

"Female doctors"   Interview.

Nurses have continued to battle . . . instructors are nurses.   See, for example, Rahul Parikh, *Salon*.

"Nursing school . . . to be a physician."   Ibid.

Kevin Pho . . . carry that attitude into the workplace."   Kevin Pho, "Theresa Brown Unfairly Blames Doctors for Hospital Bullying," *KevinMD.com* (blog), May 7, 2011.

doctor bullies blamed a heavy workload . . ."   ACPE survey; see also "Reader Consult: Does the Culture of Medicine Enable Bad Behavior?" *WSJ Health* (blog), May 25, 2011.

"Surgeons have learned . . . behavior by observation."   Alan H. Rosenstein and Michelle O'Daniel, "Impact and Implications . . ."

"culture of disrespect among healthcare providers"   "Intimidation: Practitioners Speak up About this Unresolved Problem (Part I)," *ISMP Medication Safety Alert*, March 11, 2004.

In October 2014 . . . Ebola from a patient   See, for example, Alice Par, "Nurses 'Infuriated' by Suggestion of Dallas Ebola Protocol Breach," Time.com, October 14, 2014.

"Dr. Thomas Frieden . . . breach in protocol."   Rebecca Kaplan, "CDC Chief on Second Ebola Case: There Was a Breach in Protocol," *Face the Nation*, cbsnews.com, October 12, 2014.

National Nurses United . . . to an isolation unit   See, for example, "Dallas Nurses Accuse Hospital of Sloppy Ebola Protocols," abcnews.com, October 15, 2014.

protective gear left their necks exposed   See, for example, Saeed Ahmed, "Ebola Outbreak: Get Up to Speed with the Latest Developments," *CNN Breaking News*, October 14, 2014.

Frieden later said . . . misconstrued.   See, for example, "CDC: Nurse not to blame for breach of protocols in Ebola infection." Nurse.com, Oct. 16, 2014.

"There's a lot of outrage . . . blame the nurse again."   Nancy Shute, "Nurses Want to Know How Safe Is Safe Enough with Ebola," npr.org, October 14, 2014.

At Vanderbilt Medical Center in 2013   Kimberly Curth, "Vanderbilt Medical Center to Have Nurses Cleaning Up." WSMV TV, Nashville, Tennessee, September 6, 2013.

half-and-half   "Will Work for Half-and-Half," *Emergiblog* (blog), July 14, 2012.

Nearly 40 percent of doctors   ACPE study. The Joint Commission's Sentinel Event Alert, July 9, 2008.

As of 2015 . . . to earn a doctorate.   See, for example, Gardiner Harris, "Calling More Nurses 'Doctor,' A Title Physicians Begrudge," *The New York Times,* October 2, 2011.

Nurse leaders say . . . respect in the medical field.   Ibid.

physicians have turned the debate . . . endangers patients.   See, for example, Cindy Borgmeyer, "AMA Delegates Oppose DNPs as Medical Team Leaders," *AAFP News Now,* June 25, 2008; Amy Lynn Sorrel, "AMA Meeting: Physician Supervision of Nurses Sought in all Practice Agreements," June 29, 2009.

They argue that . . . confuse patients   See, for example, "American College of Physicians Response to the Institute of Medicine's Report," *Journal of the American College of Physicians,* November 1, 2010; Jeremy Olson, "U Program Turns out 'Doctor Nurses' but the Name Ruffles Some Doctors," *St. Paul Pioneer Press,* June 21, 2008.

an attempt to equate . . . medical training.   See, for example, Cindy Borgmeyer, "AMA Delegates Oppose DNPs as Medical Team Leaders," *AAFP News Now,* June 25, 2008.

loudly protested the DNP . . . dentists, and podiatrists.   "ANA Letter to AMA on HOD Resolution 303 (A-08) Protection of Titles 'Doctor,' 'Resident,' and 'Residency.'" Targeted News Service, June 11, 2008. Interview with AMA spokesperson. See also Resolution 232, AMA Resolutions, June 2008.

Eventually . . . physician Interview with AMA spokesperson. See also Resolution 232, AMA Resolutions, June 2008.

Nurse practitioners say . . . the field.   See, for example, Mary Anne Dumas, president, National Organization of Nurse Practitioner Faculties, "Letter to the Editor," *American Medical News,* August 18, 2008.

more time to spend with patients and charge less for their services. "28 States Consider Expanding Nurse Practitioners' Duties," *American Health Line,* April 14, 2010.

"essentially the same" health See, for example, Carla K. Johnson, *The Virginian-Pilot* (Norfolk, VA), April 18, 2010. See also "Research from Drs. Linda Aiken, Carole Estabrooks, and Others Have Established a Clear Link Between Higher Levels of Nursing Education and Better Patient Outcomes." Doctor of Nursing Practice (DNP) Talking Points. American Association of Colleges of Nursing, October 2009.

nineteen states and the District of Columbia Interview with AANP spokesperson. In these areas, NPs can "evaluate patients, diagnose, order and interpret diagnostic tests, initiate and manage treatments—including prescribe medications—under the exclusive licensure authority of the state board of nursing," according to the American Association of Nurse Practitioners. Other states require oversight of NPs.

Nurse-owned practices . . . expected to grow. Peter McMenamin, "In 2011 in Every State Thousands of Medicare F-F-S Beneficiaries Were Treated by an APRN," *ANA NurseSpace,* January 2, 2013.

looming physician shortage in the United States by 2020 See, for example, Chen May Yee, "A Doctor and a Nurse, All in One Package," *Star Tribune* (Minneapolis), April 27, 2008. See also Samuel Weigley et al. "Doctor shortage could take turn for the worse." *24/7 Wall St. usatoday.com,* October 20, 2012.

"The medical profession . . . in the United States." Interview.

"code of conduct" . . . managing those behaviors. The Joint Commission *Sentinel Event Alert* 40.

"moderate improvement" Alan H. Rosenstein and Michelle O'Daniel, "A Survey of the Impact . . ." See also Julia Edwards.

In 2005 . . . quarter of these nurses. David Maxfield et al. "The Silent Treatment: Why Safety Tools and Checklists Aren't Enough to Save Lives." VitalSmarts, *AORN Journal,* and AACN.

only 41 percent . . . "greatest negative impact." Ibid.

TJC continues to receive "Workplace Bullies Can Undermine Safety," *Occupational Health Management,* March 1, 2010.

"there are still large, disconcerting" Alan H. Rosenstein and Michelle O'Daniel, "A Survey of the Impact . . ."

"Tempo!" "Workplace bullies can undermine safety."

red phones at each nurses station Interview.

Nurses in a New Brunswick, Canada, hospital . . . in support. "Needed: Happy Endings in Workplace Bullying Cases," *The Times & Transcript* (New Brunswick), May 13, 2010. Code Pink in many hospitals refers to infant or pediatric abduction.

"Code White" to the same effect. "Workplace Bullies Can Undermine Safety."

"nurse-friendly" hospitals See, for example, Terry Simpson, "Transplant or Hospice," Yourdoctorsorders.com, January 29, 2012. Emphasis in "doctor-*unfriendly*" is mine.

"it affects my entire day." Interview.

"We train, hire. . . . They are pit crews." Atul Gawande, "Commencement Address at Harvard Medical School," May 26, 2011. Accessed at newyorker.com.

"the issue boils down to . . . excellent patient care?" Guest blog by the anonymous nurse of Those Emergency Blues (blog), on *KevinMD,* February 25, 2012. This post was in reference to a specific case against a nurse who was allegedly fired after a confrontation with a doctor; however, the quote applies to the larger issue of disrespect between the professions. I did not discuss that specific case because there were some questions as to the credibility of the sources.

of the top-ten media-generated See Jacinta Kelly, Gerard M. Fealy, and Roger Watson, "The Image of You: Constructing Nursing Identities in YouTube." *Journal of Advanced Nursing* 68, no. 8 (August 2012). Also see, for example, "Study: YouTube Gives Mixed Messages About Nursing." Nurse.com, July 17, 2012. Similarly, a "study of 280 films, produced between 1900 and 2007 from across the world, showed that 26 percent depicted nurses as sex objects," in *Nursing Times,* October 2008.

2010 Dr. Oz show See, for example, Staff and Wire Reports, "Dr. Oz's Dancing 'Nurses' Draw Nurse Group's Ire." *The Oklahoman* (Oklahoma City), December 10, 2010.

nurses protested Dr. Phil See, for example, Bob Groves, "An Image Problem, from TV to Silver Screen; Nurses Want Respect from Pop Culture," *The Record* (Bergen County, NJ), May 6, 2007. See also, "Dr. Oz's sexy 'nurse' backup dancers," *The Truth About Nursing*, December 6, 2010. See also Susan Campbell, "Does Your Nurse Dance/Dress Provocatively?" Courant.com. December 8, 2010.

waitresses dressed as sexy nurses See, for example, Larissa Liepins, "World's Weirdest Restaurant Premieres Tonight on Food Network," *The Daily Gleaner,* (New Brunswick) April 4, 2012.

a sexy nurse costume with white fishnets See, for example, Sonya Padgett, "Hangover Heaven Doctor Treats the Buzz Kill on Strip," *Las Vegas Review-Journal,* April 14, 2012.

In England, a bus company advertised See, for example, Flora Drury, "Sexy Nurse Sparks Fury on the Wards," *Worcester News,* March 16, 2010; "Sexy Nurse Ad On Bus Causes Uproar," *NSW Nurses' Association,* May 3, 2010; "British Nurses: We're Not Sex Objects, Either," *Adweek,* March 18, 2010.

"You will be motivated . . . emergency department." See, for example, "Hospital Advertises for 'TV Series-Hot' Nurses." *Asian News International,* February 22, 2012. The Internet ad used the term "TV-series snygga" after a satisfied patient had praised the hospital with those words. Translated to English, "snygg" or "snygga" is the equivalent of "hot" or "good-looking." See also "Swedish Hospital Seeks 'Hot' Nurses for Summer Employment," *The Digital Journal,* February 22, 2012.

largest Emergency Care Unit in the Nordic region Ibid.

scrubs that might be stained with blood, urine Interviews.

"We're sweaty and smelly" Interviews.

Certified nursing assistant Author correspondence with Erin Gloria Ryan.

"Nothing sexier . . . bowel movements on a chart." Comment following Margaret Hartmann, "BADVERTISING: Hospitals Are Obviously Full of Sexy Nurses!" Jezebel.com, March 18, 2010.

"Some nurses do fit . . ." Interview.

"lecherous old perverts" Interview.

"People are happy to sexualize . . . " Claire Lomas, "Sexualising Nurses Could Lead to Attacks on Staff, Warns Unison," *Nursing Times,* March 23, 2010.

In 2010, a Dutch nurse union . . . sexually gratifying him. Ben Berkowitz, "Nurses' Union: Care Does Not Include Sex." Reuters, March 11, 2010.

The man . . . nurses had done the same. News Staff. "Sex Is Not Healthcare, Union Says," November, 3, 2010.

When the student refused . . . unfit for the job. Ben Berkowitz, Reuters.

"I've got to get myself a nurse in Holland." Ronan McGreevy, "Nurse Stereotypes as Sex Objects Persist on Internet, Study Finds," *The Irish Times,* July 24, 2012.

union launched a campaign . . . front of her face Victoria Thompson, "Sexy Nurses: Tongue in Cheek or Demeaning and Gratuitous?" *Nursing Times,* March 19, 2010.

patients "are free to ask. You are free to refuse." Ibid.

87 percent of them said yes. Interviews.

"actually living Grey's Anatomy*"* Interview.

"Hospital life is . . . time to eat" Interview.

"Some places . . . stressed-out people together." Interview.

Nurses have gotten intimate in on-call rooms Interviews.

equipment lockers . . . patient rooms Interviews.

offices Interviews.

parking lots Interviews.

"heady" feeling Interview.

"Sexual exploits . . . call room at night Interview.

"It's like any kind of trauma" Interview.

they hook up with Interviews.

"I wanted to be" Interview.

"residency was all-consuming . . ." Interview.

A camera captured a nurse giving oral sex   Interview.
"She became a joke"   Interview.
Louisiana oncology nurse accidentally   Interview.
"Usually it only causes issues . . . "   Interview.
nurses caught having sex . . .   *The Herald* (Glasgow), "Nurses in Sex Session Suspended,"
   January 30, 1997.
When a resident and a nurse were caught   Interview.
"As Britons, we are obsessed . . ."   Robert Gore-Langton, "Carry on Nursing our Saucy
   Fantasies." *The Express,* March 4, 2008.
When a group of nurses posed. . . ."practice into question."   "Sexy Nurse Calendar Causes
   Complaints to NMC," *Nursing Times,* October 28, 2008.
posed nude for a charity . . .   Rob Harteveldt, "The NMC Should Focus on Things that
   Really Matter - Not Sexy Nurse Calendars," *Nursing Times,* February 3, 2009.
knowingly rented out a ward . . .   "Big Budget" Porn Film Shot in London Hospital. BBC
   News, July 6, 2010.
Lord Benjamin Mancroft . . . "promiscuous."   "Mancroft's House of Lords Speech in Full."
   Bath Chronicle, March 6, 2008. See also, for example, Morag Turner, "U.K. We're No
   Angels," *The Express,* March 8, 2008; Jenny McCartney, "Nurses: The Angels Who Fell
   from Grace?" *Sunday Telegraph* (London), March 2, 2008.
His evidence was . . .   "Mancroft's House of Lords Speech . . ."
"sexual boundaries" guidelines . . . dating patients.   See, for example, "Guide to Patient
   Relationships," *The Times* (London), January 22, 2008.
One in six U.K. nurses . . .   "Nurses Risk Breaking Rules on Relationships," *Nursing Times,*
   February 25, 2008. See also, for example, Morag Turner.
A British nurse received . . . they had sex.   "Nurse Had Illicit Affair with Heart Op Patient."
   Daily Mail (London), July 29, 2010.
between 1999 and 2009 . . . "constitutes sexual misconduct."   "Practical Guidelines for
   Boards of Nursing on Sexual Misconduct Cases." National Council of State Boards of
   Nursing, 2009.
Oklahoma Nursing Board . . . broke up with him.   Nolan Clay, "Nurse Loses License Over
   Patient Sex," *The Oklahoman,* January 16, 2011.
Mayo Clinic . . . relationship was consensual.   Warren Wolfe, "Male Nurse's Sex in Psych
   Ward Didn't Break Rules," *Star Tribune,* August 3, 2009.
In Australia, a sixty-one-year-old . . . "ethical relationship."   Julia Medew, "Nurse Faces
   Disciplinary Action Over Relationship," *The Age* (Melbourne), February 18, 2006.
Nurse and Midwifery Council investigated   "NMC to Investigate Nurse Accused of
   'Inappropriate Relationships,'" *Nursing Times,* March 11, 2010.
"Cancer nurse bedded . . . "   John Kay and Alex Peake, "Cancer Nurse Bedded Three
   Victims' Husbands," *The Sun,* March 10, 2010.
divorced mother of two . . . his wife passed away.   See, for example, Andrew Levy,
   "Macmillan Nurse Sacked for Having 'Affairs' with Patients' Widowers Reveals Her
   Love for Man Whose Wife Died Last Year," *Daily Mail,* March 11, 2010.
Some states, including Maine   "Disciplinary Action and Violations of Law," *Department of
   Professional and Financial Regulation, State Board of Nursing,* Chapter 4.
Arizona   R4-19-403, Unprofessional Conduct, "Laws & Rules," *Arizona State Board of
   Nursing.*
Washington State   Washington Administrative Code, Title 246, Section 246-840-740.
Three weeks . . . sided with the hospital.   Ed Canning, "Employee-Client Relationships are
   Tricky," *Hamilton Spectator* (Ontario, Canada), May 6, 2006.
Lori Dupont tried to end . . . harassed her at work.   See, for example, Doug Schmidt,
   "Daniel Turns to Blackmail," *Windsor Star* (Ontario), November 9, 2006. Schmidt
   covered this story extensively.
When several nurses complained . . .   Doug Schmidt, "Daniel's Return Unsettling," *Windsor
   Star,* November 10, 2006.
nurses took it upon . . . bent over to speak to him   Ibid.
broke a nurse's finger   Doug Schmidt, "Daniel Turns to Blackmail."

quiet weekend day . . . then killed himself. Doug Schmidt, "A Killing At Hôtel-Dieu: How a Workplace Romance Became a Deadly Obsession." *Windsor Star,* November 4, 2006.

"an unforeseen event" Doug Schmidt, "Why?: Family, Friends Ask: Could Nurse's Death Have Been Prevented?" *Windsor Star,* November 11, 2006.

Dupont's family and coworkers . . . Colin Johnston observed. Ibid.

when Daniel was pursuing Dupont . . . "problems." Doug Schmidt, "Dupont 'Relentlessly' Pursued," *Windsor Star,* November 7, 2006.

CHAPTER 3

"The nurse takes appropriate" "The ICN *Code of Ethics for Nurses.*" International Council of Nurses, Geneva, Switzerland, 2006.

"Almost every single" Interview.

"If I had a dollar for every horny . . . " Interview.

ER nurse in Sacramento . . . Interview with Dansby.

Medics brought in . . . able to revive Interview with Dansby. See also Jessica Garrison and Molly Hennessy-Fiske, "Violence Afflicts ER Workers; Incidents Often Go Unreported, but Some Evidence Points to a Growing Problem," *The Los Angeles Times,* July 31, 2011.

Dansby left the patient . . . off of her. Interview with Dansby.

Shaken and injured . . . assailant is still free. Ibid.

When Dansby told her department Jessica Garrison and Molly Hennessy-Fiske; confirmed with Dansby.

Afraid of losing her job . . . "that hospital door." Interview with Dansby.

"ward rage" See, for example Torri Minton, "Cry for Health: Poor Working Conditions Driving Nurses out of Hospitals," *San Francisco Chronicle,* May 20, 2001.

On the rise See, for example, Staff Report, "Not in a Day's Work," *National Nurse,* November 2010; "Preventing Violence in the Healthcare Setting." *Sentinel Event Alert* 45, The Joint Commission, June 3, 2010.

nine out of ten . . . "Emergency Department Violence Surveillance Study." *Emergency Nurses Association Institute for Emergency Nursing Research,* November 2011. See also Jessica Gacki-Smith et al., "Violence Against Nurses Working in U.S. Emergency Departments," *Journal of Nursing Administration* 39, no. 7/8 (July/August 2009); and Paula Zahn, "Nurses Under Attack," *Paula Zahn Now,* CNN, July 11, 2007.

a quarter of ER nurses . . . past three years. "Emergency Department Violence Surveillance Study"; see also Jessica Gacki-Smith et al.

every nurse they know Interviews.

Experts have attributed the rise . . . crime or accident scenes. Interviews; see also, for example, "Guidelines for Preventing Workplace Violence for Healthcare and Social Service Workers." U.S. Department of Labor: Occupational Safety and Health Administration; "Workplace Violence: Assessing Occupational Hazards . . ."; Jessica Gacki-Smith et al.

third-most dangerous profession An examination of the Bureau of Labor Statistics Survey of Occupational Injuries and Illnesses reveals that nurses rank behind only police officers and correctional officers in the number of nonfatal assaults that resulted in days off from work due to illness or injury. A separate set of BLS data that more explicitly specifies professions shows that the assault incidence rates (again resulting in days off from work due to illness or injury) for RNs, LPNs, and licensed vocational nurses rank behind only health technicians and health aides.

"nurses are nearly twice as likely . . ." Lois Berry and Paul Curry, "Nursing Workload and Patient Care," Canadian Federation of Nurses Unions, 2012.

"the actual number . . ." "Guidelines for Preventing Workplace Violence . . ."

sixteen times more likely . . . See, for example, "Workplace Violence in Healthcare Settings," Center for Personal Protection and Safety, August 2011; see also Alex Rose, "Protection Sought for Healthcare Workers," *Delaware County Daily Times,* March 2, 2011.

In 2012, Douglas Kennedy . . . See, for example, Ann Curry and Carl Quintanilla, "Douglas Kennedy Speaks Out for First Time Since Confrontation with Two Nurses," *Today*, April 13, 2012.

hospital had not discharged . . . See, for example, "Statement on Northern Westchester Case Does Not Address Assault on Nurses," Targeted News Service, April 4, 2012.

concerned maternity nurses . . . *"through the air."* Ibid.

Kennedy went downstairs . . . *welfare of a child.* Ibid.

superiors told them not to report . . . Interviews.

Nurses who don't keep . . . See, for example, Elizabeth Simpson, "Danger in the ER Health," *Virginian-Pilot* (Norfolk), April 13, 2012; August Gribbin, "Hospital Health Hazard," *The Washington Times*, February 10, 2002.

Tammy Mathews . . . *hospital fired her.* Lauren Auty, "Nurses Face an Epidemic of Violence in Hospitals," Philly.com, December 1, 2011.

between 65 and 80 percent . . . "Workplace Violence in Healthcare Settings," Center for Personal Protection and Safety, August 2011; *Emergency Department Violence Surveillance Study*, November 2011.

"incidents of violence . . ." "Guidelines for Preventing Workplace Violence . . ."

a Massachusetts judge . . . Elaine Thompson, "Hurt Healing Hands: Effort to Protect Health Workers," *Telegram & Gazette* (Massachusetts), April 8, 2010.

hospitals that encourage nurses . . . See, for example, *Emergency Department Violence Surveillance Study*, August 2010; "ED Nurses Seeking Protection from Violence," *Hospital Employee Health*, July 1, 2010; *Emergency Department Violence Surveillance Study*, November 2011.

"Victims are often untrained . . ." "Preventing Workplace Violence," American Nurses Association Occupational Health and Safety Series, 2006.

In 2007, a drug-seeking patient . . . *"actually getting worse."* JoNel Aleccia, "Swearing, Spitting, Choking: ER Nurses Endure This and More." *Vitals*, msnbc.com, November 9, 2011. Nurses' tolerance is expected to be even higher than patients' tension. A New York ER nurse said that a patient scratched her, bit her, spit on her, and hit her so hard that her jaw broke. The attacker later told her, "I'm sorry. I was tired of waiting." "Workplace Violence in Healthcare Settings," Center for Personal Protection and Safety, August 2011.

"What I don't have patience for . . ." Interview.

many hospitals aren't providing . . . Interviews.

In nearly three-quarters of assaults . . ." *Emergency Department Violence Surveillance Study*.

"They want the nurses to ignore it . . ." Interview.

More assaults occur . . . See, for example, "ED Nurses Seeking Protection from Violence," *Hospital Employee Health*, July 1, 2010.

target nurses. Examination of Bureau of Labor Statistics data on assaults causing occupational illnesses and injuries involving days away from work: 64 percent of assaults against healthcare practitioners and techs were against nurses. See also "Nonfatal Occupational Injuries and Illnesses Requiring Days Away from Work, 2010." News Release. *Bureau of Labor Statistics*, November 9, 2011; "Occupational Hazards in Hospitals," *CDC Workplace Safety and Health*, National Institute for Occupational Safety and Health, April 2002; "Workplace Violence in Healthcare Settings."

hospitals don't train their staff Interviews.

"My residents get more training" Interview.

Tennessee state senators . . . five to four vote Steven Hale, "Ford Lashes Out at Nurses," Tennessee Report, February 15, 2012.

Attacking a nurse is still only a misdemeanor Ken Steinhardt, "Progress on Felony Workplace Assault Laws," *ENA Connection* 8, no. 2, February 2014.

In 2006, Brenda Coney . . . killed a pharmacist. Charles Broward, "Jury Sides with Family of Killed Shands Pharmacist," *Florida Times Union*, October 1, 2011.

trauma patient who had been stabbed Author correspondence with Paul Matera; see also August Gribbin, "Hospital Health Hazard," *The Washington Times*, February 10, 2002.

punched Matera . . . what he was doing."   Author correspondence with Paul Matera.
The American Medical Association gave him   August Gribbin
"The whole Nurse Jackie thing"   Resources for nurses trying to stop substance abuse are
   listed in Chapter 10. For ease of reference, you can find a good preliminary list of links
   and contact information on this website: http://www.peerassistance.com/links.htm

CHAPTER 4

"The nurse treats colleagues"   The ANA's *Code of Ethics For Nurses*; see http://nursingworld.org.
"Somewhere along the line"   Interview.
"I knew the minute"   Interview.
Relationship-Based Care program   Developed by Creative Healthcare Management; see
   http://chcm.com/relationship-based-care/.
"silent epidemic"   Laura A. Stokowski, "A Matter of Respect and Dignity: Bullying in the
   Nursing Profession," Medscape.com, September 30, 2010.
"professional terrorism,"   Malcolm A. Lewis, "Will the Real Bully Please Stand Up,"
   Personnel Today, May 1, 2004.
"insidious cannibalism"   Penny Sauer. "Do Nurses Eat Their Young? Truth or
   Consequences," *Journal of Emergency Nursing,* January 2012.
"the dirty little secret of nursing."   Theresa Brown, "When the Nurse is a Bully," *The New
   York Times,* February 11, 2010. Brown is also the author of *Critical Care: A New Nurse
   Faces Death, Life, and Everything in Between. HarperOne* (2010).
75 percent of nurses had been verbally   Michelle Rowe and H. Sherlock, "Stress and Verbal
   Abuse in Nursing: Do Burned Out Nurses Eat Their Young?" *Journal of Nursing
   Management* 13, 2005.
only 23 percent said no.   Shellie Simons, "Workplace Bullying Experienced by
   Massachusetts Registered Nurses and the Relationship to Intention to Leave the
   Organization," *Advances in Nursing Science* 31, no. 2 (2008).
"Most of us could probably . . . "   "Bullying in the Workplace: Reversing a Culture,"
   American Nurses Association, Nursebooks.org, Maryland (2012).
Portugal   See, for example, Luis Sa and Manuela Fleming, *Issues in Mental Health Nursing,*
   29 (2008).
Finland   See, for example, Mika Kivimäki, Marko Elovainio, and Jussi Vahtera,
   "Workplace Bullying and Sickness Absence in Hospital Staff," *Occupational and
   Environmental Medicine* 57 (2000); Cheryl A. Dellasega, *American Journal of Nursing.*
Australia   See, for example, Suzanne Lappeman, "Nurses Are the Bullies, Says Lucas,"
   Gold Coast Bulletin (Australia), November 24, 2010; Denise Cullen, "Nursing Initiative
   Pays Off," *Weekend Australian,* January 15, 2011; Penny Sauer.
New Zealand   Brian G. McKenna et al., "Horizontal Violence: Experiences of Registered
   Nurses in Their First Year of Practice," *Journal of Advanced Nursing* 42; Janette
   Curtis, Isla Bowen, and Amanda Reid, "You Have No Credibility: Nursing Students'
   Experiences of Horizontal Violence," *Nurse Education in Practice* 7, no. 3 (May 2007).
Ireland   See, for example, Eithne Donnellan, "Most Migrant Nurses Bullied—Study," *The
   Irish Times,* May 7, 2010.
Canada, Taiwan . . . Turkey.   "Bullying in the Workplace: Reversing a Culture," American
   Nurses Association; Penny Sauer.
Taiwan   See also H. C. Pai and S. Lee, "Risk Factors for Workplace Violence in Clinical
   Registered Nurses in Taiwan," *Journal of Clinical Nursing* (May 2011).
Poland   Dorota Merecz et al., "Violence at the Workplace—A Questionnaire Survey of
   Nurses," *European Psychiatry* 21 (2006).
Japan   Interviews. Thank you to Andrew Robbins and K.O. for assistance in Japan. See
   also, for example, Kiyoko Abe, "Hierarchical Models of Workplace Bullying Among
   Japanese Hospital Nurses," Unpublished Dissertation, University of Minnesota,
   Minneapolis (May 2007).
"'angels in white'"   Interview. Other nurses in Japan shared similar sentiments in interviews
   for this book.

one in three nurses quits . . . See, for example, Martha Griffin, "Teaching Cognitive Rehearsal as a Shield for Lateral Violence: An Intervention for Newly Licensed Nurses," *Journal of Continuing Education in Nursing* (November–December 2004).

bullying—not wages— See, for example, Shellie Simons, "Workplace Bullying Experienced by Massachusetts . . ."; Katrina Creer, "Nurses Scared Off," *Sunday Telegraph* (Sydney, Australia), August 31, 2003.

nurse bullying is responsible . . . three years. Martha Griffin.

"It is destroying new nurses" Interview.

more nurses experience bullying Judith Vessey, "Bullying of Staff Registered Nurses in the Workplace: A Preliminary Study for Developing Personal and Organizational Strategies for the Transformation of Hostile to Healthy Workplace Environments," *Journal of Professional Nursing* (September–October 2009); Lyn Quine, "Workplace Bullying in Nurses," *Journal of Health Psychology* (2001); Janette Curtis.

nurses are verbally abused more Michelle Rowe and H. Sherlock, "Stress and Verbal Abuse . . ."

"backbiting and unnecessary scrutiny" . . . "as my peers." Alan H. Rosenstein and Michelle O'Daniel, "Impact and Implications . . ."

"nurses eat their young" J. E. Meissner, "Nurses: Are We Eating Our Young?" *Nursing,* March 1986.

practice festers . . . no nurse is immune. See, for example, Laura A. Stokowski. Interviews.

"There is a culture of treating" Interview.

nurse-on-nurse hostility . . . lateral violence. See, for example, "Workplace Violence: Assessing Occupational Hazards . . ." Technically, experts say that "bullying" refers to repeated negative actions against a nurse by someone who has power over the victim, such as a charge nurse bullying a staff nurse, or an experienced nurse bullying a new graduate. Horizontal violence, by contrast, can characterize a single incident and occur without the hierarchy variable.

"back-door undermining . . . behaviors." Alan H. Rosenstein and Michelle O'Daniel, "A Survey of the Impact . . ."

"being given an unmanageable . . ." Shellie R. Simons, Roland B. Stark, and Rosanna F. DeMarco, "A New, Four-Item Instrument to Measure Workplace Bullying." *Research in Nursing and Health* (2011).

"to stop talking . . ." Cheryl Y. Woelfle and Ruth McCaffrey, "Nurse on Nurse," *Nursing Forum,* July 2007.

"Nonverbal innuendo . . . a negative situation." Martha Griffin; L. L. Veltman, "Disruptive Behavior in Obstetrics: A Hidden Threat to Patient Safety," *American Journal of Obstetrics and Gynecology* (June 2007).

gossip; ignore Janice E. Hurley, *Nurse-to-Nurse Horizontal Violence: Recognizing It and Preventing It,* NSNA Imprint, September/October 2006; E. Duffy, "Horizontal Violence: A Conundrum for Nursing," *The Collegian,* April 1995; C. Dunbar, "Managers Can Prevent Incidents of Horizontal Violence," *AORN Management Connections,* 2005; Cheryl A. Dellasega. *Connections,* 2005.

Several other behaviors fall . . . condescend AACN Position Statement, "Zero Tolerance for Abuse."

belittle . . . exclude a nurse from socializing. See, for example, Janice E. Hurley et al.

when nurses give hints . . . monitoring a peer's work. See, for example, Shellie Simons, "Workplace Bullying Experienced by Massachusetts Registered Nurses and the Relationship to Intention to Leave the Organization," *Advances in Nursing Science* (April–June 2008).

"manipulating . . . to turn against a nurse." Cheryl A. Dellasega.

Verbal sexual harassment . . . less prominently. See, for example, Curtis et al.

"sexual harassment . . . behaviour from patients." Brian G. McKenna, "Experience Before and Throughout the Nursing Career." *Horizontal Violence: Experiences of Registered Nurses in Their First Year of Practice.*

The Workplace Bullying Institute . . . "car she drives." Gary and Ruth Namie, *The Bully at Work,* Sourcebooks, 2000.

"the Troll" or "Bitch on wheels." Interviews.
higher body mass index Mika Kivimäki et al.
making fun of their clothes . . . Interviews.
"make themselves feel better . . ." Interview.
"Structural bullying" . . . problem in the field. S. Simons and B. Mawn, "Bullying in the Workplace—A Qualitative Study of Newly Licensed Registered Nurses," *American Association of Occupational Health Nurses Journal* (July 2010).
more than one-third of nurse respondents . . . Brian G. McKenna.
Nurses report that charge nurses . . . sick days. See, for example, S. Simons and B. Mawn, "Bullying in the Workplace;" ANA's "Bullying in the Workplace: Reversing a Culture."
"During my first pregnancy . . ." S. Simons and B. Mawn.
Virginia nurse called in sick . . . "they're going to." Interview.
"core values" Interview.
a nurse was sent . . . policies on physicians. Interview.
"nurses create a kind of hierarchy . . ." "'Thick Divide' Still Exists Between Many ED Staffs," *Hospital Access Management*, February 1, 2007.
"Real Nurse" Interviews.
LPNs See, for example, http://www.nursinglicensure.org/articles/lpn-versus-rn.html
rivalries among specialties Interviews.
psychiatric nurses "eccentric." Interviews.
because her specialty is known Interview.
"They think we don't work" Interview.
"People think I put Band-Aids" Interview.
"I think the public generally" Interview, Carolyn Duff.
"I will absolutely admit" Interview.
Reason they prefer . . . "dump and run" Interviews.
"We don't like taking patients" Interview.
For approximately half Interviews.
"We don't just take vitals." Interview.
"It's not safe to leave . . ." Interview.
Horizontal violence may be directed . . . See, for example, S. Simons and B. Mawn.
nurses have been targets because of their accents See, for example, Denise Cullen, "Nursing Initiative Pays Off," *Weekend Australian*, January 15, 2011.
or ethnicity . . . per diem nurse See, for example, S. Simons and B. Mawn.
because they received . . . undeserved. See, for example, Cheryl A. Dellasega.
puts them at a disadvantage . . . Interview.
male doctors treat male nurses . . . Susan Strauss, "A Study on Physician Bullying as Gender Harassment to Female and Male Operating Room Nurses in Minnesota (Part I)," *Minnesota Nursing Accent* (September–October 2008).
"I think I have better relationships . . ." Interview.
he is disproportionately assigned . . . Interview.
"I'm not really involved . . ." Interview.
comes from cliques . . . See, for example, C. Rocker, "Addressing Nurse-to-Nurse Bullying to Promote Nurse Retention," *OJIN: The Online Journal of Issues in Nursing*, August 29, 2008; Malcolm A. Lewis, "Will the Real Bully Please Stand Up," *Personnel Today*, May 1, 2004.
"Misuse of power . . . vulnerability of both." ANA's "Bullying in the Workplace: Reversing a Culture."
nurses have higher job See, for example, Shellie Simons, "Workplace Bullying Experienced . . ."; Michelle Rowe and H. Sherlock.
"Some places have . . ." Interview.
nurse was tormented . . . Interview.
"something straight out of Mean Girls . . ." Interview.
"subjected to a despotic set . . . comes out strong" "The Hospital Tyrants and Their Victims, the Nurses: What Doctors Say of the Oppression of Young Women in These Institutions," *The New York Times*, August 22, 1909.
"the abominable outrages . . ." Ibid.

"with statements like, 'This is typical'"   E. Duffy.

In 1970, Brazilian philosopher . . .   See, for example, Linda Kay Matheson and Kathleen Bobay, "Validation of Oppressed Group Behaviors in Nursing," *Journal of Professional Nursing* (July–August 2007).

As group members are made   Shellie Simons, "Workplace Bullying Experienced . . ."

Because the oppressed group . . ."oppressed group behavior." See, for example, Linda Kay Matheson and Kathleen Bobay.

because of a history of submissiveness . . . an oppressed group.   See, for example, Linda Kay Matheson and Kathleen Bobay; Woelfle, Y. Cheryl; Janice E. Hurley.

"The culture of the healthcare setting . . ."   Center for American Nurses (part of ANA). Lateral Violence and Bullying in the Workplace. Approved February 2008.

"Unfortunately, many nurses . . ."   Michelle Rowe and H. Sherlock.

Venting to doctors . . .   See, for example, "Workplace Violence: Assessing Occupational Hazards . . ."; Dianne M. Felblinger.

when nurses are empowered . . .   See, for example, H.K.S. Laschinger et al., "New Graduate Nurses' Experiences of Bullying and Burnout in Hospital Settings," *Journal of Advanced Nursing* 66 (December 2010).

does not empower employees . . .   Penny Sauer.

keeps nurses short-staffed—nurse bullying increases   Laurie Scudder, "Mean Nurses: Verbal Abuse of Early-Career Colleagues," *Disclosures,* July 22, 2013.

environments with volatile workloads . . . workplace bullying.   Penny Sauer.

become hostile toward . . .   Diana Reiss-Koncar, "The War Against Nurses," *Salon,* July 27, 2001.

"are more likely to vent . . ."   Michelle Rowe and H. Sherlock.

If nurses are rarely afforded . . .   See, for example, Laura A. Stokowski.

physically and emotionally worn out . . .   G. L. Vonfrolio, "End Horizontal Violence," *RN,* February 2005.

Nurses who are too drained . . .   Johns Hopkins Children's Center clinical nurse specialist Cynda Hylton Rushton has made this observation.

much higher levels of burnout . . .   See, for example, H.K.S. Laschinger et al.; S. Einarsen, S. B. Matthiesen, and A. Skogstad, "Bullying, Burnout and Well-Being Among Assistant Nurses," *Journal of Occupational Health and Safety—Australia and New Zealand* (1998); Luis Sa and Manuela Fleming.

"There is a sort of test . . ."   Interview.

"Due to the broad base . . ."   Interview.

"the fact that a new nurse . . ."   Interview.

"Nurses put their own on steep . . ."   Interview.

"sorority initiation"   Interview.

OR's tradition of initiating . . .   Interview.

"a type of initiation . . ."   The ANA's "Bullying in the Workplace: Reversing a Culture."

". . . the many challenges they will face"   Interview.

". . . I wasn't at that hospital . . ."   Interview.

". . . My experience was awful."   Interview.

"Here, a select group . . ."   Interview.

"Tolerance for some forms . . ." Martha Griffin; see also Judith Vessey.

"are usually themselves past . . ."   Janette Curtis et al.

"Why do we tear . . ."   Interview.

"new nurses to prove themselves."   Interview.

"we've coddled these new young nurses . . ."   Interview.

"Nurses take an immense . . ."   Interview.

". . . for the sake of the patients."   Interview.

a small number of nurse bullying   Brian G. McKenna, "Experience Before . . ."

"One nurse was so intimidating . . ."   Interview.

nurses tend to keep quiet . . .   See, for example, Brian McKenna; G. A. Farrell.

. . . don't realize that it is unacceptable.   See, for example, Shellie Simons, "Workplace Bullying Experienced. . ."; Martha Griffin.

when nurses confronted their aggressors . . .   Martha Griffin.

"...*explain it to her at that moment.*"   Interview.

"*It all depends on where my head . . .*"   Interview.

A nurse in Singapore said . . .   Wee Li Hong, "Nurses' Day: Rookie's Less Laudatory View," *The Straits Times* (Singapore), August 6, 2008.

"*We work hard . . .*"   Interview.

Younger nurses, new to the field . . .   Malcolm A. Lewis, "Will the Real Bully Please Stand Up," *Personnel Today,* May 1, 2004.

expected to take on massive responsibility   See, for example, Sally Nicol, "Nursing in a State of Confusion," *The Courier Mail* (Queensland, Australia), November 14, 2005.

pressured to work on critical patients   Pauline C. Beecroft et al., "Outcomes of a One-Year Pilot Program," *The Journal of Nursing Administration* (December 2001).

average nurse is forty-seven . . .   See, for example, "Nursing Shortage," American Association of Colleges of Nursing (updated April 24, 2014).

many nurses are delaying retirement   David Auerbach, Peter Buerhaus, and Douglas Staiger, "Registered Nurses Are Delaying Retirement, a Shift That Has Contributed to Recent Growth in the Nurse Workforce," *Health Affairs,* (August 2014).

"*The younger nurses have good skills . . .*"   Interview.

"*Today, baccalaureate degree nurses . . .*"   Author correspondence with Donna Yates-Adelman.

"*New nurses are lumped . . .*"   Interview.

"*older, diploma-prepared . . .*"   Linda Kay Matheson and Kathleen Bobay, citing I. Daiski, "Issues and Innovations in Nursing Practice: Changing Nurses' Dis-empowering Relationship Patterns," *Journal of Advanced Nursing* 48, no. 1 (2004). See also Judith Vessey.

"*were those with university . . .*"   Cheryl Woelfle.

"*I hate nursing students . . .*"   Interview.

just as psychologically damaging   See, for example, "Workplace Violence: Assessing Occupational Hazards . . ."

Nurse victims can suffer   See, for example, Brian G. McKenna, "Experience Before . . ."

shame   See, for example, Dianne M. Felblinger, "Incivility and Bullying in the Workplace and Nurses' 'Shame' Responses," *Journal of Obstetric, Gynecologic, and Neonatal Nursing* 37 (2008) (A CE course on bullying); "Workplace Violence: Assessing Occupational Hazards . . ."

self-blame, guilt   See, for example, "Workplace Violence: Assessing Occupational Hazards. . ."

post-traumatic stress disorder.   Ibid.; Rebecca Catalanello, "Bullying at Work Can Make You Sick, but Remedies Are Few," *St. Petersburg Times,* July 26, 2009.

eroded self-esteem.   Michelle Rowe and H. Sherlock, "Stress and Verbal Abuse . . ." (2005); Janette Curtis et al.

substantial economic consequences   See, for example, Mika Kivimaki et al.; Pauline C. Beecroft, Lucy Kunzman, and Charles Krozek, "Internship: Outcomes of a One-Year Pilot Program," *Journal of Nursing Administration* (December 2001); Martha Griffin; Brian G. McKenna, "Experiences Before . . ."

higher rates of workplace . . . thousands of dollars.   See, for example, Pauline C. Beecroft et al., "Internship . . ."; Martha Griffin and Brian G. McKenna, "Horizontal violence . . ."

between $40,000 and $100,000 per nurse   See Lois Berry and Paul Curry.

cause increased medical errors . . .   See, for example, Michelle Rowe and H. Sherlock; G. A. Farrell, "Aggression in Clinical Settings: Nurses Views," *Journal of Advanced Nursing* 25, no. 3, (1997); Cheryl Woelfle.

"*lateral violence stops" . . . provide safe care.*   Martha Griffin.

"*secret club*"   Interview.

advocates for patients . . . each other.   Cheryl Woelfle,

their transition to practice.   Penny Sauer.

"*We may be fat, old . . .*"   Interview.

"*are the foundation of hospital care . . .*"   Interview. One such description: "To explain congestive heart failure, she told us that the heart is like stretched-out underwear and, without the elasticity, cannot function properly and pump the blood throughout the body."

" *. . . It's just the way it is with nurses.*"   Interview.

CHAPTER 5

"The nurse owes the same . . ." The American Nurses Association, *Code of Ethics For Nurses*, http://nursingworld.org.

"I go home sometimes . . ." Interview.

"I love the free entertainment . . ." Interview.

Elena Uhls . . . . . . "it's better that way." Interview. This is not her real name.

nurses' top health and safety concern . . . American Nurses Association, *Nursing World 2011 Health and Safety Survey*, LCWA Research Group, August 2011.

approximately 1.8 tons A. Nelson, A. Baptiste, "Evidence-Based Practices for Safe Patient Handling and Movement," *Online Journal of Issues in Nursing*, September 30, 2004.

More nurses are concerned . . . "accident after a shift." ANA *Nursing World 2011 Health and Safety Survey*.

The number of nurses reporting . . . "a frequent occurrence." Ibid.

Other common nurse injuries . . . See, for example, Karyn Buxman, "Humor in the OR: A Stitch in Time," *AORN Journal* (July 2008).

"Most women's health nurses . . ." Interview.

"not only for the patient . . ." Interviews.

"If you can't deal with it, you leave." Interview.

nurses may be more susceptible . . . See, for example, Patrick Meadors, "Compassion Fatigue and Secondary Traumatization: Provider Self Care on Intensive Care Units for Children," *Journal of Pediatric Healthcare* (January 2008); D. Boyle, "Countering Compassion Fatigue: A Requisite Nursing Agenda," *Online Journal of Issues in Nursing*, January 31, 2011.

"Nurses are not only 'first responders'. . . . " D. Boyle.

"The patients become part . . ." Interview.

87 percent of nurses . . . Meredith Mealer et al., "The Prevalence and Impact of Post-Traumatic Stress Disorder and Burnout Syndrome in Nurses," *Journal of Depression and Anxiety* 26, no. 12 (2009).

high rates of suicide . . . See, for example, Department of Health and Human Services, Centers for Disease Control and Prevention, National Institute for Occupational Safety and Health, "Exposure to Stress: Occupational Hazards in Hospitals," July 2008.

35 percent of nurses . . . 12 percent of emergency medicine residents. Darlene Welsh, "Predictors of Depressive Symptoms in Female Medical-Surgical Hospital Nurses," *Issues in Mental Health Nursing* 30 (2009).

Occupational reasons for this depression Ibid.

Patient care can be taxing . . . people who aren't nurses. Interviews.

"People don't know . . ." Interview.

Workplace stressors . . . These are just a few of many examples.

In Quebec Brian Daly, "Rash of Suicides at a Quebec City Hospital," QMI Agency, Torontosun.com, August 12, 2010.

At least one . . . "won't be the last." Marianne White, "Union Worried About Rash of Nurse Suicides," *Postmedia News*, August 14, 2010.

82 percent of nurses . . . nurses to become ill. Charlie Cooper, "Stressed Nurses Are 'Forced to Choose Between Health of Patients and Their Own.'" *The Independent*, September 30, 2013.

South African nurses . . . Tanya Jonker-Bryce, "'Fatigued' Nurses Threat to Patients," *WeekendPost* (South Africa), June 11, 2011.

30 percent of nurses are burnt out See, for example, "Self-Care of Physicians: Strategies for Care," *Hospice Management Advisor*, August 1, 2009.

defined as a "loss of caring." M. McCreaddie and S. Wiggins, "The Purpose and Function of Humour in Health, Health Care, and Nursing: A Narrative Review," *Journal of Advanced Nursing* (March 2008).

low energy, and thoughts of quitting. See, for example, Debra Wood, "How to Manage Compassion Fatigue in Oncology Nurses," *Oncology Nursing News*, March 26, 2009.

related but lesser known condition See, for example, Laura Landro, "Informed Patient: Helping Nurses Cope with Compassion Fatigue," *The Wall Street Journal*, January 3, 2012; Caitlin Crawshaw, "Caring Workers Pay the Price; Mind and Body Compassion Fatigue Flies Under the Radar." *The Telegraph-Journal* (New Brunswick), June 20, 2009. Little research has been done on the emotional impact of patient care on nurses. See, for example, M. Bloomer, W. Cross, and C. Moss, "The Impact of Death and Dying on Critical Care Nurses," *Australian Nursing Journal* (September 2010).

secondary traumatic stress disorder See, for example, M. McCreaddie.

empathetic nurses unconsciously absorb See, for example, D. Boyle.

experience the traumas emotionally . . . "spiritual depletion" See, for example, B. Lombardo, C. Eyre, and D. Boyle; Patricia Potter et al., "Compassion Fatigue and Burnout: Prevalence Among Oncology Nurses," *Clinical Journal of Oncology Nursing* (October 2010).

"a state of psychic exhaustion." D. Boyle.

"What is to give light" "Compassion Fatigue Program Gives Staff Skills to Be Resilient Against the Cost of Caring." States News Service, January 3, 2012. Indeed, Tulane Traumatology Institute director Charles R. Figley has said, "There is a cost to caring. Professionals who listen to clients' stories of fear, pain, and suffering may feel similar fear, pain, and suffering because they care. Sometimes we feel we are losing our own sense of self to the clients we serve." See "Compassion Fatigue: Coping with Secondary Traumatic Stress Disorder in Those Who Treat the Traumatized," *Routledge Psychosocial Stress Series*, 1995.

anxiety, depression . . . loss of objectivity B. Lombardo and C. Eyre.

less able to feel empathy . . . with certain patients See, for example, Laura Landro, "When Nurses Catch Compassion Fatigue, Patients Suffer," *The Wall Street Journal*, January 3, 2012.

Burnout can lead to . . . heavy-heartedness. See, for example, Meredith Mealer et al.

"Compassion fatigue does not" Debra Wood, "The Personal Cost of Caring Can Be High," *Oncology Nursing News*, October 6, 2009.

"are associated with a sense . . ." D. Boyle.

"Doctors are demanding . . ." Interview. Experts say that if a nurse doesn't treat compassion fatigue early, the condition can permanently affect the way she/he cares for patients (see D. Boyle). Yet compassion fatigue, arguably a major occupational health and safety hazard, is still relatively little known among healthcare providers.

social workers, counselors . . . See, for example, Caitlin Crawshaw, "Caring Workers Pay the Price; Mind and Body Compassion Fatigue Flies Under the Radar," *The Telegraph-Journal* (New Brunswick), June 20, 2009.

"They often enter the lives . . ." D. Boyle.

Simpson calculated that . . . D. Wood, "The Personal Cost . . ."

some types of personalities . . . See, for example, G. C. Keide, "Burnout and Compassion Fatigue Among Hospice Caregivers," *American Journal of Hospice and Palliative Care* (May–June 2002).

     Also note, according to a 2014 study, nurses who are motivated primarily to help other people may be the most likely to burn out. Jeanette Dill, Rebecca Erickson, and Jim Diefendorff, "Motivation and Care Dimensions in Caring Labor: Implications for Nurses' Well-Being and Employment Outcomes," unpublished paper in progress, provided to the author in August 2014.

already highly empathizing people Author correspondence with Oakland University School of Nursing professor Barbara Penprase regarding a study in progress.

"We are programmed to . . ." Interview.

demands of managed care . . . Nadine Najjar et al, "A Review of the Research to Date and Relevance to Cancer-Care Providers," *Journal of Health Psychology* (March 2009).

eight to ten percent . . . terminally ill patients. See Meredith Mealer et al. "The Prevalence and Impact . . ."

Other events that could lead . . .   Meredith Mealer et al., "Prevalence of Post-traumatic Stress Disorder Symptoms in Critical Care Nurses," *American Journal of Respiratory and Critical Care Medicine*, 175, no. 7 (2007).

similar to female Vietnam veterans.   Interestingly, the ICU nurses most likely to exhibit these symptoms were night-shift nurses who were not the charge nurse. See Meredith Mealer et al., "Prevalence of Post-traumatic Stress . . ."

Twenty-four to 29 percent . . . general nurses.   Ibid.

Outpatient nurses   Meredith Mealer et al., "The Prevalence and Impact . . ."

"intense fear, helplessness"   See Darlene Welsh, "Predictors of Depressive Symptoms in Female Medical-Surgical Hospital Nurses," *Issues in Mental Health Nursing* 30 (2009).

"Often, I feel it's an impossible job"   Interview.

In 2010, Kimberly Hiatt . . . 140-milligram dose.   JoNel Aleccia, "Nurse's Suicide Highlights Twin Tragedies of Medical Errors," msnbc.com, June 27, 2011.

A ten-fold overdose . . . not necessarily be fatal.   Interview with a neonatologist at another hospital.

hospital personnel escorted Hiatt   See, for example, JoNel Aleccia. "Nurse's Suicide Highlights . . ."

(who had heart problems)   See, for example, Theresa Brown, "High Price of Mistakes Sits Heavily on Nurses," *The New York Times*, The Virginian-Pilot Edition, July 17, 2011.

Hiatt, who told staff . . . careful in the future."   Ibid.

Hiatt was stunned . . . her entire career.   JoNel Aleccia, "Nurse's Suicide Highlights . . ."

Administrators had given her . . . "leading performer."   Ibid.

The state nursing board required . . .   See, for example, "Too Many Abandon the 'Second Victims' of Medical Errors," *ISMP Medication Safety Alert*, July 14, 2011.

Hiatt had difficulty finding . . . committed suicide.   Ibid; Carol M. Ostrom, "Nurse's Suicide Follows Tragedy," *Seattle Times*, April 20, 2011.

Hiatt reportedly suffered . . . often be neglected."   See "Too Many Abandon . . ."

surgeons who thought they made . . .   See, for example, JoNel Aleccia, "Nurse's Suicide Highlights. . . ."

92 percent of doctors surveyed . . ."   Ibid.

"If we fire every person . . ."   F. Norman Hamilton, "Suicide of Nurse after Tragic Event," Letters to the Editor, *Seattle Times*, April 22, 2011.

second victims usually require . . . "time of greatest need."   "Too Many Abandon . . ."

"Of course, we will also . . ."   Tom Hansen, "Children's Hospital CEO Responds to Infant Overdose," kirotv.com, September 28, 2010.

half of nurse respondents believed . . .   Thank you to Judy Huntington, the executive director of the Washington State Nursing Association, for providing the author with survey data.

After terminating Hiatt . . .   "Patient Safety Day Strengthens Seattle Children's Efforts to Improve Medication Safety," Seattlechildrens.org, October 30, 2010.

In 2003 and 2009 . . .   See, for example, "Death Was Third Fatal Medication Error At Children's," kirotv.com, September 28, 2010.

"This was not the fault . . ."   See, for example, Q13 FOX News Web Reporter, on chicagotribune.com, October 1, 2009.

"If my mom got an insulin . . ."   JoNel Aleccia, "Nurse's Suicide Highlights. . ."

Ohio nurse Beth Jasper   CNN Wire, "Lawsuit: Nurse Who Died in Car Wreck was 'Worked to Death,'" KVDR.com, November 13, 2013.

The case was dismissed . . .   Dismissal order, James Jasper vs. Jewish Hospital, Court of Common Pleas, Hamilton County, Ohio, entered April 10, 2014.

In Massachusetts, after a newborn . . .   Scott Allen, "The 'Second Victims' of Medical Tragedies," *Boston Globe,* November 30, 2004.

"have a little cry."   Interview.

even when their hospitals . . .   Interviews.

if an average hospital RN salary . . .   T. M. Dall, "The Economic Value of Professional Nursing," *Medical Care* 47, no. 1 (2009).

staffing for hospitals is not . . .   Interview, Peter McMenamin. The author is grateful to McMenamin for spending a significant amount of time explaining the economics of nursing.

A strong nursing staff . . .   P. Miller, "Nurses Drive Hospital Revenue Too," *HCPRO, Inc.* (March 2009).

nurses could do a better . . .   Interviews; also see, for example, B. Lombardo and C. Eyre, "Care for Caregiver to Avoid Low Morale and Burnout," *Hospice Management Advisor,* August 1, 2009.

"People will just about kill . . ."   Donna Gray, "Care Providers Get Compassion Fatigue: Burnout Common Among Healthcare Professionals," *Calgary Herald* (Alberta), February 2, 2006.

nurses take self-care measures . . . their feelings.   See, for example, Patrick Meadors, "Compassion Fatigue and Secondary Traumatization: Provider Self Care on Intensive Care Units for Children," *Journal of Pediatric Healthcare* (January 2008); "Self-Care of Physicians: Strategies for Care," *Hospice Management Advisor,* August 1, 2009; "Female Nurses Reduce Burnout in ICU Teams," *Nursing Times,* August 30, 2011.

"permitting ourselves to seek support"   Interview.

Some hospitals do have programs . . .   Interviews.

Barnes-Jewish Hospital in St. Louis recently . . . staff retreats.   Interview, Patricia Potter, director of research for patient-care services. See also Laura Landro, "When Nurses Catch . . ."

with experience . . . prepare themselves accordingly.   Interview.

registered nurses younger than thirty . . . the profession's demands.   R. Erickson and W. Grove, "Why Emotions Matter: Age, Agitation, and Burnout Among Registered Nurses," *Online Journal of Issues in Nursing,* October 29, 2007.

"The greatest common risk"   Tara Parker-Pope, "A Doctor's View of Medical Mistakes," nytimes.com, March 26, 2008.

Burnout and compassion fatigue have been linked . . .   See, for example, B. Lombardo and C. Eyre; Nadine Najjar et al.

correlated with higher patient mortality rates . . .   See, for example, Lara Landro, "Informed Patient: Helping Nurses Cope . . ."; Patricia Potter et al.; D. Boyle.

prone to make mistakes.   See, for example, Brittany Hoover, "Compassion Fatigue May Cripple Health Workers, Expert Says," *Lubbock Avalanche-Journal,* March 30, 2012.

fatigue alone can cause . . .   ISMP Medication Safety Alert, "Nurse Advise–ERR," December 2005.

nurse burnout is linked to . . . $69 million a year.   Jeannie P. Cimiotti et al., "Nurse Staffing, Burnout, and Healthcare Associated Infection." *American Journal of Infection Control* (September 2012).

Michigan Health and Hospital Association implemented . . .   See, for example, Tina Rosenberg, "Speaking Up for Patient Safety, and Survival," *The New York Times,* Opinionator, April 28, 2011.

for every 10 percent . . .   "Study: Nurse Safety, Patient Safety Linked," United Press International, November 8, 2011.

a national emergency.   See, for example, Meredith Mealer, "The prevalence and impact . . ."

99.9 percent of the nurses surveyed . . .   R. Erickson and W. Grove.

"I work where kids die"   Interview.

As Georgia nurse Brittney Wilson . . .   Wilson gave the author permission to attribute the quote. Wilson posted this comment at: Kevin Pho, "Should nurses be fired for fatal medication errors?" KevinMD.com, May 2, 2011.

all but three circumstances . . .   See, for example, R. T. Penson, "Laughter: The Best Medicine?" *The Oncologist* (September 2005). Globally, the use of humor in hospitals varies by the culture. In Taiwan, for example, nursing school professors teach therapeutic humor more than U.S. faculty, but use that humor less often in clinical settings because of a reverence for illness. See Lenny Chiang-Hanisko, Kathleen Adamle, and Ling-Chun Chiang, "Cultural Differences in Therapeutic Humor in Nursing Education," *Journal of Nursing Research* 17, no. 1 (2009).

humor can help patients . . . their treatments.   Ibid.

nurses use humor with patients . . . See, for example, Howard J. Bennett, "Humor in Medicine," *Southern Medical Journal* (December 2003); R. T. Penson et al.

staging pranks . . . bejeezus out of her. Interviews.

hidden under a sheet . . . shrieking down the hallway. Jim deMaine, "Gallows Humor is Only a Temporary Release from a Traumatic Situation," KevinMD.com, November 13, 2011.

A California nurse has sprayed . . . Interview.

Nurses have awakened night shift . . . Interview.

"I am not the only nurse . . ." Interviews.

When a young Southern nurse asked . . . Interview.

"I'd been punk'd." Interview.

"It tastes infected . . ." Interview.

urologists tend to have a lewd . . . Interviews.

"We get very naughty . . . like you mean it." Interview.

A Texas nurse remembered . . . Interview.

"gallows humor. . ." tragedy or death. See, for example, Howard J. Bennett; J. Sayre, "The Use of Aberrant Medical Humor by Psychiatric Unit Staff," *Issues in Mental Health Nursing* 22 (2001); Karyn Buxman.

when a doctor calls out . . . die in one night. http://themountainsarecalling.blogspot. com/2010/06/thoughts-on-death.html. Used with the nurse blogger's permission.

"circling the drain" . . . "Eternal Care Unit." Karyn Buxman.

"donor-cycles." Ibid.

"the departure lounge." "Gallows Humour in Hospitals Can Help Doctors and Patients Feel Better," *Daily Mail*, September 27, 2011.

Gunshot wound . . . Celestial transfer. "Tragedy, Black Humor, and Coping," *Health Beat*, November 1, 2012.

In the middle of the night . . . they ate the pizza." Katie Watson, "Gallows Humor in Medicine," *The Hastings Center Report*, September–October 2011.

nearly 90 percent used it . . . exercising (30 percent). Anne Villeneuve, "Why Paramedics Go for the Punch(line)," *Dartmouth Medicine*, Spring 2005.

In 2014, a Virginia patient . . . up a rectum. See, for example, Evan Bleier, "Colonoscopy Patient Sues Doctors for Making Fun of Him While He Was Unconscious," Upi.com, April 22, 2014.

more than $5 million in damages Elizabeth Waibel, "Patient Says Bethesda Practitioners Mocked Him During Colonoscopy," Gazette.net, May 13, 2014.

derogatory humor, in which . . . Delese Wear et al., "Derogatory and Cynical Humour Directed Towards Patients: Views of Residents and Attending Doctors," *Medical Education*, January 2009.

make fun of patients' names . . . locker. Interviews.

"Status Dramaticus" . . . "into the Hilton." Interview.

hummed the Jaws theme. Interview.

"only one joke per patient." J. Sayre.

targeted more than others . . . were removing. R. H. Coombs, S. Chopra, D. R. Schenk, and E. Yutan, "Medical Slang and Its Functions," *Social Science and Medicine* (April 1993).

trade anecdotes . . . hospital urban legends." Ibid.

"whose illnesses and health problems . . ." Delese Wear et al., "Making Fun of Patients: Medical Students' Perceptions and Use of Derogatory and Cynical Humor in Clinical Settings."

"difficult" patients . . . "us all look good." See R. H. Coombs et al.

they usually intend . . . A lot. Interviews.

"There's nothing potentially funny . . ." Ibid.

some ERs keep an orifice box . . . Interviews.

glass perfume bottles . . . an entire apple Interviews.

After Indiana nurses pulled a . . . Interview.

he had swallowed "something . . ." Interview.

required surgery to remove. Interview.

phone pictures of amusing X-rays. Interviews.

in meetings See, for example, Delese Wear et al. "Derogatory . . ."

"difference between whistling" Ibid.

humor helps medical professionals Ibid.

"Sometimes when something happens" Interview.

"find the bright side . . ." Interview.

shown to improve doctors' . . . See, for example, Howard J. Bennett.

It allows them to express See, for example, R. T. Penson et al.

"having a common sense . . ." R. H. Coombs.

"How does it feel to be . . ." R. T. Penson et al.

"stray bullet effect" . . . type of patient. See, for example, Delese Wear et al. "Derogatory . . ."

"Critics of backstage gallows . . ." See Katie Watson.

medical students use derogatory . . . See, for example, R. H. Coombs.

"a safety valve for 'letting off steam.'" These arguments are more persuasive than the idea that people who need to fill long stretches of silence in the Operating Room resort to gossip and jokes. (One medical student reasoned, "What else are you going to do? Oh yeah, that's a nice tibia . . . ? You have to say something." See Delese Wear et al. "Making Fun of Patients . . .").

"It's almost more depressing . . ." Interview.

"scandalous" . . . Interview.

can empower healthcare workers . . . locate joy or playfulness See, for example, Linda Caputi. "Humor in the Healthcare Workplace: A Cure for Stress." Presented at the Healthcare Educators' Conference, June 22, 2012; Karyn Buxman.

"Nurses need to blow off . . ." Interview.

nursing school educators who used humor . . . to combat burnout. See, for example, M. McCreaddie and S. Wiggins, "The Purpose and Function of Humour in Health, Health Care, and Nursing: A Narrative Review," *Journal of Advanced Nursing* 61, no. 6 (2007).

"Start a collection . . ." Karyn Buxman.

"When is behind-the-scenes . . . death won." Katie Watson.

CHAPTER 6

"The nurse promotes . . ." The American Nurses Association's *Code of Ethics For Nurses*: http://nursingworld.org.

"Hospitals tend to focus . . ." Interview.

base 30 percent of hospitals' Medicare HCAHPS Fact Sheet (CAHPS Hospital Survey), May 2012.

"Delivery of high-quality . . ." Department of Health and Human Services. *Federal Register*, Vol. 76, No. 160, August 18, 2011.

Beginning in October 2012 . . . See, for example, Jordan Rau, "Patients to Affect Hospital Bonuses," *Kaiser Health News*, in partnership with the *Washington Post*, April 28, 2011.

percentage will double in 2017 See, for example, Laura Landro, "The Informed Patient: A Financial Incentive for Better Bedside Manner," *The Wall Street Journal*, November 8, 2011.

Blue Cross Blue Shield See, for example, Liz Kowalczyk, "Nurses Balk at Bid to Guide Dealings with Patients," *The Boston Globe*, March 21, 2012.

Hospital Value-Based Purchasing Program "Administration Implements New Health Reform Provision to Improve Care Quality, Lower Costs," Healthcare.gov, April 29, 2011.

thirty-two-question survey . . . improved the patient's medical issue. See HCAHPS Survey: http://www.hcahpsonline.org, March 2014.

"my roommate was dying" See "Scrubs Contributor," Scrubsmag.com, July 4, 2012.

"This somehow became the fault . . ." Interview.

"Many patients have unrealistic . . ." Interview.

Medicare calculates scores . . . Not an average rating. "Always." Confirmed with a CMS spokesman; See also, for example, Cheryl Clark, "Top 12 Healthcare Quality Concerns in 2011," *HealthLeaders Media*, January 4, 2012.

Medicare awards bonuses . . . See, for example, "Administration Implements New Health Reform Provision to Improve Care Quality, Lower Costs," Healthcare.gov, April 29, 2011: "Hospitals will be scored based on their performance on each measure relative to other hospitals."

Washington, DC, and New York patients . . . lower ratings. See, for example, Jordan Rau, "Patients to Affect Hospital Bonuses."

either call or mail . . . See, for example, Jordan Rau, "Test for Hospital Budgets: Are the Patients Pleased?" *The New York Times*, November 7, 2011.

a patient asked Molly . . . Interview.

patients who reported being most . . . J. Fenton, A. Jerant, K. Bertakis, and P. Franks, "The Cost of Satisfaction: A National Study of Patient Satisfaction, Healthcare Utilization, Expenditures, and Mortality." *Archives of Internal Medicine,* March 2012.

results could reflect that doctors . . . Ibid.; see also "Patient Satisfaction Linked to Higher Healthcare Expenses and Mortality," UC Davis Health System Press Release, February 13, 2012. In an email to the author, Fenton clarified, "Most of our work on satisfaction pertains to outpatients, although some have generalized it to hospital care."

"Focusing on what patients want . . ." Theresa Brown, "Hospitals Aren't Hotels," *The New York Times*, March 14, 2012.

hospitals that perform worse . . . "definitely recommend the hospital." This is a conservative tally. I did not include hospitals that scored better than the national average on any one category, even if they had multiple categories in which they scored worse than average, because of the low but still possible likelihood that patients responding to the surveys fell into the "better" categories. I also excluded hospitals that did not have enough data in any one category for Medicare to rank them, in case highly satisfied patients filling out the surveys could have fallen into those categories.

"Patients can be very . . ." Interview.

In 2012, when a white father . . . JoNel Aleccia, "Hospital Granted Dad's Request: No Black Nurses, Lawsuit Says," NBCNews.com, February 23, 2013.

Hurley settled. . . $41,250 apiece. Gary Ridley, "Hurley Paid Nearly $200,000 to Settle No-Black-Nurses Lawsuit, Records Show," MichiganLive.com, March 20, 2013.

more than 61 percent of patients . . . in the bottom half. See Saket Girotra, Peter Cram, and Ioana Popescu, "Patient Satisfaction at America's Lowest Performing Hospitals," *Circulation: Cardiovascular Quality and Outcomes* (May 2012). Some caveats: The 61 percent who would recommend low-performing hospitals is compared to 66 percent of patients at hospitals with high scores, Girotra noted in correspondence with the author. He added, "Although the difference between low and high performing HF hospitals was statistically significant, it was small. . . . Lastly, it is important to remember that the patient satisfaction ratings were provided by a sample of all patients discharged from the hospital and not just heart failure patients." In addition, Girotra said that on average, patients treated at consistently low-performing heart failure hospitals were less likely to give high marks to those hospitals compared to patients treated at high-performing hospitals.

"is part of an ongoing national effort" Sample Initial Cover Letter for the HCAHPS Survey, March 2013.

valet parking See, for example, Nina Bernstein, "Hospitals Aren't Waiting for Verdict on Healthcare Law," *The New York Times*, June 10, 2012.

live music See, for example, Laura Landro, "The Informed Patient: A Financial Incentive . . ."

custom-order room-service . . . televisions. See, for example, Melissa Burden, "Stakes High for Hospital Service," *Detroit News*, March 19, 2012.

". . . loyalty programs." Ibid.

spent approximately $50 million . . . executive chef. Todd Sloane, "The University of Patient Satisfaction," *Partners*, January–February 2012.

Beaumont Hospital spent half a million . . . score." Ibid.

scripting nurses' patient interactions. See, for example, Nina Bernstein, "Hospitals Aren't Waiting . . ."; Nina Bernstein, "Walkouts by Nurses Loom as Hospitals Seek to Cut Costs," *The New York Times*, December 15, 2011; Liz Kowalczyk; Todd Sloane.

use particular phrases . . . See, for example, Jordan Rau, "Test for Hospital Budgets . . ."

Posters hang in break rooms Interviews.

cue cards in their pockets See, for example, Todd Sloane.

wear laminated cards . . . "in your room." Liz Kowalczyk.

at least three times per shift. Ibid.
more than 800 healthcare organizations See, for example, https://www.studergroup.
com/what-we-do/institutes/upcoming-institutes/hcahps-summit/hcahps-nashville-tn/
post-event-page/.
"coaching" https://www.studergroup.com/what-we-do/coaching/.
A.I.D.E.T. stands for Acknowledge . . . Competency Assessment. Accessed through
the Studer Group tools page. Used also in The Nurse Leader Handbook. www.
firestarterpublishing.com/NurseLeaderHandbook.
have to undergo "remediation" See, for example, Bridget Ward, "Dumbing Down
Disrespects Nurses," Letter to the Editor, *Berkshire Eagle* (Pittsfield, MA), June 7, 2011.
"improvement plan." Competency Assessment.
assessed by "A.I.D.E.T. auditors." "Tool 9: Aidet Interaction Assessment," Taking You and
Your Organization to the Next Level, Studer Group Tools, 2009.
health systems are now using . . . bonuses. Interviews; See also, for example, "Better Bedside
Manners; Customer Service Comes to Healthcare." *Indianapolis Business Journal*, March
21, 2011; Franklin Michota, "Adviser's Viewpoint Patient Satisfaction Is No Simple
Thing," *Hospitalist News*, April 2012.
auditioned and hired professional actors . . . See, for example, "Hospitals Hire Actors to
Improve Patient Satisfaction, Communication," FierceHealthcare.com, August 30, 2012.
"an open-book test . . ." "Quick-E! Pro Scripting: A Guide for Nurses," HCPro.com, 2009.
. . . do not approve of these tactics. "Hospitals are not permitted to attempt to influence or
encourage patients to respond in a particular way," Ellen B. Griffith, a spokeswoman for
the Centers for Medicare and Medicaid Services, emailed *Boston Globe*'s Liz Kowalczyk.
"hospitals must not use . . ." CAHPS Hospital Survey (HCAHPS) Quality Assurance
Guidelines, Version 9.0, March 2014.
"Stepford nurse" Liz Kowalczyk.
ten-page laminated guide . . . "Uh-huh." "Better Bedside Manners: Customer Service
Comes to Healthcare," *Indianapolis Business Journal*, March 21, 2011.
"If you haven't found a way . . ." Rebecca Hendren, "Top 5 Challenges Facing Nursing in
2012," *HealthLeaders Media*, November 15, 2011.
Oh, they get it. See, for example, "A Message from 'Rank and File, RN,'" from
Emergiblog.com, November 16, 2011.
"In our staff meetings . . ." Interview.
"good customer service skills . . ." Amy Bozeman, "Wanted: Good Customer Service Skills,"
Scrubsmag.com, July 6, 2011.
evaluates staff members on "customer satisfaction." Todd Sloane.
"Now we are told . . ." Amy Bozeman.
representatives give warm blankets . . . marks to the nurses. Ibid.
at a hospital that switched its "A Message From 'Rank and File, RN.'"
The University of Toledo Medical Center . . . "true belief." Todd Sloane.
"patients are more satisfied . . ." Liz Kowalczyk.
UTMC is among the worst performers . . . At the time of this writing, UTMC scored worse
than the national average on five categories of Hospital Readmissions, Complications
and Deaths Data. See Data.Medicare.gov for current data.
UTMC made headlines . . . See, for example, Susan Donaldson James, "Toledo Hospital
Threw Out Donor Kidney, Now Denies Negligence," Abcnews.com via *Good Morning
America*, August 29, 2013.
study comparing patient satisfaction . . . patient per nurse. Ann Kutney-Lee, et al. "Nursing:
A Key to Patient Satisfaction." *Health Affairs*, July/August 2009. The study authors
caution: "A limitation of the research is the cross-sectional design, which does not
inform us about causation."
good work environments . . . "throughout the world." Linda H. Aiken et al., "Importance of
Work Environments on Hospital Outcomes in Nine Countries," *International Journal
for Quality in Healthcare* (August 2011).

Higher staffing of registered nurses . . . assigned eight. Linda H. Aiken et al., "Hospital Nurse Staffing and Patient Mortality, Nurse Burnout, and Job Dissatisfaction," *Journal of the American Medical Association* (2002).

failure-to-rescue rates drop . . . to die See, for example, Arminee Kazanjian et al., "Effect of the Hospital Nursing Environment on Patient Mortality: A Systematic Review," *Journal of Health Services Research and Policy* (April 2005); Linda H. Aiken, "Investments in Nursing Save Lives," Center for Health Outcomes and Policy Research. A PowerPoint presentation supported by National Institute of Nursing Research; Ann Kutney-Lee et al.

readmitted to the hospital. See, for example, Jonathan Gruber and Samuel L. Kleiner, "Do Strikes Kill? Evidence from New York State," National Bureau Of Economic Research Working Paper Series (March 2010).

stay is shorter . . . error is lower. See, for example, Rebecca Hendren, "Nurse Staffing Costs Must Be Weighed Against Cost of Errors," *HealthLeaders Media*, August 30, 2011.

the fewer the nurses, the higher . . . Jeannette Rogowski et al., "Nurse Staffing and NICU Infection Rates," *JAMA Pediatrics* (May 2013).

hospitals could earn . . . and fewer tests. See, for example, Linda H. Aiken, "Investments in Nursing . . ."

in poor nurse working environments . . . saved every year. Linda H. Aiken, "Investments in Nursing . . ." In correspondence with the author, Aiken, a leading nurse researcher, clarified that "frequently" is defined as "once a month or more often."

"the single most critical . . ." "HCAHPS: Hardwiring Your Hospital for Pay-for-Performance Success," Studer Group webinar, 2011.

check in with patients every hour Ibid.

"The Most Bang for Your Buck" Ibid.

"to promote higher quality . . ." Federal Register, Department of Health and Human Services 76, no. 160, August 18, 2011.

"building a culture of healthcare excellence" Disneyinstitute.com.

CHAPTER 7

"I will abstain . . ." Florence Nightingale Pledge at the American Nurses Association: http://nursingworld.org.

"It's insanely easy . . ." Interview.

"one of the most devastating . . ." See, for example, T. Monroe, "Addressing Substance Abuse Among Nursing Students: Development of a Prototype Alternative-to-Dismissal Policy," *Journal of Nursing Education* (May 2009).

"code of silence" Interviews; see also, for example, Debra Dunn, "Home Study Program: Substance Abuse Among Nurses—Defining the Issue." *AORN Journal* (October 2005).

"don't talk rule" Debra Dunn,

"bend rules or . . . can be difficult." Ibid.

nurses worry that . . . Ibid.

quick to stigmatize . . . Ibid. See also "Substance Use Disorder in Nursing," *National Council of State Boards of Nursing*, 2011.

"Society, in general . . . grandmother's pain pills." Ibid.

army medical center nurse . . . hepatitis C. Darren Meritz, "Former Nurse at Beaumont Army Medical Center Given 3½ Years," *El Paso Times*, December 2, 2009.

Nurses across the world have stolen narcotics See, for example, Clair Weaver, "Nurse Stole Pills off Elderly," *Sunday Telegraph* (Australia), August 10, 2008; Myra Philp, "Missing Drugs: 6 Nurses Axed; Staff Suspended in Morphine 'Theft' Probe," *Sun*, August 17, 2009.

replaced or diluted it . . . during surgery See, for example, "Fentanyl Replaced With Saline Solution During Surgical Procedures," *US Fed News*, November 29, 2006; Pat Grossmith, "Indictment: Nurse Diluted Drugs," *Union Leader* (Manchester, NH), July 18, 2008; Roxanna Hegeman, "Kansas Nurse Gets 3 Years in Drug Tampering Case," *Capital-Journal*, February 3, 2012; "Nurse gets 3 years for drug tampering," *Capital-Journal*, February 25, 2012; "Woman Sentenced to Probation for Stealing Painkillers," August 6, 2005; "Pain Medication Thefts: Nurse's Drug Problem Was Recorded," *Daily Camera* (Boulder, CO), July 9, 2009.

nurse at a nursing home . . . for her migraines. "Former care home worker is struck off nursing register," *Wells Journal,* April 28, 2011. She was accused of killing other patients, but was cleared. See "Nurse accused of murdering two of the elderly residents she was stealing drugs from." *Wells Journal,* January 28, 2010.

6 to 8 percent of nurses Author correspondence with an ANA representative. Also see, for example, Cynthia Clark and Judy Farnsworth,"Program for Recovering Nurses: An Evaluation," *Medsurg Nursing* (August 2006). See also Patricia Welch Dittman, "Male Nurses and Chemical Dependency: Masterminding the Nursing Environment," *Nursing Administration Quarterly* (October–December 2008); Madeline Naegle, "Nurses and Matters of Substance," *NSNA Imprint* (November–December 2006).

same rate as the general population See, for example, Thomas Zambito, "High Anxiety in Hospitals: Nurses in Drugs, Drink Crisis," *Daily News* (NY), March 14, 2004; "What To Do When Confronting an Impaired Colleague," *Medical Ethics Advisor,* June 1, 2005.

between five and 100 times greater. T. Monroe, "Addressing Substance Abuse Among Nursing Students: Development of a Prototype Alternative-to-Dismissal Policy," *Journal of Nursing Education,* May 2009.

skilled, achieving, respected See, for example, Matthew F. Shaw et al., "Physicians and Nurses with Substance Use Disorders," *Journal of Advanced Nursing* 47, no. 5; Jane Hedrick; Debra Dunn.

67 percent of nurse anesthesia students . . . the bottom third. Jane Hedrick and Stephanie Luck, "The Alarming Trend of Substance Abuse in Anesthesia Providers," *Journal of PeriAnesthesia Nursing* (October 2004).

"intelligent, calm" . . . from their supervisors. Patricia Welch Dittman.

"believe they have the knowledge" Jane Hedrick and Stephanie Luck.

are much more likely . . . downward spirals in time. See, for example, Debra Dunn.

ER, OR, PACU . . . cope with these traumas. Ibid. See also "Substance Use Disorder in Nursing."

"who enjoy a high degree" http://www.aana.com/ceandeducation/becomeacrna/pages/default.aspx.

may be even more vulnerable . . . at more than 15 percent. Jane Hedrick and Stephanie Luck.

"they're playing with rocket fuel . . ." Interview with Art Zwerling by Eaves. Some researchers have suggested that "exposure to trace quantities of these agents in the workplace sensitizes the reward pathways in the brain and promotes substance abuse." Heather Hamza and E. O. Bryson, "The Drug Seeking Anesthesia Care Provider," *International Anesthesiology Clinics* 49, no. 1 (2011).

Jan Stewart, a CRNA . . . a friend to all." http://www.aana.com/resources2/health-wellness/Pages/Jan-Stewart-In-Memoriam.aspx.

back pain so intense . . . Sarah Ruth Gomes, Foreword, in Paula Davies Scimeca, *Unbecoming a Nurse: Bypassing the Hidden Chemical Dependency Trap.* Sea Meca, 2008.

died at age 50 . . . www.aana.com/resources2/health-wellness/Pages/Jan-Stewart-In-Memoriam.aspx.

opioid hundreds of times . . . See, for example, M. A. Clotz and M. C. Nahata, "Clinical Uses of Fentanyl, Sufentanil, and Alfentanil," *Clinical Pharmacology* (August 1991).

That's how many nurses . . . See, for example, Blythe Bernhard, "On Drugs, on Duty: Doctors, Nurses with Easy Access Can Be Vulnerable to Addiction." *St. Louis Post-Dispatch,* March 26, 2008.

. . . get most easily See, for example, Jane Hedrick and Stephanie Luck. See also "Substance Use Disorder in Nursing."

. . . abuse them more often See, for example, A. M. Trinkoff et al., "Workplace Access, Negative Proscriptions, Job Strain, and Substance Use in Registered Nurses," *Journal of Nursing Research* (March–April 2000).

Doctors' substance abuse . . . Ibid.

the nurses' familiarity . . . the general population. See, for example, A. M. Trinkoff et al.

tend to get sicker . . . See, for example, Blythe Bernhard.

take patients' doses . . . gave only one. See, for example, Brandi Watters, "Prescription Pill Abuse Surpasses Street Drugs," *Herald Bulletin* (Anderson, IN), January 26, 2010; Debra Dunn.

might sign out drugs See, for example, Anne Geggis, "2 Lose Nursing Licenses Over Missing Drugs," *News-Journal* (Daytona Beach, FL), April 1, 2006; Debra Dunn,

can steal prescription pads . . . didn't actually give See, for example, Blythe Bernhard.

or otherwise falsify hospital records See, for example, "Seattle Nurse Pleads Guilty to Unlawful Theft, Diversion of Controlled Substances," *US Fed News*, May 19, 2009.

take advantage when coworkers . . . Interviews; See, for example, David C. Shampine, "Nurse Charged with Supporting Her Vicodin Addiction with Forged Electronic Prescriptions," *Watertown Daily Times* (NY), June 8, 2012.

ate the gel . . . placebos Robin Stein, "Did Nurse Take Patients' Painkillers?" *St. Petersburg Times* (FL) South Pinellas Edition, December 3, 2005.

"Often, it's our best people" . . . "What to Do When Confronting . . ."

don't necessarily act immediately See, for example, Jason Blevins, "Addicts in Health Professions Flock to Get Peers' Help," *Denver Post*, July 23, 2009.

"should incorporate prevention . . ." Interview with AACN spokesman.

AACN doesn't monitor whether schools comply. Interview with AACN spokesman, who said there is too much variability between nursing programs to comment further.

"enables an abusing nurse . . . there was a problem." Debra Dunn.

license suspension . . . penalties are possible. See, for example, S. Trossman, "Nurses' Addictions: Finding Alternatives to Discipline," *American Journal of Nursing* 103 (September 2003).

again work in healthcare See, for example, "Nurse Gets 3 Years for Drug Tampering."

Nursing boards are . . . out of the field. Debra Dunn.

"The good news is . . . problem it becomes." Interview, Al Rundio.

Los Angeles Times and Pro Publica investigation . . . "impose discipline." Tracy Weber, Charles Ornstein, and Maloy Moore, "Loose Reins on Nurses in Drug Abuse Program," ProPublica and *Los Angeles Times*, July 25, 2009.

California eventually imposed stricter rules Tracy Weber, Charles Ornstein, and Maloy Moore, "California Adopts Stricter Rules for Drug Abusers in the Health Industry," ProPublica, November 20, 2009.

ended an anonymous . . . surgeries. See, for example, Blythe Bernhard.

forty-one have non-disciplinary . . . "Discipline/Continued Competency/Assistive Personnel Practice," National Council of State Boards of Nursing.

fewer resources than doctors . . . severe professional sanctions. See, for example, M. F. Shaw et al., "Physicians and Nurses with Substance Use Disorders," *Journal of Advanced Nursing* 47, no. 5 (2004). Despite the discrepancies between services for nurses and physicians, by focusing on treating a healthcare professional and getting her back to work, these programs at least encourage more people to seek help, rather than to continue to cover up their abuse and put patients at risk by working while under the influence.

"The rate at which nurses . . . representation." Ibid.

fewer than 1.5 percent of nurses See Cynthia Clark.

140,000 nurses . . . what they're doing. Interview with Douglas McLellan by Eaves.

compassionately mentioning the topic See, for example, "What to Do When Confronting . . ."

"The best recommendation is . . ." Interview with Julie Rice by Eaves.

"It is every nurse's responsibility . . ." "ANA Unveils Bill of Rights for RNs," American Nurses Association, cited in Debra Dunn.

legally responsible to turn in . . . See, for example, Jane Hedrick and Stephanie Luck.

"the nurse becomes [the] nursed." See Patricia Welch Dittman.

CHAPTER 8

"Nurses are frequently put" The American Nurses Association's *Code of Ethics For Nurses*.

"Somewhere along the line" Interview.

"So many things are just simply . . ." Interview.

"on day one new interns . . ."   Robert S. Huckman and Jason R. Barro, "Cohort Turnover and Productivity: The July Phenomenon in Teaching Hospitals." NBER Working Paper Series 11182, National Bureau of Economic Research.

"The July Effect" . . . in August.   See, for example, John Q. Young et al., "'July Effect': Impact of the Academic Year-End Changeover on Patient Outcomes: A Systematic Review," *Annals of Internal Medicine*, September 6, 2011.

harms patient care . . . hospital stay.   Ibid.; See also Robert S. Huckman.

U.S. death rates . . . 2,750 deaths.   Robert S. Huckman.

"spike by 10 percent in July"   David P. Phillips and Gwendolyn E. C. Barker, "A July Spike in Fatal Medication Errors: A Possible Effect of New Medical Residents," *Journal of General Internal Medicine* (August 2010).

August mortality rates   See, for example, Simon Rogers, "Will Patients Really Die This Week Because of New NHS Hospital Doctors?" *The Guardian* (London), August 1, 2012.

"beyond their capabilities."   Rebecca Smith, "Thousands of Juniors Start Jobs in NHS 'Killing Season,'" *Telegraph* (London), August 1, 2012.

in English hospitals . . . previous Wednesday.   M. H. Jen et al., "Early In-Hospital Mortality Following Trainee Doctors' First Day at Work," PlosOne.org, September 23, 2009.

"Nurses are correcting . . ."   Interview.

not the problem here   Interviews.

"I have had doctors . . ."   Interviews.

25 percent of the hospitals   Author correspondence with American Hospital Association spokesperson.

checking the "About Us" page   Author correspondence with Association of American Medical Colleges spokesperson.

"My reflex was as if . . ."   Interview.

"box shape . . ."   Interview.

"tell you the truth."   Interview.

"Sometimes physicians practice . . . but staff knew."   Interviews.

. . . wagered on patients . . . arriving via ambulance.   Interviews.

"games of chance . . ."   See, for example, R. T. Penson et al.

Different "codes" mean . . .   Interviews.

Some hospitals further . . .   Interviews.

Mr. Firestone . . . unresponsive patient   Interviews.

Ohio's Cleveland Clinic . . . take it easy.   Interview, Rev. Amy Greene. See also, for example, Carolyn Gregoire, "The Amazing Way This Hospital Is Fighting Physician Burnout," *Huffington Post*, December 2, 2013; Katie Sullivan, "Hospitals Try Holistic Approach to Treat Docs' Stress, Burnout," FierceHealthcare.com, December 3, 2013.

Cleveland Clinic's healing . . . in times past.   Ibid.

Code Brown . . . a break to eat.   Interviews.

"Parents call to ask . . ."   Interview.

several props . . . down hospital hallways.   Interviews.

Plenty of nurses admit . . . "something with poop."   Interviews.

occasionally use larger needles . . .   Interviews.

If breaking a rule . . .   Interviews.

". . . few rings is a mistake."   Interview.

personal interaction is against policy   Interview.

"We are working fourteen to sixteen hours"   Lois Berry.

without a strong support system.   Interview.

Even if I haven't.   See Michelle Crouch, "50 Secrets Your Nurse Won't Tell You," *Reader's Digest*, November 2011.

"We usually know the results . . ."   Interview.

toilet humor . . .   Interviews.

"Nurses are gross."   Interview.

"happens all the time."   Interviews.

The most common . . . plan of care.   Interviews.

". . . lose-lose scenario."   Interview.

"and not really. . . . counts the same." Interview with Arthur Caplan.
If there is time . . . choose differently. Interviews.
slow codes Interviews.
"There are lots of unsavory . . ." Interview.
"Code 55" Interview.
Some physicians will unofficially call . . . Interviews.
"Responders literally walk" Interview.
"It's often for the sake . . ." Interview.
"not ethically appropriate" Interview.
". . . as comfortable as possible." Interview.
Respectful patients might get . . . Interviews.
"I'm always happy . . ." Interview.
"rest assured that every single . . ." Interview.
Many hospitals also treat VIPs . . . Interviews.
John's Hopkins Marburg Pavilion. www.hopkinsmedicine.org/the_johns_hopkins_hospital/
    planning_visit/room/marburg_enhanced_amenities_program.html.
Nurses described accommodations . . . "because they aren't famous." Interviews.
"The doctor is at your bedside . . ." Interview.
"Half of the hospital is unavailable . . ." Interviews.
If a hospital's technicians . . . "it can be bad." Interviews.
Nurses have strong opinions . . . Interviews.
"Studies show that patients . . ." Interview.
patient with a history Interviews
If you say something . . . "getting better service." Interviews.
"Sadly, doctors and doctors' offices . . ." Interview.
"If I could talk to" Interview.
nurses do cry . . . "home from work." Interviews.
don't portray hospital . . . "make orders, and leave." Interviews.
"make their rounds in the morning." Interview.
patients who survive . . . "Even in a hospital." Interviews.
"Doctors and nurses". . . she has insurance. Interviews.
"After that talk . . ." Interview.
appreciate the fragility . . . "holy profession." Interviews.
California nurse Jared Axen Interview.
transplant nurse Allison Batson Alicia Tejada, "Atlanta Nurse Donates Kidney to Hospital Patient," ABCNews.com, January 17, 2012; Helena Oliviero, "Nurse Donates Kidney to Patient," *Atlanta Journal-Constitution*, January 29, 2012.
Batson saved his life . . . to help people. Interview with Clay Taber.

CHAPTER 9
"Nursing is a calling" See, for example. www.hhsnalumnae.org/TheNightingaleTribute.pdf.
"Nurses are the glue" Interview.
At six feet two inches . . . "sisterhood without any issues." Interviews with Dean Visk.
330,000 are male U.S. Census Bureau, "Men in Nursing Occupations: American Community Survey Highlight Report," February 2013.
41 percent of CRNAs are male Ibid.
lingering public stereotypes Interviews. See also Eve Tahmincioglu, "Men Are Much in the Sights of Recruiters in Nursing," *The New York Times*, April 13, 2003.
"hold a high degree of masculinity." Kenny Thompson, L. Lee Glenn, and Daren Vertein, "Comparison of Masculine and Feminine Traits in a National Sample of Male and Female Nursing Students," *American Journal of Men's Health* (May 2011).
gay, feminine or "not man enough" Interview.
stereotypes don't bother them Interviews.
"I realized after seeing" Interview.
"It insults my profession . . . proud to be a nurse." Interview.
disproportionately assigned Interviews.

"glass escalator"... *across other fields.* "Men in Nursing Occupations."
"Yes, I'm in a job... *end of the day."* Interview.
"It is incredibly fulfilling." Interview.

CHAPTER 10

"Nurses can work individually..." American Nurses Association's *Code of Ethics For Nurses.*
"Our clinical skills are essential..." Interview.
"Hospital finance people... expected to retire." Interview with Peter McMenamin. The Bureau of Labor Statistics estimates that 555,000 RNs and APRNs will retire over the next several years, but the occupational projections do not specify how many of those nurses are working specifically at hospitals.
"A hospital that now... sound long-term strategy." Ibid.
patient-to-nurse ratios... and patient satisfaction. See, for example, "Workplace Violence: Assessing Occupational Hazards..."; Lois Berry and Paul Curry. For length of stay, infections, upper gastrointestinal bleeding, pneumonia, and failure to rescue rates, see also Jack Needleman et al.,"Nurse-Staffing Levels and the Quality of Care in Hospitals," *New England Journal of Medicine* 346, no. 22, May 30, 2002.
Most trusted profession. http://www.gallup.com/poll/1654/honesty-ethics-professions.aspx
Directly involving nurses... these strategic meetings. See, for example, Robert Wood Johnson Foundation, "Nurses Are Key to Improving Safety," April 28, 2011.
One strategy to curb bullying... C. Rocker, "Addressing Nurse-to-Nurse Bullying to Promote Nurse Retention," *Online Journal of Issues in Nursing*, August 29, 2008.
  Steering committee: see, for example, *ISMP Medication Safety Alert*, March 25, 2004.
"no retribution" policy See, for example, *ISMP Medication Safety Alert*, April 24, 2014.
Some hospitals have trained Interviews.
a quiet room... B. Lombardo and C. Eyre.
soothingly colored walls... Ibid.
Advocate Lutheran General Hospital... "Three-Tiered Emotional Support System Generates Positive Feedback From Providers Who Become 'Second Victims' of an Unanticipated Clinical Event," Agency for Healthcare Research and Quality (March 2009).
"Using a colleague's first name..." See *ISMP Medication Safety Alert*, March 25, 2004.
Hospitals have had success See, for example, Emergency Department Management, "Take Steps to Curb Violence, Improve Safety for ED Personnel," October 1, 2011.
... or conducting bag checks. "Preventing Violence in the Healthcare Setting," Sentinel Event Alert, *The Joint Commission* 45, June 3, 2010.
consider installing metal detectors. See, for example, "OSHA Guidelines for Preventing Workplace Violence for Healthcare and Social Workers," 2004.
Within six months after... "Workplace Violence in Healthcare Settings," Center for Personal Protection and Safety, August 2011.
By requiring staff to report See, for example, Jessica Gacki-Smith et al., "Violence Against Nurses Working in U.S. Emergency Departments," *Journal of Nursing Administration* (July–August 2009).
"The program helped reduce..." "Occupational Hazards in Hospitals," CDC Workplace Safety and Health, National Institute for Occupational Safety and Health, April 2002.
"at a minimum, workplaces should" OSHA Guidelines for Preventing Workplace Violence for Healthcare and Social Workers (2004).
The most important step... getting harmed." Interview with Douglas McLellan by Eaves.
illness, not willful misconduct See, for example, Debra Dunn and T. Monroe.
nurses with chemical dependency issues Some helpful links can be found at http://www. peerassistance.com/links.htm. For resources searchable by state, visit http://webapps. aana.com/Peer/directory.asp. (While the AANA's directory is intended for nurse anesthetists, many of the resources and state assistance programs are for all nurses. Peer advisors volunteer only for CRNAs and student nurse anesthetists.) The ANA's Impaired Nurse Resource Center also includes some links to organizations specializing in addiction: http://www.nursingworld.org/MainMenuCategories/WorkplaceSafety/

Healthy-Work-Environment/Work-Environment/ImpairedNurse/Impaired-Nurse-Resources.html.

administrators could tap them... See, for example, Kevin Pho, "Should Nurses Be Fired for Fatal Medication Errors?" *KevinMD.com*, May 2, 2011.

"A mistake does not mean..." David Maxfield et al., "The Silent Treatment: Why Safety Tools and Checklists Aren't Enough to Save Lives."

Montreal's Jewish General Hospital... See, for example, Aaron Derfel, "Jewish General Dramatically Cuts Bed-Sore Cases," *Gazette* (Montreal), July 20, 2012.

Designate one family member... Interviews. See also "Total Disregard for Visiting Hours," allnurses.com, comment, September 19, 2012.

"Even if you're worried about annoying..." Interview.

maintain a written medical history... pain or complaint. Interviews.

Your hospital is not as clean... Interviews.

"It is really important..." Interview.

at least sixteen hours per day. Interview.

Not all doctors and nurses remember... Interviews.

Bring or find your own... love them most? Interviews.

Even if your hospital medications... "abused by a drunk," Interviews.

"Most nurses bust their ass... deal with them." Interview.

fastest-growing occupation Bureau of Labor Statistics' Employment Projections 2012–2022, released in December 2013. See also Bureau of Labor Statistics. Occupations Projected to Add Most New Jobs, 2012 to 2022 (January 27, 2014).

"The profession is exciting..." Interview, Terri Weaver.

"Campaign for Nursing's Future." Interview with spokesman; see also www.discovernursing.com.

"Choosing nursing as a profession..." Author correspondence with Joan Shaver.

scientists, engineers... Interviews with several deans of nursing schools.

"gives you a chance..." Interview.

"consider no less..." Kathleen Potempa.

"They have the same..." Interview, Bobbie Berkowitz.

lifelong goal. Interview, Mary Kerr.

"Be avid readers..." Interview, Linda Norman.

"We've got to get away..." Ibid.

"Never give advice..." Interview, Judith Karshmer.

"The best coping resource..." Interview.

"It's a platform for nurses..." Interview, Brian Short.

"The point of the profession is to provide patient care..." Interview, Terri Weaver.

"To be a good nurse..." Interview.

"Many times patients wanted..." Interview.

Nurses nationwide told me... "identify the possible options." Interviews.

"After a bad day..." Interview.

"I am not asking you to confirm..." *Impaired Practice in Nursing: A Guidebook for Interventions and Resources,* Massachusetts Nurses Association. National Nurses United, 2011.

"... positive effect on the nurse as well." Author correspondence with Beth Perry. See also Beth Perry, "Why Exemplary Oncology Nurses Avoid Compassion Fatigue," *Canadian Oncology Nursing Journal* 18, no. 2 (2008).

taught a group of new nurses... bullying by peers. Martha Griffin.

"Experienced nurses do feel threatened..." Interview.

exercise in which participants share... Interview with Patricia Potter, Barnes-Jewish director of research for patient-care services. See also States News Service, "Compassion Fatigue Program Gives Staff Skills To Be Resilient Against the Cost of Caring," January 3, 2012.

"I absolutely"... "who love what they do." Interviews.

ABOUT THE AUTHOR

ALEXANDRA ROBBINS, winner of the 2014 John Bartlow Martin Award for Public Interest Magazine Journalism, is the author of four *New York Times* bestsellers. Her previous book was voted the Goodreads Best Nonfiction Book of the Year. She has written for *The New Yorker*, *Vanity Fair*, *The New York Times*, and other publications, and has appeared on numerous television shows, from *60 Minutes* to *The Colbert Report*.

For lectures: alexandrarobbins.com